D1350328

Regional Anesthesia

An Illustrated Procedural Guide

Third Edition

Michael F. Mulroy, M.D.

Staff Anesthesiologist
Department of Anesthesiology
The Virginia Mason Medical Center
Clinical Professor
Department of Anesthesiology
University of Washington
Seattle, Washington

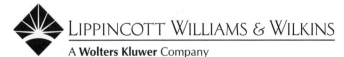

LIPPINCOTT WILLIAMS & WILKINS
A **Wolters Kluwer** Company
Philadelphia · Baltimore · New York · London
Buenos Aires · Hong Kong · Sydney · Tokyo

Acquisitions Editor: R. Craig Percy
Developmental Editor: Julia Seto
Production Editor: Thomas J. Foley
Manufacturing Manager: Colin J. Warnock
Cover Designer: Mark Lerner
Compositor: Lippincott Williams & Wilkins Desktop Division
Printer: Data Reproduction Corporation

© 2002 by LIPPINCOTT WILLIAMS & WILKINS
530 Walnut Street
Philadelphia, PA 19106 USA
LWW.com

Printed in the USA

Library of Congress Cataloging-in-Publication Data
Mulroy, Michael F.
  Regional anesthesia : an illustrated procedural guide / Michael F. Mulroy.—3rd ed.
    p. ; cm.
  Includes bibliographical references and index.
  ISBN 0-7817-3645-5
  1. Conduction anesthesia—Handbooks, manuals, etc. I. Title.
  [DNLM: 1. Anesthesia, Conduction—Handbooks. WO 231 M961r 2002]
RD84.M85 2002
617.9'64—dc21

                                        2002017857

10 9 8 7 6 5 4 3 2

To Brian and Lauren, who reminded me that there are more important accomplishments than writing a book.

To my predecessors at the Mason Clinic; especially to L. Donald Bridenbaugh, who has done so much for others in building the department, encouraging his staff, and teaching his staff and residents alike the art of regional anesthesia and medicine; and to Dan Moore, who founded the department and established the tradition of regional anesthesia at Virginia Mason.

Contents

Contributing Authors

James D. Helman, M.D.
Staff Anesthesiologist
Department of Anesthesiology
The Virginia Mason Medical Center
Seattle, Washington

Linda Jo Rice, M.D.
Director of Pain Medicine
All Children's Hospital
St. Petersburg, Florida; and
Professor of Clinical Anesthesia
University of South Florida
College of Medicine
Tampa, Florida

Preface

This is a practical manual of regional anesthesia for both students and practitioners. It is a "how to" guide for common regional techniques to be used and referred to in the operating room. It provides information to justify the reasons and purposes of the techniques. It also provides the pharmacologic and physiologic data to support the choices of drugs and doses and to avoid common complications. The manual presents commonly performed techniques for all regions of the body, while discussing their application in the subspecialty areas of pediatrics, obstetrics, and pain management. In a practical manual of this breadth, however, encyclopedic depth is not the goal. For definitive texts on any of the subjects discussed, the reader should consult standard texts and original reports listed in the references at the end of each chapter.

Familiarity with the first five chapters of the manual supplements the procedural chapters that follow. Discussions of premedication, equipment, and common complications are presented in this introductory section, but are referred to only briefly in subsequent chapters. The discussions of specific techniques are organized into chapters on axial blockade and techniques involving the upper and lower extremities, head, and trunk. In addition to detailed step-by-step description of block techniques, each chapter reviews relevant anatomy, drug considerations, and specific complications. The final chapters deal with the application of regional techniques in the subspecialty areas of pediatrics, obstetrics, and acute and chronic pain management. Greater detail is available in subspecialty texts, but the practitioner who is called on only occasionally to provide pain management or pediatric regional anesthesia will find helpful guidelines in these final chapters. These chapters will be particularly useful to the novice.

The manual is designed to be used as a practical guide where anesthesia is performed. Successful regional anesthesia, however, requires more than the use of a simple map at the time of the procedure. The reader, especially the novice, is encouraged to review the anatomy in more detailed standard anatomy texts and atlases before approaching the patient. Three-dimensional visualization and appreciation of anatomy is essential for successful regional anesthesia, and review of the landmarks on a skeleton or a live model is helpful. Knowledge of the drugs to be used and their potential complications is also essential before approaching the patient.

The techniques described here are those generally used at the Virginia Mason Medical Center. Where scientific data are available to substantiate a preference for a specific approach or technique, they are included in the references. Much of regional anesthesia, however, remains an art. Personal experience and preference still dictate many of the approaches described. There is substantial variation, even within our department, in the performance of common techniques. All of the individual variations cannot be included, but it would be unfortunate if medicine of any kind were practiced by the use of a "cookbook" formula accepted by all. The art of regional anesthesia is dynamic, as reflected in the new drugs, equipment, and techniques included in this new edition and there is no doubt that further changes lie ahead.

This manual would not have been possible without the contributions and support of the entire Anesthesia Department of the Virginia Mason Clinic. The final product reflects the contributions of each staff member (though not necessarily expressing opinions that everyone will agree with!). The resident staff and the graduates have also made invaluable suggestions regarding content and clarity over the years; as always, we learn as much from our students as they learn from us. Specific appreciation goes to Linda Jo Rice, M.D., for her contribution on the application of regional techniques to the pediatric population, which we do not serve at Virginia Mason, and to James Helman, M. D., for his expertise in approaching the management of chronic pain. I thank Iris Nichols for her patient efforts in providing the original illustrations that support the text, and Jennifer Smith for her additions and modifications in the art for this edition. Finally, Craig Percy deserves the credit for nurturing this third edition. It is hoped that these efforts have produced a manual that will help the novice and graduate alike in improving their regional anesthesia skills.

Michael F. Mulroy, M.D.

Regional Anesthesia

An Illustrated Procedural Guide

1 Local Anesthetics

Local anesthetic compounds produce temporary blockade of neural transmission when applied to nerve axons. Today's useful local anesthetics are chemical descendants of cocaine, the plant alkaloid extracted from the leaves of the coca plant. This poorly water-soluble, weak base is a benzoic acid derivative joined by an ester linkage to a tertiary amine compound. The synthetic descendants generally possess the same three essential functional units: a *hydrophilic* chain joined to a *lipophilic* portion by an ester or amide *linkage* (Fig. 1.1). These descendants also are poorly water-soluble, weak bases that are used as aqueous solutions of the hydrochloride salts of the tertiary amine. The local anesthetic is present in equilibrium as both the ionized (cationic) salt and the uncharged base. The presence of ionized and un-ionized forms, combined with the intrinsic lipophilic and hydrophilic portions of the parent compound, confers an ability to traverse both aqueous and lipid membranes, a property that is essential in allowing these compounds to reach their neural cell wall target and produce anesthesia. The balance of these physicochemical properties in the specific structure of each compound is important in determining the potency, duration, and clinical characteristics of each drug. The ester or amide linkage between the two ends of the compound determines the route of metabolism and indirectly influences the specific toxicities of the compounds.

History

Cocaine, the first local anesthetic, was imported into Europe from South America in the mid-19th century (1). Koller in Vienna was the first to discover the advantages of cocaine's properties as a topical ophthalmologic anesthetic. His report in 1884 was a great step forward in surgical anesthesia, and enthusiastic experimentation with the drug ensued. However, cocaine's problems of neurotoxicity, systemic toxicity, and addiction potential soon became apparent. These limitations led to experimental exploration for more potent and less toxic chemical derivatives. This early era of research coincided with a vibrant period of development of regional anesthetic techniques. Wider use of new local anesthetics soon relegated cocaine to a minor role as a topical anesthetic, because of its unique vasoconstrictive properties.

The first successor to cocaine was developed in Germany. Procaine is an ester-linked benzoic acid derivative (an amino-ester) similar to cocaine. Although an improvement over cocaine in toxicity, procaine still had problems with short duration, systemic toxicity, and occasional allergic sensitivity. The development of tetracaine improved the duration but still left problems with toxicity. A

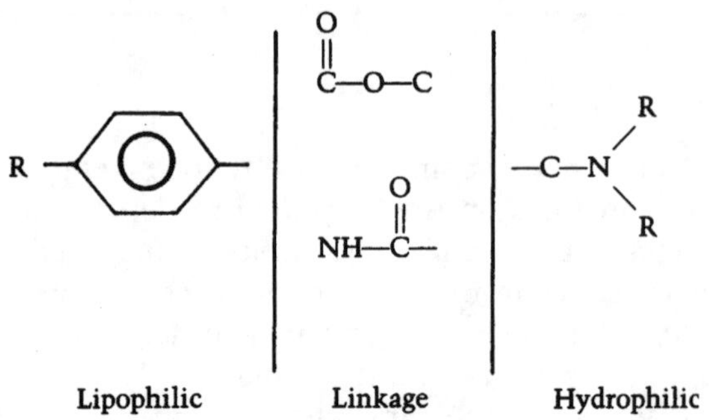

Figure 1.1   **Typical Structure of Local Anesthetic Molecule**

second era of development occurred in Sweden between 1930 and 1960, introducing the *amide* linkage for local anesthetics with the formulation of lidocaine. The amino-amides are chemically more stable and have less allergic potential than the esters. Subsequent development has produced variations on this structure, which have expanded the spectrum of potency and duration of local anesthetic drugs (Table 1.1).

Activity   Despite the enthusiasm for chemical development in the beginning of this century, little was known about the mode of action of these drugs until experimental techniques in the 1960s allowed a clearer understanding of the cellular effect of local anesthetics. The structural similarities of these drugs indicate a similar mechanism and site of action. Although the precise mechanism of molecular action is still debated (2), much has been learned about the essential steps in the process of nerve-conduction blockade by these drugs.

Application of local anesthetics to isolated nerve fibers produces a disruption of function associated with a blockade of membrane depolarization. Cellular integrity and metabolism are unaffected, but when a sufficient concentration of anesthetic is achieved in the perfusing solution, electrical conduction (depolarization) does not occur in response to an electrical stimulus. The conductance of sodium into the cell (which normally produces the depolarization) is blocked. The repolarization associated with potassium flux through the potassium-specific channels remains unimpeded. Physical blockade or conformational change in the sodium channels themselves by the cationic form of the local anesthetics appears to produce this temporary dysfunction.

The external opening of the sodium-specific channel is not the site of action. Local anesthetic application to the *external* opening of the sodium channel alone is ineffective in blocking conduction,

Table 1.1 Physiochemical Properties of Local Anesthetics

Drug (Brand Name)	Type (Year Introduced)	Chemical Structure	Relative Potency		pK$_a$	Lipid Solubility	Protein Binding
			Frog Sciatic Nerve	Rat Sciatic Nerve			
Cocaine	—	CH$_2$—CH——CHCOOCH$_3$ / NCH$_3$—CHOOC$_6$H$_5$ / CH$_2$—CH——CH$_2$	—	—	—	—	—
Procaine (Novocaine)	Ester (1905)	H$_2$N——COOCH$_2$CH$_2$N(C$_2$H$_5$)(C$_2$H$_5$)	1	1	8.9	0.6	5.8
Benzocaine	Ester (1900)	H$_2$N——COOC$_2$H$_5$	—	—	3.5	—	—
Tetracaine (Pontocaine)	Ester (1930)	H$_9$C$_4$—N(N)——COOCH$_2$N(CH$_3$)(CH$_3$)	16	8	8.5	80	75.6
2-Chloroprocaine (Nesacaine)	Ester (1952)	H$_2$N——(Cl)COOCH$_2$N(C$_2$H$_5$)(C$_2$H$_5$)	4	1	8.7	—	—
Lidocaine (Xylocaine)	Amide (1944)	(CH$_3$)(CH$_3$)—NHCOCH$_2$N(C$_2$H$_5$)(C$_2$H$_5$)	4	2	7.72	2.9	64.3
Mepivacaine (Carbocaine, Polocaine)	Amide (1957)	(CH$_3$)(CH$_3$)—NHCO—N(CH$_3$ piperidine)	2	2	7.6	0.8	77.5
Prilocaine (Citanest)	Amide (1960)	(CH$_3$)—NHCOCH—NH—C$_3$H$_7$ / CH$_3$	3	2	7.7	0.8	55
Ropivacaine (Naropin)	Amide (1995)	(CH$_3$)(CH$_3$)—NH—CO···N(H)(C$_3$H$_7$ piperidine)	—	—	8.1	14	95
Bupivacaine (Marcaine, Sensorcaine) Levobupivacaine (Chirocaine)	Amide (1963)	(CH$_3$)(CH$_3$)—NHCO—N(C$_4$H$_9$ piperidine)	16	8	8.1	27.5	95.6
Etidocaine (Duranest)	Amide (1972)	(CH$_3$)(CH$_3$)—NHCOCHN(C$_2$H$_5$)(C$_2$H$_5$)(C$_3$H$_7$)	16	8	7.74	141	94

Adapted from Covino, B. G., Vasallo, H. G. *Local Anesthetic: Mechanism of Action and Clinical Use.* New York: Grune & Stratton, 1976, and from deJong, R. H. *Local Anesthetics.* St. Louis: Mosby-Year Book, 1993.

as demonstrated by experiments bathing the nerve with permanently charged lidocaine molecules. This charged (*cationic*) form of the local anesthetic cannot penetrate the lipid cell wall or enter the channel directly from the external orifice. The un-ionized (lipid soluble) base form of the molecule must first penetrate the cell wall and reach the axoplasm (Fig. 1.2). Once inside, the molecule again can exist as both the ionized and un-ionized forms in equilibrium, and it appears that the cationic form of the molecule most readily enters the channel during depolarization and disrupts sodium conductance. Blockade is concentration-dependent, and it also requires disruption of several contiguous channels to overcome the natural reserve of conduction ability in mammalian nerves (Fig. 1.3). Interaction of the local anesthetic with the channel is reversible, and it ends when the concentration of local anesthetic falls below a critical minimum level.

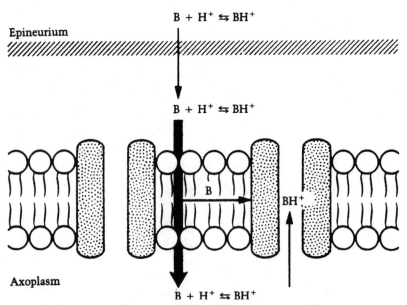

Figure 1.2   **Equilibration of Local Anesthetics Across the Cell Membrane**
The local anesthetic exists in tissue in equilibrium between the ionized salt and the poorly soluble base (*B*). The uncharged base diffuses most readily through the lipid barriers of the epineurium and the cell wall, and at each level reestablishes equilibrium with its ionized counterpart in a ratio dependent on the tissue acidity and the pK_a of the compound. The base may reach the sodium channel by direct diffusion through the axolemma interior, but is more likely to enter the sodium channel and bind to its receptor as the ionized form from within the axoplasm. (From Barash, P. G., Cullen, B. F., Stoelting, R. K., Eds. *Clinical Anesthesia.* Philadelphia: Lippincott, 2001, with permission.)

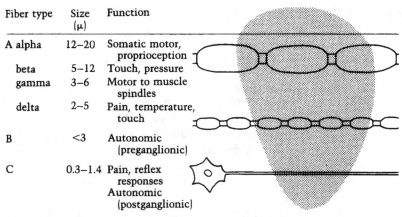

Fiber type	Size (μ)	Function
A alpha	12–20	Somatic motor, proprioception
beta	5–12	Touch, pressure
gamma	3–6	Motor to muscle spindles
delta	2–5	Pain, temperature, touch
B	<3	Autonomic (preganglionic)
C	0.3–1.4	Pain, reflex responses Autonomic (postganglionic)

Figure 1.3

Classification of Nerve Fiber Types
The large myelinated fibers require blockade of three adjacent nodal regions to block conduction. Although these fibers have been reported to be equally or even more sensitive to local anesthetics than the smaller fibers in the laboratory, clinically blockade is usually manifest first in the small (pain and sympathetic) nerve fibers. This may be due to variable penetrance of the local anesthetic into the fatty tissues surrounding the various nerves, or may reflect some component of frequency-dependent blockade.

These general features of local anesthetic action are well known. The specific clinical performance of each compound varies considerably because several factors affect each of the steps of nerve block anesthesia. Several physicochemical properties of the specific molecules determine how well and how long they each perform tissue penetration, cell wall transfer, and reversible conduction blockade (Table 1.2). Knowledge of these properties is helpful in understanding some of the clinical actions of the drugs, as well as in predicting the performance of new compounds that may be developed.

Table 1.2.

Properties of Local Anesthetic Compounds

Characteristic	Correlate
Chemical linkage	Metabolism
Lipid solubility	Potency
Dissociation constant	Speed of onset
Protein binding	Duration of action
Frequency-dependent blockade	Sensorimotor dissociation
Vasodilation potential	Duration, apparent potency
Tissue penetrance	Speed of onset

Physical Properties

Lipid Solubility

The neural cell wall target of these drugs is a lipid structure. It is not surprising that the local anesthetics are more lipid soluble than water soluble. In general, as in the gaseous general anesthetic agents, these drugs show some correlation between *lipid solubility and potency* (see Table 1.1). This relationship is not simply linear. Even the determination of solubility is variable, and the establishment of potency is an empirical determination that has not been accomplished with the same reproducibility as with the inhalation anesthetic drugs.

The unit of potency used for local anesthetics is the *minimum concentration* (C_m) of local anesthetic necessary to block impulse conduction in a nerve of a given diameter within a "reasonable" period of time. This is usually determined by bathing an isolated portion of animal peripheral nerve in an anesthetic solution while stimulating it at one end and recording the compound action potentials produced distal to the bathed portion of nerve. Unfortunately, this is not a satisfactory equivalent to the concept of *minimum alveolar concentration* (MAC) for measuring equipotent doses of general anesthetic gases in humans because the C_m for local anesthetics varies considerably based on the experimental conditions. Confounding variables in various experimental reports include the criteria for degree of blockade, the time allowed for blockade, electrolyte concentration of the bath, presence or absence of a sheath, and rate of stimulation. The variability of individual types of nerves (large fibers versus small, myelinated versus unmyelinated) adds to the confusion (3) (Fig. 1.3). The concentration of drug and the pH of the perfusate used also produce variations. All of these variables make a reproducible value between studies and laboratories difficult to obtain and have led to conflicting data regarding potency. The two scales of relative potencies described in Table 1.1 were obtained under specific laboratory conditions in different preparations. Other values might be obtained under different circumstances. Although these values demonstrate the crude relationship to lipid solubility, they also underscore the variability in measurement and the difficulty in extrapolating laboratory data to clinical practice of regional anesthesia.

A further limitation of the C_m concept is the absence of a means of measuring tissue concentrations of local anesthetics in the clinical setting. Even if there were such a method, the presence of "tissue effects" *in vivo* introduces yet another set of variations between laboratory isolated nerve data and clinical experience. The most notable discrepancy here is the frequent laboratory observation that large myelinated A fibers are more readily blocked than small C fibers, whereas in the intact animal the opposite is generally the case. Other examples of this are the "reduced" potency of lidocaine because of its vasodilator property, and the "enhanced" potency of chloroprocaine because of its tissue penetrance.

Clinically, there are many exceptions to predictions based on laboratory potencies. Many of the well-known exceptions ("greater" potency of mepivacaine, "lesser" potency of etidocaine) are explained in detail in Chapter 2. These exceptions make clinical experience more relevant in regional anesthesia than in comparable discussions of general anesthesia. Although the laboratory determinations of potency serve as guidelines, the choice of drug and concentration are usually based on clinical experience (see Tables 2.1 and 2.2).

Dissociation Constant

Another factor that influences the ability of the local anesthetic to penetrate lipid membranes is the variable proportion of each drug that is present in the lipid-soluble (uncharged) form versus the water-soluble (cationic, protonated) form. Because they are weak bases, local anesthetics in solution exist in equilibrium between these two forms (Fig. 1.4). The tendency to exist as the base or the charged

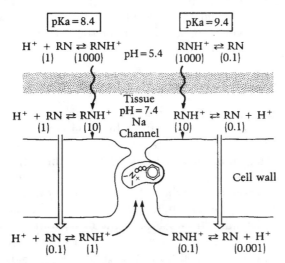

Figure 1.4

Effect of Ionization on Activity
The proportion of local anesthetic in the base (un-ionized) form will depend on its own pK_a and the pH of the solution. A drug with a pK_a of 8.4 is 3 pH units (10^3) away from its 50% equilibrium point when prepared in a commercial solution at pH 5.4, producing roughly the ratio shown. When injected into body tissue, the pH increases and the ratio approaches equality, but is still a factor of ten away. For a solution with a pK_a that is higher, the ratio is even further from equality. Because only the un-ionized form will penetrate lipid membranes, the higher pK_a solutions will usually have slower onset because of less effective drug at the site of action.

form depends on the ambient hydrogen ion concentration and is described by the specific *dissociation constant* (pK_a) for each drug. Specifically, the pK_a is the pH at which 50% of the drug molecules are in the charged quaternary nitrogen state and 50% are in the uncharged tertiary form. A pK_a of 7.4 designates a compound that at normal body pH has an equal number of molecules in the charged and uncharged forms. The pK_a value of most local anesthetics is higher than 7.4. Usually, commercial local anesthetic solutions are "acidic" relative to their pK_a, as is normal body tissue. This produces a dominance of local anesthetic molecules in the ionized form. The higher the pK_a (the further away from body pH), the more of the local anesthetic that exists as charged molecules at body pH.

The un-ionized base is necessary for nerve penetration, while a dominance of the charged (cationic) form on the outside delays onset of anesthetic action. Regardless of intrinsic lipid solubility, drugs with pK_a values closer to body pH are expected to have more rapid *onset of action*, whereas drugs with high dissociation constants will have less base available at tissue pH and should appear slower in onset, or "weaker." The dominance of the nondiffusible cationic form also explains the apparent reduced efficacy of most local anesthetics in the presence of local inflammation (tissue acidosis). Commercial preparations of local anesthetics that contain epinephrine buffered to a low pH (to preserve the epinephrine) also appear slower in onset because of the presence of relatively little diffusible base form.

Protein Binding

Although the lipid membranes represent the most significant obstacle to a local anesthetic's diffusion, the site of action in the sodium channel is a protein structure. The affinity of the drug for the protein unit appears to be related to the length of the aliphatic chains on the compound. The *duration of action* of local anesthetics appears related to their affinity to these protein compounds. The greater the protein-binding characteristics of the compound, the longer the time to "wash out" the drug from the sodium channel. This is particularly evident in the cases of bupivacaine and etidocaine, where the addition of a slightly longer chain to the amine portion of the respective parent compounds mepivacaine and lidocaine increases both lipid solubility and protein binding, producing compounds that are four times more potent and act twice as long (see Table 1.1).

Protein binding is also an important consideration affecting toxicity. The high protein binding of bupivacaine is useful in obstetrics because it reduces the free drug in the plasma in normal patients, and thus little diffusible drug is available to cross the placental circulation. If plasma protein-binding sites are saturated or interfered with by other compounds, such as bilirubin or propranolol, central nervous system toxicity may be seen at unexpectedly low blood levels of local anesthetic (see Chapter 3).

Other Properties

Several other properties influence clinical activity, but they may not be readily quantified in the laboratory setting.

Vasodilation

All local anesthetics, except for cocaine, produce some degree of biphasic vasoactivity. The effect is dose-dependent and varies for each drug. Bupivacaine is a vasoconstrictor at low concentrations, and it dilates arterioles only at concentrations higher than those seen clinically. Lidocaine is a constrictor at low concentrations, but at clinical levels it is usually a vasodilator. The resulting increase in local blood flow tends to increase the vascular uptake of the anesthetic, producing an apparent decrease in potency and duration of action. Lidocaine is twice as potent as mepivacaine in the laboratory, but equipotent clinically because of greater local vasodilation. This effect can be antagonized by the addition of vasoconstrictors to the local anesthetic, which may partially explain the apparent enhanced potency of epinephrine-containing solutions. Duration is affected by vasodilation as well as apparent potency. Local anesthesia can be short-lived in the highly vascular epidural or intercostal space, but it can last four to six times longer in less vascular peripheral nerves, such as the sciatic nerve.

Frequency Dependence

For most drugs, entry into the sodium-conducting channels is achieved when the channel is open during the period of membrane depolarization. Some of the drugs, particularly lidocaine, ropivacaine, and bupivacaine, exhibit an interesting characteristic of producing a degree of blockade proportional to the amount of time the channel is open. Specifically, they produce more rapid and denser blockade in nerves with higher frequencies of conduction (where the sodium channels are open more times per second). In the laboratory, this difference can be demonstrated by stimulating nerve preparations at various frequencies and observing the degree of blockade at various anesthetic concentrations. Clinically, this *frequency-dependent blockade* produces a greater decrement of pain/sensory (high frequency) transmission than of motor (low frequency) conduction (4) (Fig. 1.5). These anesthetics appear to produce more analgesia per increment of motor blockade than do similar compounds with less frequency discrimination. This *sensorimotor dissociation* is usually desirable clinically. It explains why lidocaine and bupivacaine are often favored over drugs such as

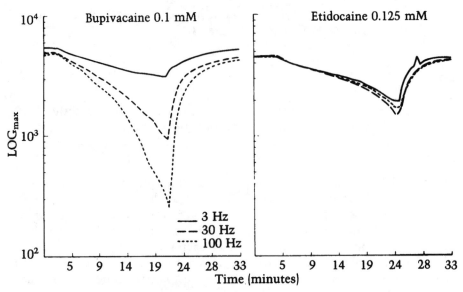

Figure 1.5   **Frequency-Dependent Blockade**
The local anesthetics lidocaine and bupivacaine produce a more intense blockade of nerve fibers when the fibers are stimulated at higher frequencies. In contrast, etidocaine produces a similar degree of blockade regardless of frequency of stimulation. This frequency dependence may account for the sensorimotor dissociation seen with blockade with certain local anesthetics. (From Scurlock, J. E., Meymaris, E., Gregus, J. The clinical character of local anesthetics: A function of frequency-dependent conduction block. *Acta Anaesthesiol. Scand.* 22: 601, 1978, with permission.)

tetracaine and etidocaine, which possess otherwise similar physico-chemical properties.

Tissue Penetrance

Another variable and unpredictable property of the local anesthetics is their ability to penetrate perineural tissue and reach the cell membrane. This property is not well quantified and has not been studied extensively. One evaluation of lidocaine found no variation in potency if perineural tissue were removed or left intact, but there are many examples of dramatic clinical differences between drugs, particularly in the case of chloroprocaine. In contrast to predictions of a slow onset based on its high pK_a, this drug has one of the fastest clinical onsets.

Summary   In summary, local anesthetics act by producing reversible blockade of sodium channels in nerve membranes, thus disrupting electrical nerve transmission. Some of the physical properties of the local anesthetics can explain and predict their clinical action. Lipid solubility is associated with relative potency, pK_a is associated with onset of action, and protein binding is associated with duration. Because of the often-overriding effects of vasodilation, frequency-dependent blockade, and variable tissue penetrance, accurate predictions of clinical activity are difficult. Each chapter of this manual contains specific suggestions as to appropriate drugs, dosages, and expected durations for each unique clinical situation. The next chapter describes some of the specific idiosyncrasies of the currently available local anesthetics.

References

1. Fink, B. R. Leaves and needles: The introduction of surgical local anesthesia. *Anesthesiology* 63: 77, 1985.
2. Strichartz, G. Molecular mechanisms of nerve block by local anesthetics. *Anesthesiology* 45: 421, 1976.
3. Gissen, A. J., Covino, B. G., Gregus, J. Differential sensitivities of mammalian nerve fibers to local anesthetic agents. *Anesthesiology* 53: 467, 1980.
4. Courtney, K. R., Kendig, J. J., Cohen, E. N. Frequency-dependent conduction block: The role of nerve impulse pattern in local anesthetic potency. *Anesthesiology* 48: 111, 1978.

2 Clinical Characteristics of Local Anesthetics

The physical properties of the local anesthetics (described in Chapter 1) help determine much of their clinical performance. Unique individual clinical characteristics, however, make exact predictions of potency, onset, and duration on a theoretical basis difficult. This chapter will discuss empirical clinical properties of the commonly used local anesthetics.

General Principles

Some general principles apply to the use of all of these drugs.

Minimal Effective Dose

All of the local anesthetics produce local and systemic toxicity when used in excessive amounts. The diagnosis and treatment of toxicity are discussed in Chapter 3, but prevention by careful selection of drug, concentration, and volume is a more desirable goal. Many practitioners believe they are avoiding toxicity by using less than the maximum recommended dose published by the manufacturer, as listed in Table 2.1 and in the *Physicians' Desk Reference* (PDR). In fact, clinically toxic blood levels can be achieved with much smaller quantities if intravascular injection occurs or under circumstances that promote rapid absorption. Exposure of the patient to risk can be minimized by using the *minimal effective dose* of local anesthetic drug. To achieve this, the *lowest effective concentration* of local anesthetic is desirable for any block. Penetration of epidural layers may require the highest commercial drug concentrations, but the use of such concentrations on peripheral nerves is unnecessary. High concentrations may increase motor blockade and may increase duration of block, but their use increases the total milligram dose of drug and limits the total amount of solution that can be employed. The potential problem of nerve or tissue damage is also associated with higher concentrations.

Concentration Effect

Opposing this need to employ the lowest effective concentrations is the advantage of faster onset and "denser" block with higher concentrations. As with the inhalation agents, the initial concentration of local anesthetic may be increased to speed the onset (penetrance) of the anesthetic. The most striking example is penetration of mucous membranes, which is generally quite slow for the local anes-

Table 2.1 Local Anesthetic Drug Clinical Doses

Drug (brand name)	Clinical Concentrations	Maximum Recommended Doses (PDR)					Toxic Blood Levels (µg/mL)	
		Plain (Total Milligrams)	Milligrams per Kilogram of Body Weight	With Epinephrine		Other	CNS	CV
				Total	Milligrams per kilogram			
Cocaine	1%–4%	200	1.5	—	—	—	—	—
Procaine (Novocaine)	1%–10%	500	—	—	—	1,000	—	—
Benzocaine	14%–20%	—	—	—	—	—	—	—
Tetracaine (Pontocaine)	1%	—	—	200	—	—	—	—
2-Chloroprocaine (Nesacaine)	1%–3%	800	11	1,000	14	1,000	—	—
Lidocaine (Xylocaine)	0.5%–5%	300	4.5	500	7	500	18–21	35–50
Mepivacaine (Carbocaine, Polocaine)	1%–2%	400	—	550	7[a]	500	22	—
Prilocaine (Citanest)	—	—	—	500	—	—	20	—
Ropivacaine (Naropin)	0.25%–1.0%	250	—	250	3	—	4	?10
Bupivacaine (Marcaine, Sensorcaine)	0.25%–0.75%	175	—	225	3	400	4.5–5.5	6–10
Levo-bupivacaine (Chirocaine)								
Etidocaine (Duranest)	1%–1.5%	300	4	400	6	400	4.3	—

PDR, *Physicians' Desk Reference*; CNS, central nervous system; CV, cardiovascular.
[a]Specific dose for epinephrine-containing solution not identified; this is maximum described dose.

thetics that exist primarily in the cationic form in solution. Using two to four times the usual concentration can overcome this slow onset by providing more molecules in the base form at the point of diffusion, so that actual penetration will appear equal to that seen in exposed nerves. Another example is the use of higher concentrations in the epidural space, where the fatty tissue, dura, and cerebrospinal fluid (CSF) present extensive barriers to penetration. Here the use of 0.75% bupivacaine produces much more rapid onset than an equivalent milligram dose of 0.25%. Another common clinical example is the use of 3% chloroprocaine. Although the high pK_a of this drug would suggest a slow onset, the low toxicity allows the use of a high concentration, so that clinical onset is rapid. The advantages of using higher concentrations can be offset by the risk that systemic blood levels may increase rapidly to the toxic range.

Volume

Volume of local anesthetic solution for a given block also should be kept at a minimum to reduce total dose. The volume requirement is often inversely proportional to the reliability of the anatomic landmarks, and certain procedures inherently require large volumes. If precise localization (as with a nerve stimulator or paresthesia) is obtainable, smaller volumes are effective. With neurolytic agents, precise localization is essential, because even small volumes of these agents may cause significant tissue damage.

Duration

Duration of local anesthetic block is determined by many factors. The primary determinant is the drug employed. The specific lipid affinity and the protein binding of each drug determine how long it will remain in its effective position in the lipid nerve membrane. Other factors make it difficult to predict the clinical duration of a specific drug for a specific block in a specific patient. Local blood flow is critical. Regions with high flows (such as the face and the epidural space) will produce shorter durations than areas with less vascular supply (such as the sciatic nerve or other peripheral nerves). Patient age also will contribute to this effect, because blood flow in many areas declines with age. The addition of vasoconstrictors or the local anesthetic's inherent vasodilator properties also will have an effect.

Differential Sensitivity

Differential sensitivity of nerve fibers has already been mentioned (see Fig. 1.3). Clinically, small or unmyelinated fibers (the B and C fibers in the physiologist's categorization of conduction speed) appear most sensitive to local anesthetic blockade. Their small diameter and lack of myelin sheaths allow the local anesthetic to block a sufficient band of contiguous sodium channels rapidly. In contrast, the large myelinated A fibers require that a much larger surface area and longer length be blocked before conduction is interrupted. Although these fibers have fewer sodium channels per unit of surface area and can be blocked more easily in certain laboratory situations, clinically, the small temperature- and pinprick-sensitive fibers are anesthetized before proprioception and motor function (A fibers).

Differential blockade is seen in a temporal sense during the onset of spinal anesthesia, as temperature sensation and pinprick discrimination disappear early. It also occurs in a concentration effect, whereby low concentrations of local anesthetics may produce analgesia without motor blockade. This difference is accentuated with the drugs demonstrating frequency-dependent blockade.

On individual fibers, there is a related phenomenon of *transition blockade*, as originally described by Wedensky. This occurs during onset and regression of neural blockade when the concentration of local anesthetic at the membrane is just below the C_m. At this point, single-impulse transmission may be blocked, but a series of impulses may result in every third or fourth impulse being transmitted. Apparently, the first few impulses are insufficient to produce depolarization, but they sensitize (or partially depolarize) the sodium channel to allow depolarization with the next impulse. Clinically, this may produce distorted sensation, such as "crawling" or "itching," in a partially anesthetized area. It may explain why an area numb to a single pinprick may still perceive a skin incision (multiple stimuli) as partially painful. It also may explain the occasional observation of apparent "hyperesthesia" as blocks spread and recede. Fortunately, this transition state is a temporary phase in the development of total anesthesia and is more of an intellectual curiosity than a significant clinical factor in regional anesthesia.

Another form of differential blockade occurs during epidural blockade as a result of variable penetrance of some of the local anesthetics in specific regions of the spinal nerves. Specifically, bupivacaine and chloroprocaine produce good anesthesia of the dorsal root entry fibers, whereas etidocaine penetrates into the spinal cord itself to produce anesthesia of the long nerve tracts (1). The result is a more segmental block with the former drugs, whereas etidocaine can provide some anesthesia distal to the site of injection.

Finally, the phenomenon of *tachyphylaxis* has been described (2), where subsequent injections (or infusions) of local anesthetics become less effective, either in the form of decreased duration or extent of blockade. This has been seen with spinal, caudal, and epidural anesthesia. The mechanism is unclear. Changes in the pH of tissues do not explain the phenomenon. The addition of epinephrine to local anesthetic solutions appears to reduce or prevent tachyphylaxis. It does not appear to be a problem with low concentrations of local anesthetics, such as the 0.05% to 0.125% bupivacaine infusions delivered for postoperative analgesia. Infusions of opioids also tend to eliminate this problem. In current practice, where low concentrations of local anesthetics plus opioids are the standard in obstetrics and pain management, tachyphylaxis is more of a curiosity than a clinically relevant problem.

Mantle Effect

A "mantle" effect has been described when anesthesia is performed on peripheral nerves to an extremity. The highest concentration of local anesthetic occurs on the outside of the peripheral nerve bundle. The onset of anesthesia will be perceived first on these outer (mantle) fibers, which are usually the fibers innervating the more proximal structures of a limb. The fibers to the distal limb structures tend to lie in the "core" of the nerve; therefore, anesthesia of the hand or foot may occur more slowly because the concentration of local anesthetic rises (by diffusion) more slowly here than on the outside of the nerve bundle. The regression of block may then proceed in the opposite fashion, because the concentration of anesthetic decreases first in the core area of the nerve.

These subtle distinctions may be observed if careful attention is paid to the onset of regression of blockade, but, generally, they do not affect the clinical course of neural blockade.

Specific Drugs

Cocaine

Cocaine fell into disfavor with early regional anesthetists because of local neural toxicity and the problem of abuse. It is still a useful topical anesthetic because of its inherent vasoconstrictor property. This is due to its blockade of the reuptake of catecholamines in sympathetic nerve terminals, and it contrasts with the direct vasodilation associated with clinical concentrations of other local anesthetic drugs. Cocaine's primary application is in the nasopharynx prior to nasal intubation or surgery (Table 2.2). The customary 4% solution will give onset of anesthesia in 4 to 5 minutes, but this

Table 2.2 Local Anesthetic Drug Clinical Uses

Drug (Brand Name)	Topical	Spinal	Epidural Surgical Obstetric ("Preservative Free")		Peripheral Nerve Block	Intravenous Regional
Cocaine	4%	NA	NA	—	NA	NA
Benzocaine	5%–20%	NA	NA	—	NA	NA
Short duration						
Procaine (Novocaine)	NA	10%	NI	NI	1%	NI
2-Chloroprocaine (Nesacaine)	NI	NA	2%–3%	2%–3%	1%–2%	NI
Intermediate duration						
Lidocaine (Xylocaine)	4%	5%	1.5% 2%	1.5% 2%[a]	0.5% 1%	0.5%
Mepivacaine (Carbocaine, Polocaine)	NA	NA	1% 1.5% 2%	NI	1%	NA
Prilocaine (Citanest)	NA	NA	2%–3%	NI	1%	0.5%
Long duration						
Ropivacaine (Naropin)	NA	0.5%[b]	0.75%, 1%[c]	0.2%	0.5%	NA
Bupivacaine (Marcaine, Sensorcaine) Levobupivacaine (Chirocaine)	NA	0.5% 0.75%	0.5% 0.75%[c]	0.125%[d] 0.25% 0.5%[a]	0.25% 0.5%	0.25%[b]
Etidocaine (Duranest)	NA	NA	1% 1.5%	NI	1%	NI
Tetracaine (Pontocaine)	1%–2%	1%	NA	NA	NA	NA

Note: Drugs are grouped in general duration of action. Concentrations listed are those recommended for particular application.
NA, not available, NI, not indicated.
[a]Produces motor blockade suitable for cesarean delivery.
[b]Not approved for this use.
[c]For single injection only; lower concentrations should be used for follow-up injections of catheters.
[d]Not prepared commercially; must be diluted at time of use.

can be shortened by use of higher concentrations or direct preparation of fresh crystals. The maximum recommended dose is 200 mg, or 5 mL of the 4% solution. The systemic toxicity of local anesthetics is additive, so that the common practice of using cocaine in the nose followed by liberal quantities of lidocaine or tetracaine for pharyngeal or tracheal anesthesia increases the hazard of a systemic reaction. Fortunately, systemic absorption from the mucosal surfaces is relatively poor and systemic reactions are rare despite the common practice of ignoring additive toxic doses.

Because of the abuse potential and the current illegal market problems, the use of lidocaine combined with a vasoconstrictor has been advocated as a substitute for this sole remaining clinical use of cocaine.

Benzocaine

Benzocaine was the first synthetic local anesthetic. Despite its similarity to cocaine as a benzoic acid derivative, it is not clinically effective. It is an exception to the general form of the local anesthetic molecule because of the absence of the tertiary amine group. This limits the compound to the uncharged state. Even though this form may penetrate lipid layers well, it is poorly soluble in water and thus can only be marketed in low concentrations. Its low water solubility also means that very little of the drug will enter the axoplasm. Although it appears to be able to reach the sodium channels by direct diffusion through the cell membrane (another exception to local anesthetic activity), it is clinically poorly effective. Use of benzocaine today remains limited to anesthesia of mucous membranes and (in higher concentrations) skin. Methemoglobinemia has been reported with absorption of excessive doses.

Procaine

As the first commercially successful synthetic descendant of cocaine, procaine was, for many years, the standard local anesthetic. Its rapid hydrolysis by plasma cholinesterases makes it one of the safest drugs in terms of systemic blood levels. Its effectiveness is limited by poor tissue penetrance and short duration. Procaine is primarily used for subcutaneous infiltration, where 1% solutions are very effective. It is not effective as a topical agent, and it gives unreliable anesthesia when used in the epidural space. For spinal anesthesia, the block is similar in duration to lidocaine, but with a higher failure rate and frequency of side effects (nausea especially). If used, the commercial 10% solution must be diluted to either hypo- or hyperbaric 5% mixtures. Interestingly, if fentanyl is added to improve reliability, the severity of itching is greater than when this opioid is combined with other local anesthetics (3). The aminoester compounds may have a different interaction with mu opioids at the spinal cord level.

A concern with procaine, as with the other esters, is the incidence of sensitization and allergy, usually to the metabolite *para*-aminobenzoic acid (PABA). The frequency of this problem is not documented, but this allergic sensitivity (along with the greater chemical stability of the amide drugs) favors the continued popularity of the amino-amide local anesthetics over procaine. In addition, previous suggestions that the amino-esters were safer than the amino-amides in the presence of malignant hyperthermia have not been substantiated.

Tetracaine

Another benzoic acid ester derivative, tetracaine, was synthesized in 1930. Its high pK_a is associated with a slower onset, but it provides the long duration of anesthesia that procaine lacks. Although more potent, toxicity also is proportionately increased. Until the arrival of the long-acting amino-amides, it was the drug of choice (in 0.25% or 0.5% concentrations) for long-acting peripheral nerve blocks. The maximum dose of 100 mg and its slow onset limit its use. Currently, it is used for spinal anesthesia, where small milligram doses are quite effective. It can be prepared as a hypobaric, isobaric, or hyperbaric solution. It is currently marketed as both a 1% solution and as niphanoid crystals.

Tetracaine also is used as an excellent topical anesthetic, primarily in the eye and the upper airway. Absorption from the mucosa provides rapid anesthesia, but the potential for systemic toxicity is high.

2-Chloroprocaine

The last of the esters introduced, chloroprocaine, is also one of the safest of local anesthetics in terms of systemic toxicity. Its rapid hydrolysis by plasma esterases can allow infiltration of up to 1,000 mg without signs of toxicity. This safety is obviously absent in patients with ineffective plasma cholinesterase. The duration of anesthesia is 45 to 60 minutes for an epidural and may be an advantage in ambulatory surgery. The 2% and 3% solutions are effective for epidural anesthesia. This level of potency is greater than would be expected from laboratory and physicochemical properties alone and presumably reflects greater tissue penetrance by this drug. The rapid onset of chloroprocaine anesthesia has made it popular both in outpatient procedures and in obstetrics. In the latter situation, the rapid hydrolysis also makes it the least likely drug to cross the placenta and produce neurobehavioral effects in the newborn. In conjunction with its rapid onset, chloroprocaine is characterized by a rapid termination of effect, which may provide a rude onset of discomfort before the end of surgery or delivery. Chloroprocaine also is used in peripheral nerve blocks, but here its short duration is limiting.

There have been several problems with the formulation of chloro-procaine. The stigma of neurotoxicity associated with the commercial formulation of chloroprocaine hydrochloride (Nesacaine) in the 1970s (see Chapter 3) was due to the presence of the antioxidant chemical bisulfite in 0.2% concentration at an acid pH of 3.5. A reformulation with a 0.07% bisulfite has not been associated with neurotoxicity. Another preparation (with 0.01% ethylenediaminetetraacetic acid [EDTA] as an antioxidant) has been removed from the market and replaced with a preservative-free alternative. The issue of back muscle irritation with large quantities of this drug has not been totally resolved, but appears to be infrequent (see Chapter 3). Chloroprocaine as a single-injection epidural anesthetic is ideal when rapid recovery is desired, as in ambulatory anesthesia (4).

One other problem with chloroprocaine is that it appears to interfere with the action of spinal cord opiates, which also limits its utility for inpatient procedures. When it is injected, even in small quantities, the potency and duration of the mu opioid agonists are decreased.

Dibucaine

This local anesthetic is probably most famous in the United States for its use as an inhibitor of plasma cholinesterase in testing patients for a defect in this enzyme. It is manufactured in the United States only for topical use as a cream, although it finds use outside the United States as a spinal anesthetic, particularly in the hypobaric form. It is an amide drug with relatively high potency.

Lidocaine

The first of the amide-linked local anesthetics, lidocaine soon replaced the esters in popularity following its clinical introduction in the early 1950s. It has a longer duration than procaine and a greater safety margin than tetracaine. It also avoids the incidence of allergic sensitization seen with the esters. To date, true allergy to any of the amino-amide class of anesthetics is rare. Lidocaine in 1% and 1.5% solutions became the standard drug for peripheral nerve blocks, as 1.5% and 2% concentrations became the norm for epidural anesthesia. The phenomenon of frequency-dependent block also created the appearance of greater sensory blockade in proportion to motor blockade than was seen with tetracaine. Lidocaine represented such a significant improvement that all subsequent developments in local anesthetics have been modifications of its amino-amide structure, and all local anesthetics have been compared to it as a standard.

Lidocaine is well absorbed topically and is frequently used for upper airway and tracheal anesthesia. Higher concentrations (4%) are required for topical use because the penetration is still not as great as in local infiltration. Lidocaine works well in local infiltration and in peripheral nerve blockade. In 0.5% concentration, it is also effective for intravenous regional anesthesia. In addition to epidural anesthesia, lidocaine also has been shown to be effective as a subarachnoid drug. It produces 45 to 90 minutes of spinal anesthesia. A 2% solution can be used as an isobaric injection, or it can be diluted to a hypobaric concentration. A commercial hyperbaric preparation has been used extensively for years, but recent concern about transient neurologic symptoms (see Chapter 3) suggest that this drug should be used in small doses and diluted concentrations.

Substantial experience with the systemic toxic effects of the drug is available because of its extensive use as a continuous-infusion antiarrhythmic. Inappropriate infusion rates have helped to demonstrate the onset of progression of central nervous system (CNS) toxicity, especially in the presence of decreased hepatic clearance resulting from hepatocellular dysfunction or impaired hepatic blood flow. Anesthetic doses of amino-amide drugs must be reduced in these situations.

Considered by many as the "standard" local anesthetic drug today, lidocaine does suffer in some comparisons. Although apparently free of the implication of cardiotoxicity, it is slower in onset than chloroprocaine and shorter in duration than bupivacaine. Attempts to improve onset have led to extensive work with carbonation of the drug (see Adjuvants, this chapter), and the attempts to improve duration have led to the synthesis of the next generation of local anesthetics by modification of the basic lidocaine molecule (see Table 1.1).

Eutectic Mixture of Local Anesthetics

One unusual application of lidocaine is in combination with prilocaine as a topical cream. The mixture of the crystalline bases of each of these compounds produces a new entity, a eutectic mixture of local anesthetics (EMLA) that has a lower melting point and behaves as a unique local anesthetic. As a mixture of bases, it contains a higher percentage of the active base form, which is also capable of diffusing through the skin. This mixture has a slow onset, but it has been very effective in producing topical anesthesia of the skin. It has been most widely applied in pediatric patients to provide anesthesia for intravenous line placement. There has not been significant toxicity with the cream, but its slow onset (it needs to be applied 45 to 60 minutes in advance with an occlusive dressing) has limited its application.

Mepivacaine

The aliphatic portion of this compound is a cyclical tertiary amine like ropivacaine and bupivacaine, but its shorter side chain confers lipid solubility and other characteristics very similar to those of lidocaine. Clinically, it is also very similar to lidocaine. Mepivacaine is less of a vasodilator than lidocaine and thus appears to possess slightly greater potency and somewhat greater duration of action. In epidural use, 1.5% mepivacaine will last 4 hours, compared to 3 hours for 1.5% lidocaine.

Mepivacaine is useful for epidural anesthesia, peripheral nerve block, and local infiltration. It is not well absorbed by mucous membranes, and thus it is not useful topically. Metabolism by the fetus and newborn is slow; for this reason, it appears unsuitable for obstetric analgesia. Mepivacaine has been reported to accumulate in plasma as a result of its protein binding, and thus it may not be suitable for prolonged intermittent epidural administration.

Prilocaine

This compound represents an attempt to improve on lidocaine, but it has had mixed success. It is the most rapidly metabolized amino-amide local anesthetic. This reduction in toxicity potential is offset by the unique toxicity of the metabolite, the *ortho*-toluidine ring, which produces methemoglobinemia (see Chapter 3). Unfortunately, there is no current commercial preparation available for surgical anesthesia in the United States.

Bupivacaine

Bupivacaine represents a similar attempt to improve on a good compound, with better results. Its structure represents the addition of a four-carbon aliphatic side chain to the mepivacaine molecule. The resulting dramatic increase in lipid solubility and protein binding produces a much greater duration of action compared to the previous amide local anesthetics. Its introduction was the first significant change in this class. The duration increase was achieved at the expense of speed of onset (latency of 15 to 20 minutes), but this is generally recognized as an acceptable price for the dramatic improvement in duration.

Clinically, bupivacaine is used in concentrations ranging from 0.05% to 0.75%. The lowest concentrations are used as epidural infusions to provide analgesia (or potentiation of opioid analgesia) for obstetrical or postoperative pain relief. Slightly higher concentrations (0.125% and 0.25%) provide only partial epidural analgesia and negligible motor blockade and are particularly useful in obstetric analgesia. Good sensory anesthesia can be attained with local infiltration of the 0.25% solution. The intermediate concentration of 0.5% provides excellent anesthesia for peripheral nerves and in epidural anesthesia. The 0.75% concentration produces excellent epidural anesthesia with rapid onset and profound motor blockade. The higher concentration also increases the potential for toxicity, and its use is not recommended in obstetrics or for reinjection of epidural catheters (see Chapter 3). Bupivacaine 0.75% is also an excellent spinal anesthetic, comparing favorably to tetracaine. It can be used as an isobaric or hyperbaric solution. Although epinephrine is usually added to all these concentrations to reduce systemic absorption and enhance blockade, its effect on the (already long) duration of bupivacaine is minimal.

Bupivacaine, like lidocaine, possesses significant frequency-dependent blocking properties (see Chapter 1) and thus has acquired a reputation for excellent sensory anesthesia compared to its motor-blocking properties. This is highly satisfactory to patients, who are reassured by the early return of movement in their extremities while analgesia persists. This effect is particularly useful in obstetric analgesia.

The major concern about bupivacaine currently is cardiac toxicity associated with unintentional high systemic blood levels (see Chapter 3), which has resulted in the introduction of two safer amino-amide alternatives.

Ropivacaine

Concern about the cardiotoxicity of bupivacaine has led to the development of ropivacaine, a compound chemically and clinically intermediate between mepivacaine and bupivacaine. Its side chain is a propyl group (compared to methyl for mepivacaine and butyl for bupivacaine). It is manufactured as the L-enantiomer only, in contrast to previous local anesthetics, which were produced as racemic mixtures. The L-form of the amino-amides is less cardiotoxic. As might be expected, ropivacaine is slightly less potent (5,6) and slightly shorter in duration than bupivacaine when used for epidural anesthesia. It appears to be more clinically equal in peripheral nerve block, and has been used in every situation where bupivacaine has been employed (7,8). Concentrations of 0.75% and 1% provide good epidural anesthesia, whereas 0.5% concentrations are effective for peripheral blockade. It appears to have slightly greater sensory–motor dissociation, though this difference is obscured by variances in potency and the extent of the difference is still unclear. This property has supported the use of ropivacaine alone (without opioids) in obstetrical and analgesic infusions. It is safer from the cardiotoxicity viewpoint, and may be, despite its higher cost, an appropriate choice for regional anesthetic techniques associated with a higher risk of systemic toxicity.

Levobupivacaine

Levobupivacaine is the pure L-enantiomer of bupivacaine, and, like ropivacaine, possesses less cardiotoxic potential. Introduced in 2000, it appears to have clinical characteristics similar to the racemic mixture in onset, potency, and duration of analgesia and motor block (9,10). It also has similar potentiation of opioids and sensory-motor dissociation to bupivacaine. Again, it is a more costly alternative, but may be appropriate for the anesthetic techniques associated with a higher risk of systemic toxicity.

Etidocaine

Etidocaine is a derivative of the lidocaine structure, with a longer, more lipid-soluble side chain. The increased lipid solubility and protein binding results in duration similar to that of bupivacaine. In contrast to bupivacaine, though, etidocaine has a rapid onset of action.

Although its potency should be similar to that of bupivacaine (based on physicochemical properties), twice the concentration is actually required for clinical applications. Epidural anesthesia is usually performed with 1.5% solutions, whereas a 1% solution is available for peripheral nerve block. There is an absence of frequency-dependent block with this compound and thus an apparently more profound (and sometimes disconcerting) motor blockade. It is thus not useful in obstetric analgesia or postoperative pain relief.

Etidocaine does have greater ability to penetrate the spinal cord itself when used for epidural analgesia. It produces profound blockade of the long nerve tracts within the cord like spinal anesthesia, rather than anesthesia of the nerves at their entry point or at the dorsal root ganglia (as seen with bupivacaine and 2-chloroprocaine) (1). Despite this greater extent of anesthesia, etidocaine has remained unpopular because of the disproportionate motor block.

Adjuvants   ### Vasoconstrictors

Vasoconstrictors are frequently added to local anesthetic solutions, most often to prolong the anesthetic effect. They also reduce the *peak blood levels* of local anesthetics by slowing absorption. The peak blood levels may occur slightly later when epinephrine is added, but they also will be lower. Epinephrine may be added to essentially every local anesthetic solution for peripheral nerve block except for "end" arteries, such as the digits or penis, where blood-flow compromise is undesirable.

Vasoconstrictors also improve the *quality* and *reliability* of the block, especially with spinal anesthesia. This has been demonstrated with tetracaine, lidocaine, and bupivacaine spinal anesthesia as well as with epidural blockade. The mechanism of this phenomenon is unclear. Epinephrine may simply increase the amount of local anesthetic available by reducing vascular uptake. There is also a suggestion that it may have intrinsic anesthetic properties in the subarachnoid space, perhaps by affecting pain receptors. One negative effect of the addition of subarachnoid epinephrine is the potential prolongation of the return of normal urination, which may delay discharge from ambulatory surgical units (11).

Another reason for inclusion of epinephrine in local anesthetic solutions is its effectiveness in detecting unintentional intravenous injection when used appropriately in a *test dose* (see Chapter 3).

Phenylephrine is another vasoconstrictor used to prolong spinal anesthesia. With equipotent doses, (0.1 mg epinephrine = 1 mg phenylephrine), equivalent prolongation can be achieved. Phenylephrine is best limited to subarachnoid injection, because its systemic absorption from other locations is capable of producing systemic vasoconstriction and reduction of cardiac output.

The epinephrine injected in tissues outside the subarachnoid space is absorbed systemically and may produce adverse effects on the cardiovascular system if large quantities are used. In small doses, the beta-adrenergic effect is usually beneficial, and epinephrine in epidural anesthetic solutions will help maintain the cardiac output by increasing myocardial contractility and heart rate. Quantities more than 0.25 mg total dose may be associated with arrhythmias or other undesirable cardiac effects (12). The concentration of epinephrine should be reduced if this total dose is exceeded. In practical terms, this means that if more than 50 mL of solution is to be used, the epinephrine must be reduced to less than 1:200,000 (5 µg/mL).

Opioids

The addition of short-acting opioids such as fentanyl and sufentanil to spinal anesthetics appears to intensify the block and prolong the duration of anesthesia in a degree similar to epinephrine but without prolongation of time to urination (13). They also provide residual analgesia beyond the duration of the local anesthetic in many cases. These combinations have been especially useful in ambulatory anesthesia in reducing the total local anesthetic dose and allowing rapid discharge. As with epidural analgesia, however, there are side effects such as pruritus (see Chapter 24).

Clonidine

Alpha$_2$-agonists have been shown to have analgesic properties when injected on nerves or in the subarachnoid space. Side effects limit their application as a sole agent, but small doses of clonidine have been shown to significantly prolong local anesthetic effects in spinal (14), epidural (15), intravenous regional (16), and peripheral nerve block (17,18) applications, both when injected with the drugs and when given orally (19). It is a useful combination in obstetrics (20) and pain therapy (21) as well as surgery. The effect is limited by systemic side effects such as hypotension and bradycardia with larger doses, but the use of small doses (50 to 75 µg) appears to be effective in prolonging duration without significant side effects. The high cost of clonidine in its current preparation is the major factor limiting its more widespread application in the United States.

Table 2.3   **Doses for Alkalinization of Local Anesthetics**

Local Anesthetic	Dose of Bicarbonate	pH of Final Solution
Chloroprocaine	1 cm^3 for each 30 cc	6.8
Lidocaine, mepivacaine	1 cm^3 for each 10 cc	7.2
Bupivacaine	0.1 cm^3 for each 10 cc	6.4

Alkalinization

Alkalinization of commercial local anesthetic solutions has been advocated to increase the pH of the solution closer to the pK$_a$ and thus drive more of the extracellular local anesthetic into the un-ionized base form. This more diffusible form then exists at relatively "higher" concentrations at the cell membrane and penetrates faster. More rapid onset is seen with lidocaine and mepivacaine, and to a lesser extent with bupivacaine (22). Although increased duration has been demonstrated with bupivacaine, the risk of precipitation is greatest and the benefit for onset is least with this drug.

An appropriate amount of an 8.4% commercial solution (1 mEq per mL) of sodium bicarbonate can be added to the local anesthetic solution just before injection. Care must be taken to avoid overenthusiastic alkalinization; these poorly soluble bases will precipitate in highly alkaline solutions. An amount of bicarbonate adequate to increase the pH to 6.5 to 7.5 is sufficient to improve speed of onset. Exceeding the levels listed in Table 2.3 may be associated with precipitation of local anesthetic base from solution, leaving a clinically ineffective preparation. Once alkalinized, these solutions should be used within 6 hours.

Carbonation

Carbonate salts of the local anesthetic base have been available in Canada as another means of speeding the onset of action. Although there are conflicting clinical efficacy results regarding this preparation, both laboratory and clinical data indicate that carbonation can reduce the onset time and the time to maximum anesthetic levels. The carbonate salt is technically difficult to manufacture and is unlikely to be available in the United States.

Compounding

Compounding of local anesthetic solutions also has been a popular means of attempting to improve onset and duration. Generally, a shorter-acting drug such as chloroprocaine or lidocaine is added to a long-acting drug such as bupivacaine to produce the best of both effects—rapid onset and long duration (23). When mixing solutions, the final concentration of each anesthetic will obviously be diluted by the addition of the other. The activity of each drug will be in proportion to its final concentration.

This process is not without risk. The toxicity of the drugs is at least additive, and care must be taken not to exceed maximum recommended doses. Unexpected interactions also may cause synergistic toxicity. Bupivacaine has been shown to increase the levels of free mepivacaine to almost twice the expected concentrations and to interfere with the serum hydrolysis of chloroprocaine. The addition of chloroprocaine to bupivacaine in obstetric anesthesia has been shown to decrease the duration of the bupivacaine when compared to the use of bupivacaine alone (24). The mechanism of these interactions is not fully understood or readily predictable from the physicochemical characteristics of the drugs. It would seem prudent to proceed with caution (if at all) when using compounded mixtures and be particularly aware of potential additive or synergistic toxicity. The use of other techniques, such as alkalinization or the use of an induction area for performance of blocks, may be more safe and effective in speeding onset.

Hyaluronidase

Hyaluronidase has been recommended in peripheral nerve block solutions. This enzyme breaks down collagen bonds and allows greater spread of solutions along tissue planes usually restricted by fine collagenous septa. Although it might be expected to improve the spread of local anesthetic, this has not been proven to be the case; it has actually been shown to impair the quality of anesthesia, at least in epidural use. Its use appears limited to retrobulbar injections.

Dextran

Dextran and other high-molecular-weight compounds have been advocated as adjuvants that might potentially increase the duration of local anesthetic mixtures. Despite some positive reports, the prolongation of anesthesia by either dextran or hyaluronic acid does not appear to be consistent or reliable. The encapsulation of local anesthetics in polymer microspheres appears to have greater potential for creating a long-acting preparation, but this work is experimental at this time.

References

1. Cusick, J. F., Myklebust, J. B., Abram, S. E. Differential neural effects of epidural anesthetics. *Anesthesiology* 53: 299, 1980.
2. Bigler, D., Lund, C., Mogensen, T., Hjortso, N. C., Kehlet, H. Tachyphylaxis during postoperative epidural analgesia—new insights. *Acta Anaesthesiol. Scand.* 31: 664, 1987.
3. Mulroy, M. F., Larkin, K. L., Siddiqui, A. Intrathecal fentanyl-induced pruritus is more severe in combination with procaine than with lidocaine or bupivacaine. *Reg. Anesth. Pain Med.* 26: 252, 2001.
4. Mulroy, M. F., Larkin, K. L., Hodgson, P. S., Helman, J. D., Pollock, J. E., Liu, S. S. A comparison of spinal, epidural, and general anesthesia for outpatient knee arthroscopy. *Anesth. Analg.* 91: 860, 2000.

5. Capogna, G., Celleno, D., Fusco, P., Lyons, G., Columb, M. Relative potencies of bupivacaine and ropivacaine for analgesia in labour. *Br. J. Anaesth.* 82: 371, 1999.
6. Polley, L. S., Columb, M. O., Naughton, N. N., Wagner, D. S., van de Ven, C. J. Relative analgesic potencies of ropivacaine and bupivacaine for epidural analgesia in labor: Implications for therapeutic indexes. *Anesthesiology* 90: 944, 1999.
7. McClellan, K. J., Faulds, D. Ropivacaine: An update of its use in regional anaesthesia. *Drugs* 60: 1065, 2000.
8. Owen, M. D., Dean, L. S. Ropivacaine. *Expert Opin. Pharmacother.* 1: 325, 2000.
9. Foster, R. H., Markham, A. Levobupivacaine: A review of its pharmacology and use as a local anaesthetic. *Drugs* 59: 551, 2000.
10. McLeod, G. A., Burke, D. Levobupivacaine. *Anaesthesia* 56: 331, 2001.
11. Chiu, A. A., Liu, S., Carpenter, R. L., Kasman, G. S., Pollock, J. E., Neal, J. M. The effects of epinephrine on lidocaine spinal anesthesia: A crossover study. *Anesth. Analg.* 80: 735, 1995.
12. Katz, R. L., Bigger, J. T., Jr. Cardiac arrhythmias during anesthesia and operation. *Anesthesiology* 33: 193, 1970.
13. Liu, S., Chiu, A. A., Carpenter, R. L., Mulroy, M. F., Allen, H. W., Neal, J. M., Pollock, J. E. Fentanyl prolongs lidocaine spinal anesthesia without prolonging recovery. *Anesth. Analg.* 80: 730, 1995.
14. Bonnet, F., Buisson, V. B., Francois, Y., Catoire, P., Saada, M. Effects of oral and subarachnoid clonidine on spinal anesthesia with bupivacaine. *Reg. Anesth.* 15: 211, 1990.
15. Eisenach, J. C., Lysak, S. Z., Viscomi, C. M. Epidural clonidine analgesia following surgery: Phase I. *Anesthesiology* 71: 640, 1989.
16. Reuben, S. S., Steinberg, R. B., Klatt, J. L., Klatt, M. L. Intravenous regional anesthesia using lidocaine and clonidine. *Anesthesiology* 91: 654, 1999.
17. Casati, A., Magistris, L., Fanelli, G., Beccaria, P., Cappelleri, G., Aldegheri, G., Torri, G. Small-dose clonidine prolongs postoperative analgesia after sciatic-femoral nerve block with 0.75% ropivacaine for foot surgery. *Anesth. Analg.* 91: 388, 2000.
18. Singelyn, F. J., Gouverneur, J. M., Robert, A. A minimum dose of clonidine added to mepivacaine prolongs the duration of anesthesia and analgesia after axillary brachial plexus block. *Anesth. Analg.* 83: 1046, 1996.
19. Liu, S., Chiu, A. A., Neal, J. M., Carpenter, R. L., Bainton, B. G., Gerancher, J. C. Oral clonidine prolongs lidocaine spinal anesthesia in human volunteers. *Anesthesiology* 82: 1353, 1995.
20. D'Angelo, R., Evans, E., Dean, L. A., Gaver, R., Eisenach, J. C. Spinal clonidine prolongs labor analgesia from spinal sufentanil and bupivacaine. *Anesth. Analg.* 88: 573, 1999.
21. Eisenach, J. C., DuPen, S., Dubois, M., Miguel, R., Allin, D. Epidural clonidine analgesia for intractable cancer pain. The Epidural Clonidine Study Group. *Pain* 61: 391, 1995.
22. Capogna, G., Celleno, D., Laudano, D., Giunta, F. Alkalinization of local anesthetics. Which block, which local anesthetic? *Reg. Anesth.* 20: 369, 1995.
23. Seow, L. T., Lips, F. J., Cousins, M. J., Mather, L. E. Lidocaine and bupivacaine mixtures for epidural blockade. *Anesthesiology* 56: 177, 1982.
24. Cohen, S. E., Thurlow, A. Comparison of a chloroprocaine–bupivacaine mixture with chloroprocaine and bupivacaine used individually for obstetric epidural analgesia. *Anesthesiology* 51: 288, 1979.

3 Complications of Regional Anesthesia

Each regional anesthetic technique has specific complications associated with the related anatomy or procedure. Several general problems can arise whenever needles and local anesthetic drugs are employed. The general complications will be reviewed in this chapter.

Local Anesthetic Toxicity

Local anesthetics can cause adverse drug reactions in three different ways.

Allergy

Allergy to the drugs is rare and almost always associated with the amino-ester preparations. True sensitivity reactions to the amino-amides are extremely rare. Cross-reactivity to an amino-amide drug has not been shown with allergy to an amino-ester. The amide class can be used with safety in patients who give a history of true allergy to an amino-ester local anesthetic (hives, bronchospasm, hypotension). Skin testing is available (1), but rarely does the anesthesiologist obtain the history sufficiently before the scheduled surgery to allow a complete investigation. If testing is done, the amino-ester compounds have a high incidence of skin reactivity and may produce suspicious reactions on skin testing that must be differentiated from true allergy.

Most patients who are tested following a report of a "reaction" are not truly allergic, and most frequently the symptoms are related to an anxiety or adrenaline reaction. The most common source of confusion is the patient who describes a previous unpleasant experience in a dentist's office. These symptoms are usually due to systemic absorption of epinephrine and should be distinguished from true allergy.

The *para*-aminobenzoic acid (PABA) liberated by the hydrolysis of the amino-ester anesthetics is believed responsible for the allergic reactions. Patients with a known allergy to sunscreens containing PABA are best treated with an amino-amide drug.

Tissue Neurotoxicity

Local tissue neurotoxicity is possible with any drug injection. Muscle damage is known to occur after injection of local anesthetics, but it is usually mild and resolves spontaneously (2). Neurotoxicity has been reported rarely following injection of every local anesthetic (3–5). Needle trauma and intraneural injection are the most commonly associated events (see Neuropathy, this chapter). High concentrations of the local anesthetics and the inclusion of epinephrine have been implicated in nerve damage with intraneural injection. The clinical local anesthetic solution that contains concentrations of potential concern is the 5% lidocaine used for spinal anesthesia. Although this preparation is toxic to nerves in the laboratory, the absence of extensive clinical problems suggests that the dilution in cerebrospinal fluid (CSF) is sufficient to avoid perilous toxicity. There is, however, a syndrome of transient neurologic symptoms (TNS) that presents more frequently after lidocaine spinal anesthesia (4). Symptoms, which include back pain radiating to the buttocks or legs, emerge 6 to 24 hours after resolution of block, with no motor or sensory deficit, and usually resolve spontaneously in 3 to 10 days. The syndrome is more frequent in outpatients, especially those having knee arthroscopy or lithotomy positions, but occurs significantly more frequently when lidocaine is the local anesthetic used (6). The frequency is 15% to 30% with lidocaine, but this may be reduced to the 3% to 5% incidence seen with bupivacaine if very low doses (20 to 25 mg) are used. Until the mechanism of this syndrome is clarified, it may be prudent to avoid large doses (greater than 100 mg) of lidocaine for spinal anesthesia, and to select alternative drugs or lower doses (20 to 25 mg) for lithotomy or arthroscopy procedures. Dilution of the 5% solution before injection is currently recommended.

When injecting any local solution, the lowest effective concentration should be used on peripheral nerves. This not only reduces the potential for local and systemic toxicity, but also may allow larger volumes to be used, which may promote wider areas of analgesia. Higher concentrations (0.75% bupivacaine, 1.5% etidocaine, 2% lidocaine, etc.) are reserved for initial epidural injection.

Other factors may explain cases of local toxicity. Preexistent nerve damage should always be excluded. Improper dilution of crystalline preparations may produce toxic concentrations of drug. Contamination of local anesthetic solutions with sterilizing agents or skin cleansing agents is another possible source of neurotoxicity. Detergents used to clean regional-block equipment may leave toxic residues and should be avoided (see Chapter 5).

Systemic Toxicity

Systemic (central nervous system [CNS]) toxicity due to excessive cerebral local anesthetic blood levels is the most serious and frequent adverse outcome of local anesthetic use. Toxic levels are most often produced by unintentional intravenous or intraarterial injection. Toxicity also can result from the slow absorption of drug following peripheral injection. Historically, local anesthetic seizures were most commonly associated with intravenous injection during epidural anesthesia, with a frequency approaching 1% in large reported series (7). The use of safety steps after 1980 has significantly reduced this frequency (8), and the addition of test doses has reduced the frequency even further, but not to zero (9,10) (Table 3.1). Currently, systemic toxicity appears to be a higher risk with peripheral nerve blocks, where the incidence in large series is still low (3,10).

Significant blood levels due to absorption are obtained after any regional block except spinal anesthesia, with the highest levels following intercostal and epidural blocks. These peaks are delayed until 20 minutes following injection and are related to the total dose of drug employed, the presence of a vasoconstrictor, and the relative blood supply at the site of injection. Toxic symptoms are dose related and all local anesthetics have similar toxic–therapeutic ratios for central toxicity. Increasing arterial blood levels of local anesthetic produce progressive depression of CNS function. Once the seizure threshold is reached (Fig. 3.1), tonic–clonic convulsions occur and are followed by coma if blood levels continue to increase. The early stages involve inhibitory–excitement imbalances that produce unpleasant subjective sensory symptoms, followed by muscle twitching prior to actual seizures. Symptoms are protean. They may include the classic "ringing in the ears" or "tingling around the mouth," but they also may present as one of many other sensory phenomena or simply as a general change in sensorium. A decreased responsiveness may be the only prelude to tonic–clonic convulsions.

The local anesthetics themselves do not produce direct permanent damage to the CNS. The depression, as on the peripheral nerves, reverses rapidly as the blood levels fall below the seizure threshold. The major risk to the patient is from cerebral hypoxia during the period of seizures and coma. Hypoxemia is extremely rapid in onset because of the severe muscle activity in conjunction with apnea. Acidosis and hyperkalemia ensue quickly. Treatment consists of oxygenation and support until the blood levels are lowered by redistribution of the anesthetic. Ventilation can be achieved by mouth-to-mouth or bag-and-mask resuscitation or by endotracheal intubation. If the seizures are severe enough to interfere with

Table 3.1   **Risk of Systemic Toxicity**

Author	Epidurals	STRs	Risk	PNBs	STRs	Risk
Tanaka[a]	17,439	20	11 in 10,000			
Brown	16,870	2	1.2 in 10,000	7,532	15	19 in 10,000
Auroy	30,413	4	1.3 in 10,000	21,278	16	7.5 in 10,000

STR, systemic toxic reactions; PNB, peripheral nerve blocks.
[a]Tanaka did not use epinephrine test doses.

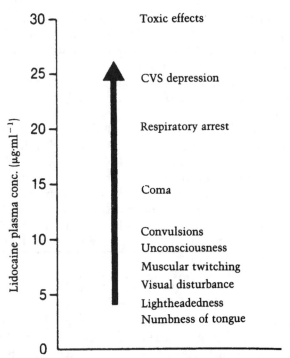

30 ‒ Toxic effects

25 ‒ CVS depression

Lidocaine plasma conc. (μg·ml^{-1})

20 ‒ Respiratory arrest

15 ‒ Coma

10 ‒ Convulsions
    Unconsciousness
    Muscular twitching
    Visual disturbance
5 ‒ Lightheadedness
    Numbness of tongue

0

Figure 3.1   **Progressive Continuum of Symptoms of Lidocaine Local Anesthetic Toxicity**
These symptoms are seen in roughly the same progression and proportion with the other local anesthetics, except that cardiovascular system (CVS) toxicity may be seen with some of the more potent amino-amides at blood levels closer to the convulsion threshold. (From Barash, P. G., Cullen, B. F., Stoelting, R. K., Ed. *Clinical Anesthesia.* Philadelphia: Lippincott, 2001, with permission.)

ventilation, they should be terminated with a rapid-acting intravenous antiseizure medication. Thiobarbiturates, benzodiazepines, propofol and succinylcholine have all been advocated; the drug of choice is the one most readily available. The doses of the barbiturates and benzodiazepines required are lower than those required for anesthesia and should be titrated to avoid excessive postictal depression, which makes neurologic assessment difficult. Generally, 1 to 3 mg per kg thiopental is sufficient to stop seizure activity. Succinylcholine is obviously not an anticonvulsant, but it is nevertheless useful in stopping motor seizure activity to allow ventilation, especially if intravenous access is lost. Regardless of the drug chosen, emphasis must remain on the need for oxygenation more than the need to abolish the seizure activity itself.

The seizure threshold varies for each drug, but, since the toxic–therapeutic ratio for the CNS is similar for all the local anesthetics, there is not any one drug that is more or less likely to produce seizures in the normal clinical doses. Several factors influence the actual seizure threshold in a given individual. Any factor that interferes with normal plasma clearance (such as liver failure with the amino-amides or plasma pseudocholinesterase deficiency with the amino-esters) will markedly increase the expected toxicity. Pretreatment with barbiturates or benzodiazepines will raise the threshold but usually only in doses sufficient to produce heavy sedation. The effect of usual anesthetic premedication cannot be relied on to protect the patient from carelessly produced high blood levels. Hypercarbia as well as metabolic acidosis also will lower the seizure threshold for all drugs. This is another reason that ventilation is essential in treatment, even to the point of mild hyperventilation. Lowering the arterial carbon dioxide level will raise the seizure threshold and speed recovery. Patient factors also influence toxicity, although controlled studies in this area are not available in humans. Renal clearance has not been a demonstrated factor. Body mass does not affect blood levels in the normal adult range.

Toxicity of the local anesthetics is additive. This is true for drugs of the same class, as well as for combinations of amino-esters and amino-amides. Practically speaking, this means that once the maximum recommended dose of an amino-amide has been used, the block cannot be supplemented with an amino-ester drug without increasing the chance for toxicity. The question of a "safe" interval between large doses has not been resolved.

There are several implications for clinical practice. First, major local anesthetic procedures should never be undertaken without resuscitation equipment immediately at hand. This includes an oxygen supply and delivery system, intravenous resuscitation drugs, and nearby cardiac monitors. An intravenous access should be in place in any patient receiving significant quantities of local anesthetic, especially if intravascular injection is a possibility.

Second, precautions must be taken to avoid high blood levels. Although the blood levels associated with seizures are known for many of the anesthetics, it is difficult to correlate or predict blood levels from clinical dosages. Manufacturers list maximum recommended doses for peripheral nerve block (see Table 2.1) based on blood levels extrapolated from animal data obtained from slow subcutaneous or intraperitoneal absorption. These maximum doses are difficult to remember, and the simplified guidelines of Table 3.2 may be more useful. The presence or absence of vasoconstrictors will influence the rate and extent of these levels. Smaller quantities of local anesthesia can, as stated, produce blood levels above the seizure threshold if injected intravenously or intraarterially in the cerebral circulation. Frequent aspiration, careful fixation of the needle, careful test doses, and incremental injections are clearly indicated whenever injections are made near blood vessels.

A *test dose* is the injection of a quantity of drug sufficient to produce some reliable subtoxic clinical sign if injected intravenously. To date, the most reliable indicator of intravascular injection is the

Table 3.2   **Simplified Maximum Doses**

| Duration of Action | Chemical type | | Maximum Doses |
	Esters	Amides	
Short	Procaine Chloroprocaine		1000 mg
Intermediate		Lidocaine Mepivacaine Prilocaine	500 mg
Long		Bupivacaine Levobupivacaine Ropivacaine	250 mg
	Tetracaine	Etidocaine	100 mg

tachycardia produced by 15 μg epinephrine injected intravenously (11). The pulse rate will increase 30% (from 80 to 110 beats per minute) 20 seconds following injection and return toward normal within 60 seconds (Fig. 3.2). The increase is transient, and a mechanical beat-to-beat pulse-counting device is essential rather than a manual count. There are several limitations to the test, and multiple safety steps are always important (7) (Table 3.3). Patients receiving beta-blocking drugs will not respond with a tachycardia, and changes in systolic blood pressure (15 mm Hg increase) will need to

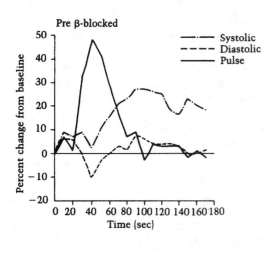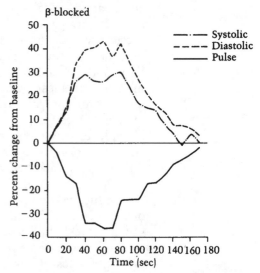

Figure 3.2   Percent change in heart rate, systolic blood pressure, and diastolic blood pressure after epinephrine test dose in normal subjects prior to beta blockade and after acute beta blockade.

Table 3.3   **Criteria for Epinephrine Test Doses**

Situation	Hemodynamic Criteria
Normal patient	HR increase >20 bpm
	SBP increase >15 mm Hg
Beta blockade	SBP increase >15 mm Hg
Advanced age	HR increase >9 bpm
	SBP increase >15 mm Hg
General anesthesia	HR increase >8 bpm
	SBP increase >13 mm Hg

HR, heart rate; bpm, beats per minute; SBP, systolic blood pressure.

be monitored or an alternative test used. Elderly patients may also have a reduced response to epinephrine. Premedicated patients cannot be relied on to report subjective clinical signs, and general anesthesia will also reduce the response to epinephrine by 50%.

Alternative tests are available. Larger doses of local anesthetic and the omission of premedication may be required if epinephrine is contraindicated or if beta blockade is present. Doses of 100 mg chloroprocaine, 100 mg lidocaine, or 25 mg bupivacaine injected intravenously will produce subjective signs and may be a reliable substitute in this situation. Another alternative is the injection of 1 mL of air while monitoring the heart sounds with a precordial Doppler stethoscope. This has been used in obstetrical anesthesia, but it may not be practical in the operating room. The inclusion of dose limitation, aspiration, and incremental injection are critical.

A third implication of CNS toxicity is the necessity for close monitoring following even a negative test dose. Blood levels will continue to increase from venous absorption (Fig. 3.3). Appropriate monitoring for local anesthetic toxicity involves frequent assessment of the patient's *mental status*. We are in an era of technologic dependence on mechanical and electronic devices to ensure patient safety. Unfortunately, no monitor can give early warning of increasing local anesthetic blood levels. Frequent conversation with and observation of the patient by the anesthesiologist is the only effective monitor of cerebral function in the postblock period. Barbiturate and benzodiazepine sedation may increase the perception threshold for local anesthetic toxicity.

Early detection of increasing blood levels and rapid treatment with oxygen will prevent hypoxic CNS sequelae following systemic toxicity of local anesthetics. Despite ideal technique, toxic reactions will occur in any practice where enough regional anesthetics are administered, and appear more likely after peripheral nerve block. These reactions should not produce any residual disability if recognized early and treated appropriately.

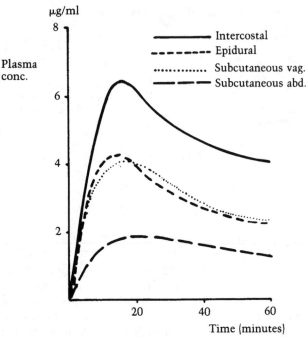

μg/ml

Plasma
conc.

———— Intercostal
------- Epidural
.... Subcutaneous vag.
— — — Subcutaneous abd.

Time (minutes)

Figure 3.3   Plasma concentrations of lidocaine continue to increase for 20 minutes
following injection, and are higher following intercostal blockade than
after epidural or subcutaneous injection. (From Cousins, M. J.,
Bridenbaugh, P. O., Eds. *Neural Blockade in Clinical Anesthesia and
Management of Pain.* Philadelphia: Lippincott, 2001, with permission.)

Special Toxicity Considerations

Prilocaine and Benzocaine

Both benzocaine and the metabolite of prilocaine (*ortho*-toluidine)
produce methemoglobinemia and a distressing cyanosis in humans.
This occurs only with high doses (around 500 to 600 mg). Prilocaine
is no longer commercially available, but this reaction is seen with
some frequency after use of large doses of topical benzocaine for
topical airway anesthesia.

2-Chloroprocaine

In 1980, several case reports described neurotoxicity following
epidural or caudal anesthesia with a chloroprocaine preparation
containing 0.2% bisulfite as the preservative. One current preparation of chloroprocaine contains no preservative and does not appear
to be neurotoxic. However, there is a syndrome of back pain when
large quantities (greater than 40 cm³) are injected (12). This pain
ensues immediately on resolution of the block, and may be related

to spasm of the paraspinous muscles. It is uncommon with single injection doses, and usually responds to opioid analgesics, but may be severe in some cases. It appears prudent to limit this drug to situations where less than 30 to 35 mL total dose will be injected.

Bupivacaine

Several cases of cardiac arrest resistant to resuscitation following systemic toxic reactions with the long-acting amino-amides bupivacaine and etidocaine have been described. These cases frequently involved obstetric patients and usually followed an unintentional intravenous injection. Although bupivacaine is no more depressant to the cardiovascular system than lidocaine when blood pressure and cardiac output are considered, bupivacaine does have a prolonged effect on the cardiac conduction system compared to lidocaine. Bupivacaine delays conduction and increases the frequency of reentrant arrhythmias at serum concentrations slightly above the seizure threshold. Thus, ventricular arrhythmias (or asystole) are more common with high blood levels of bupivacaine and may appear more frequently in the setting of acidosis and hypoxemia associated with seizures. Resuscitation is not impossible, but it does require rapid oxygenation, higher than normal epinephrine doses to treat electromechanical dissociation, and probably the use of drugs other than lidocaine to treat reentrant arrhythmias. Pregnant patients represent a particular challenge because the gravid uterus impedes venous return in the classic supine position for resuscitation, and early delivery of the fetus is desirable if maternal resuscitation is prolonged. Appropriate precautions of test dosing and incremental injection are particularly desirable during epidural administration, and appear to have reduced the frequency of these events (7) (see Chapter 7). The risk of systemic toxicity remains higher with peripheral nerve injections (3,10), and the use of alternative long-acting drugs such as ropivacaine or levobupivacaine may be advisable in this situation.

Mechanical Complications

Neuropathy

Neuropathy may result from the anesthetic itself, but more often it is due to mechanical trauma to the nerve. The overall occurrence of neuropathy is not well documented. In the United States Closed Claims experience, 16% of lawsuits against anesthesiologists involved nerve injury, but 28% of these cases involved ulnar nerve injury that was associated with general anesthesia. Spinal anesthesia and lumbosacral nerve blocks were more often associated with regional anesthesia related nerve injuries (13). This is consistent with the Finnish Closed Claim experience of 23 neurologic claims associated with 720,000 spinal and epidural anesthetics (14). A large prospective series from France reported that nerve injury was rare (34 cases in more than 100,000 anesthetics), and was most often associated with a paresthesia during performance of the block or pain on injection (3).

The issue of the safety of eliciting paresthesias is unclear. Although permanent deficits are frequently preceded by a paresthesia, many large series have reported a high frequency of deliberate or accidental paresthesias without consequences (15). Selander et al. have shown that needles with long, sharp bevels will produce more direct trauma to isolated nerves than will short-beveled needles (16), and this may explain some of the neuropathies seen after peripheral nerve blockade when paresthesias (direct nerve contact) are elicited. Direct nerve trauma can be reduced by using infiltration techniques or nerve stimulators that avoid paresthesias, although even then an unintentional nerve contact may occur, and short-term and long-term dysesthesias have been reported after brachial plexus block with a nerve stimulator (17). With either of these approaches (or with the conventional search for paresthesias), the use of a short-beveled needle also appears to be a reasonable precaution. Unfortunately, there are no prospective comparative studies that document the efficacy of any of these theoretical precautions in reducing nerve injury.

Intraneural injection is associated with a higher incidence of residual dysfunction. This is usually signaled by a cramping pain during the actual injection. Whether it is the increased intraneural pressure or the excessively high local concentration of anesthetic drug that produces the damage is not known, but injection should be halted immediately if the patient reports pain at the time of injection.

Hematoma Formation

Hematoma formation is also occasionally seen after peripheral nerve block. This is more likely if the patient has a preexisting coagulopathy. In normal patients, arteries and veins are frequently punctured during blocks without complications. A hematoma is a nuisance because the extravasated blood may interfere with the spread of local anesthetic or subsequent identification of landmarks. Later calcification of an organized hematoma may present a further inconvenience for the patient, but the incidence of this situation is extremely rare. It is appropriate to inquire about the patient's bleeding history before a block and to use the smallest practical needle and due care when near vessels.

A hematoma in the epidural or subarachnoid space is more serious, where nerve compression can lead to permanent nerve injury (18). In spontaneous spinal hematomas, the presenting symptom is usually pain followed by a neurologic deficit. With spinal or epidural anesthesia, the presentation may be limited to an inordinately prolonged motor blockade (the early pain is masked by the anesthesia). Early diagnosis and treatment are essential, and the use of these techniques (or any regional block) in the fully anticoagulated patient is inadvisable. This applies to patients on full systemic heparinization or therapeutic coumadin preoperatively, or thrombolytic infusions postoperatively. The use of low-dose coumadin before orthopedic procedures does not preclude the use of spinal anesthesia or short-term epidural analgesia (19). Placement of epidural catheters in patients who will be transiently heparinized during surgery appears to be safe (20). The use of regional block techniques in the face of "minidose" heparin therapy also appears to involve a low risk of hematoma formation. Patients receiving aspirin or nonsteroidal antiinflammatory drugs do not appear at higher risk for hematoma formation (21). Although obtaining a bleeding time has been advocated for these patients, it does not predict intraoperative hemostasis and does not appear to be useful. There is insufficient information to comment on the safety of regional techniques in the presence of other antiplatelet medications such as clopidogrel.

The major problem with regional anesthesia currently is the use of low-molecular-weight heparin preparations as thromboprophylaxis in the perioperative period. These compounds act in a manner similar to heparin, but do not affect the partial thromboplastin time (PTT) or the activated clotting time (ACT), which are commonly used to measure heparin activity. Their use in the United States has been associated with a disturbing number of epidural hematomas, and caution should be used in inserting or removing an epidural catheter or performing a neuraxial block in their presence (22). Catheter insertion should precede dosing by 2 hours, or follow at least 12 hours after dosing.

Infection

Passage of regional-block needles through infected tissues and introducing infection into deeper tissues or the subarachnoid space has been a concern, and the presence of local infection is considered a contraindication to performance of regional techniques. The question has been raised whether spinal anesthesia is safe in patients with distant infections or systemic sepsis. Animal data suggest that spinal injection is safe if appropriate systemic antibiotics are used in this situation (23). With the increasing use of long-term epidural and spinal catheters, there has been the inevitable incidence of infection. Diagnosis and treatment can be difficult in the terminally ill, chronic-pain patient, and may require removal of catheters if there is evidence of epidural infection. Epidural abscess itself is rare. A more complex question is the use of regional techniques in the presence of human immunodeficiency virus (HIV) infection. These patients may develop CNS infections early and should be evaluated for such signs before a block is performed. There is no evidence that spinal or epidural anesthesia aggravates HIV infection and related syndromes, and regional techniques are often preferable in these complicated patients. It appears safe to perform epidural blood patch in the presence of HIV infection.

References

1. Incaudo, G., Schatz, M., Patterson, R., Rosenberg, M., Yamamoto, F., Hamburger, R. N. Administration of local anesthetics to patients with a history of prior adverse reaction. *J. Allergy Clin. Immunol.* 61: 339, 1978.
2. Foster, A. H., Carlson, B. M. Myotoxicity of local anesthetics and re-generation of the damaged muscle fibers. *Anesth. Analg.* 59: 727, 1980.
3. Auroy, Y., Narchi, P., Messiah, A., Litt, L., Rouvier, B., Samii, K. Serious complications related to regional anesthesia: Results of a prospective survey in France. *Anesthesiology* 87: 479, 1997.
4. Hodgson, P. S., Neal, J. M., Pollock, J. E., Liu, S. S. The neurotoxicity of drugs given intrathecally (spinal). *Anesth. Analg.* 88: 797, 1999.
5. Kane, R. E. Neurologic deficits following epidural or spinal anesthesia. *Anesth. Analg.* 60: 150, 1981.
6. Freedman, J. M., Li, D. K., Drasner, K., Jaskela, M. C., Larsen, B., Wi, S. Transient neurologic symptoms after spinal anesthesia: An epidemio-logic study of 1,863 patients. *Anesthesiology* 89: 633, 1998.
7. Mulroy, M. F., Norris, M. C., Liu, S. S. Safety steps for epidural injection of local anesthetics: Review of the literature and recommendations. *Anesth. Analg.* 85: 1346, 1997.
8. Tanaka, K., Watanabe, R., Harada, T., Dan, K. Extensive application of epidural anesthesia and analgesia in a university hospital: Incidence of complications related to technique. *Reg. Anesth.* 18: 34, 1993.
9. Hawkins, J. L., Koonin, L. M., Palmer, S. K., Gibbs, C. P. Anesthesia-related deaths during obstetric delivery in the United States, 1979–1990. *Anesthesiology* 86: 277, 1997.
10. Brown, D. L., Ransom, D. M., Hall, J. A., Leicht, C. H., Schroeder, D. R., Offord, K. P. Regional anesthesia and local anesthetic-induced systemic toxicity: Seizure frequency and accompanying cardiovascular changes. *Anesth. Analg.* 81: 321, 1995.
11. Moore, D. C., Batra, M. S. The components of an effective test dose prior to epidural block. *Anesthesiology* 55: 693, 1981.
12. Stevens, R. A. Back pain following epidural anesthesia with 2-chlorop-rocaine. *Reg. Anesth.* 22: 299, 1997.
13. Kroll, D. A., Caplan, R. A., Posner, K., Ward, R. J., Cheney, F. W. Nerve injury associated with anesthesia. *Anesthesiology* 73: 202, 1990.
14. Aromaa, U., Lahdensuu, M., Cozanitis, D. A. Severe complications as-sociated with epidural and spinal anaesthesias in Finland 1987–1993. A study based on patient insurance claims. *Acta Anaesthesiol. Scand.* 41: 445, 1997.
15. Horlocker, T. T., Wedel, D. J. Neurologic complications of spinal and epidural anesthesia. *Reg. Anesth. Pain Med.* 25: 83, 2000.
16. Selander, D., Dhuner, K. G., Lundborg, G. Peripheral nerve injury due to injection needles used for regional anesthesia. An experimental study of

the acute effects of needle point trauma. *Acta Anaesthesiol. Scand.* 21: 182, 1977.

17. Borgeat, A., Ekatodramis, G., Kalberer, F., Benz, C. Acute and nonacute complications associated with interscalene block and shoulder surgery: A prospective study. *Anesthesiology* 95: 875, 2001.

18. Vandermeulen, E. P., Van Aken, H., Vermylen, J. Anticoagulants and spinal-epidural anesthesia. *Anesth. Analg.* 79: 1165, 1994.

19. Enneking, F. K., Benzon, H. Oral anticoagulants and regional anesthesia: A perspective. *Reg. Anesth. Pain Med.* 23: 140, 1998.

20. Liu, S. S., Mulroy, M. F. Neuraxial anesthesia and analgesia in the presence of standard heparin. *Reg. Anesth. Pain Med.* 23: 157, 1998.

21. Urmey, W. F., Rowlingson, J. Do antiplatelet agents contribute to the development of perioperative spinal hematoma? *Reg. Anesth. Pain Med.* 23: 146, 1998.

22. Horlocker, T. T., Wedel, D. J. Neuraxial block and low-molecular-weight heparin: Balancing perioperative analgesia and thromboprophylaxis. *Reg. Anesth. Pain Med.* 23: 164, 1998.

23. Carp, H., Bailey, S. The association between meningitis and dural puncture in bacteremic rats. *Anesthesiology* 76: 739, 1992.

4 Premedication and Monitoring

Premedication and intraoperative sedation are important components of regional techniques. Although "pure" regional anesthesia can be performed without supplementation, especially in ambulatory surgery, only the rare inpatient enjoys such an exercise or chooses it again. Omission of sedation is appropriate in the obstetric suite or the emergency room, where systemic medications must be carefully limited. However, in the operating room, successful regional anesthesia requires skillful use of adjuvants to produce cooperation and acceptance. This may include sedation and analgesia for the performance of the block, as well as sedation during the surgical procedure.

Goals

Basically, supplemental medication is given to attain one of three objectives:

1. To decrease apprehension and increase the degree of cooperation in the anxious patient
2. To provide analgesia and thus reduce the degree of discomfort associated with the procedure, particularly with insertion of needles or search for paresthesias
3. To produce amnesia or lack of awareness of the intraoperative and perioperative events

A fourth motive is sometimes mentioned: the hope of raising the seizure threshold to local anesthetic drugs. This is not attained with the conventional sedative doses of benzodiazepines or barbiturates, but only with doses sufficient to produce unconsciousness in most patients [1]. This approach is not warranted because it carries its own risk of respiratory and cardiac depression, and such sedation may mask the response to a test dose [2,3] or the early warning signs that usually precede bupivacaine cardiotoxicity [4].

A wide range of sedation can be produced depending on the patient and the situation (Table 4.1). There are different stages in the execution of a regional anesthetic: the performance of the block itself and the intraoperative management. Each stage requires appropriate tailoring of sedation. The outpatient having a minor procedure with little anxiety attached will require little sedation; the use of excessive amounts will negate the advantages of rapid recovery and discharge. The patient undergoing axillary block where paresthesias are sought will require a moderate amount of opioid to ease the discomfort, but not enough to blunt the perception of nerve con-

Table 4.1 Common Sedative Medications Used to Supplement Regional Anesthetic Techniques

Drug (Brand Name)	Dose Range	Applications	Comments
Benzodiazepines			
Midazolam (Versed)	1–4 mg i.v.	Outpatient premedication Inpatient intramuscular premedication	Amnesia potential
Lorazepam (Ativan)	1–2 mg p.o.	Inpatient premedication	Amnesia, postoperative sedation
Narcotics			
Fentanyl (Sublimaze)	25–200 μg i.v.	Outpatient premedication	Short duration
Sedative/hypnotics			
Propofol	25–50 μg/kg/ min i.v.	Sedation during block or surgery	Rapid recovery, antiemetic effect
Methohexital	50–100 μg/kg/ min i.v.	Sedation during block or surgery	Rapid recovery, antianalgesic effect

i.v., intravenous; p.o., by mouth.

tact. The anxious inpatient for upper abdominal surgery will require sedation and an amnestic agent for insertion of an epidural catheter, as well as intraoperative supplementation with a light general anesthetic. Most children require a general anesthetic for the performance of the block itself. [Although the use of a general anesthetic to facilitate regional block in children is accepted as reducing the chance of injury, in the adult such a practice may increase the risk of unwanted nerve injury (5).] In a teaching situation, heavy sedation and an amnestic agent are often appropriate.

Unfortunately, depressant medications increase the risk associated with regional techniques. This must always be weighed against the benefits provided.

Drugs

Opioids

The opioid class of drugs is ideal for regional-technique supplementation because these drugs in appropriate doses produce analgesia and sedation without loss of consciousness. Thus, they are excellent in enhancing patient cooperation and in reducing the discomfort associated with needle insertion or paresthesias. They also possess the desirable feature of easy reversibility with naloxone. Respiratory depression is the main drawback of the opioids, and doses must be individually titrated and the patient monitored appropriately. All of the opioids share the propensity to stimulate the chemoreceptor trigger zone and induce nausea. This is dose related and rarely occurs in the sedative dose range, but pretreatment with antiemetics may be indicated in the susceptible patient.

Fentanyl is the most popular opioid sedative because of its rapid onset, short but adequate duration, and easy titratability. It is most appropriate for the ambulatory surgery setting, but is also very effective for sedation while performing blocks in an inpatient induction area. Increments of 25 to 50 μg will give rapid analgesia and sedation for 20 to 30 minutes, usually waning as the block is completed. Dosage is a function of patient vitality, not body size; milligram per kilogram schedules should be avoided. Some respiratory depression will occur, and pulse oximetry and supplemental oxygen are appropriate.

Derivatives of fentanyl are available. Sufentanil is similar, although roughly ten times as potent; suitable dilution is advisable. Alfentanil is similar in effect but shorter in duration and less potent than fentanyl. Although perhaps ideal as an intravenous infusion anesthetic for outpatients, its sedative properties after a bolus injection may be too short to facilitate regional techniques. Remifentanil is even shorter in duration and is really suitable for use only as an infusion. The expense and need of a pump for these two drugs make bolus fentanyl doses more often the drug of choice.

Morphine and meperidine are long acting and provide good sedation as well as analgesia. Their duration is longer and the onset slower than fentanyl. These drugs were popular as inpatient intramuscular premedicants in the past, but the ease of titration of the newer intravenous opioids has made their use less common.

There are also several opioids with both agonist and antagonist properties that are intended to reduce the potential for respiratory depression. These drugs are useful, particularly as intramuscular premedication for inpatients, although they have not been shown to have significant advantages in efficacy or safety.

Benzodiazepines

Benzodiazepines are extensively used as premedicants or sedatives. They are effective, centrally acting anxiolytics, and they have the additional property of producing amnesia. Although they do not prevent seizures in the usual clinical doses (1), these drugs are effective in the treatment of local anesthetic toxicity and thus are useful to have in induction areas in the event of a toxic reaction. The amnestic property, especially of the longer-acting lorazepam (1- to 2-mg doses), is advantageous for inpatients desiring to be unaware of procedures. Like morphine, it may require 30 to 60 minutes to reach peak effect, and care must be used when titrating intravenous supplemental sedation during this period of increasing blood levels. Prolonged sedation in the recovery room is seen frequently, particularly in the elderly patient. With the increasing use of epidural analgesic regimens, there is less need for prolonged sedation or analgesia in the immediate recovery period, and long-acting drugs are not as useful.

The most popular benzodiazepine is midazolam, which has replaced diazepam for parenteral use because of its predictable dose response and absence of venous irritation. Midazolam is rapid and short acting and produces less respiratory depression than opioids. It is useful for intraoperative sedation once an adequate block has been achieved. It is also useful in producing amnesia for the block itself, although it is not analgesic in this situation and requires opioid supplementation. The amnestic effect can be a disadvantage by producing unwanted confusion and lack of cooperation in patients if excessive doses are used. Sedation can be long lasting, so the dosage should be kept to a minimum (1 to 3 mg intravenously, titrated intravenously in 0.5- to 1-mg increments). Its duration of sedation is short with these doses, lasting about 30 minutes. The amnestic effect is unpredictable, and occurs at doses lower than those required to produce sedation, which may present a problem in outpatients. Postoperative instructions may not be remembered by an apparently alert outpatient. Nevertheless, midazolam is an excellent anxiolytic, and the amnestic effect is useful both during performance of blocks and for intraoperative sedation. Larger doses may prolong recovery. The availability of the specific antagonist drug flumazenil has increased the safety margin, but it is more reasonable to shift to a shorter-acting infusion if prolonged sedation is necessary.

Barbiturates

Barbiturates have been used as sedative agents in the induction room. They are less useful than the previous two classes because they are not true analgesics or amnestics; they produce these effects only in doses sufficient to produce unconsciousness. At lower doses, they are actually "antianalgesic" and may produce exaggerated responses to pain and decreased cooperation. The rapid-acting barbiturates (such as an infusion of 0.2% methohexital) require careful titration to produce sufficient "anesthesia" while avoiding respiratory depression and airway obstruction.

For intraoperative sedation (after a block is established), an infusion of methohexital is an inexpensive sedative, as long as no painful stimuli are present. It provides more rapid recovery than a midazolam infusion, with less frequent oxygen desaturation (6).

Propofol

Propofol is primarily a general anesthetic drug, but also an excellent sedative in lower doses. Although it (like the benzodiazepines) does not have analgesic properties, it is not an antianalgesic like the barbiturates. It also lacks the predictable amnestic properties of the benzodiazepines, but it provides more rapid recovery and an apparent antiemetic effect that is beneficial, especially in outpatients. It can be used as a bolus for deep sedation during performance of some selected blocks (such as retrobulbar block) where consciousness is not necessary. As an infusion during surgical procedures, it provides anxiolytic, sedative, and amnestic properties, with the best results in the dose range of 30 to 60 μg/kg/minute (7). It is expensive for longer cases, but its rapid recovery, antiemetic effect, and easy titratability make it ideal for sedation in short outpatient procedures. The combination of small doses of midazolam and fentanyl to enhance the performance of a regional block, followed by a propofol infusion for sedation, provides an ideal formula for patient satisfaction and rapid recovery.

Ketamine

Ketamine has been used in low doses (20 to 30 mg intravenously) as a sedative during performance of regional blockade because of its analgesic properties in this dose range. Larger doses are associated with hallucinations on emergence. This drug has the advantage of maintaining cardiovascular stability and producing less respiratory depression and obtundation of airway reflexes. It is most useful for sedation during spinal anesthesia for fractured hip repair in the elderly, where the analgesia and cardiovascular support are beneficial.

Oxygen

Although not a sedative drug, oxygen is appropriate as a supplemental drug when most of these sedatives and analgesics are used. Opioids particularly produce respiratory depression, and this is potentiated by the addition of benzodiazepines. Oxygen desaturation is frequent (8), and nasal prongs or a facemask are useful, especially in the elderly.

Other Adjuvants

The preoperative visit has been shown to be extremely effective in reducing anxiety in patients. Kind attention to the patient's concern and situation will reduce the need for any of the preceding medications. Small gestures, such as comfortable positioning of the table and the offer of a warm blanket, are greatly appreciated.

Music also has sedative properties. Selected tapes can be provided through a portable cassette player or a piped-in music system. This will not only distract and pacify most patients, but the headphones also will eliminate many of the anxiety-provoking sounds and conversations of the operating room.

General Anesthetic Agents

General anesthetic agents are sometimes helpful and occasionally necessary. When upper abdominal surgery is being performed under intercostal, spinal, or epidural block, supplemental general anesthesia with an endotracheal tube is advisable to obtund diaphragmatic sensation, protect the airway, and provide controlled ventilation. The presence of a regional block reduces the minimum alveolar concentration (MAC) of inhalational anesthesia, and when the endotracheal tube is the most significant stimulus the patient may perceive, a fraction of MAC is usually sufficient.

In pediatric practice, the use of general anesthesia is common to facilitate placement of regional blocks. In this situation of more predictable anatomy and less predictable cooperation, this practice may be justified. In adults, however, performance of a regional block, even with a nerve stimulator, under general anesthesia may increase the risk of nerve or spinal cord injury (5).

Among the general anesthetics, nitrous oxide can provide sedation for a patient with an adequate block who is restless or anxious, particularly if, like propofol, it is added after intravenous opioids and sedatives have already been given. Nitrous oxide offers the advantage of rapid reversibility at the end of the procedure, in contrast to the longer-lasting effects of large quantities of intravenous agents.

Monitoring

Intraoperatively, patients undergoing regional anesthesia require the same standards of monitoring as those receiving general anesthesia. General anesthesia should be monitored with an electrocardiogram (ECG), a blood pressure device, and a pulse oximeter, but the regional anesthesia patient also must be monitored for the signs of potential systemic toxicity. Specific monitoring to detect increasing blood levels of local anesthetic must focus on the patient's mental status and thus requires constant verbal contact. The anesthetist or assistant should engage in conversation with the patient and be alert for the first signs of a change in mental concentration or slurring of speech, especially in the first 20 minutes following injection. The use of excessive sedation will hinder the early detection of impending toxicity.

A pulse oximeter is the most frequently applied monitor in the induction area. Providing information about heart rate as well as oxygen saturation, it is useful during regional anesthesia, particularly when sedation may produce respiratory depression. It is also an effective pulse counter for monitoring heart-rate changes with a test-dose solution.

Blood pressure monitoring is essential following spinal, epidural, or sympathetic blocks. An automatic noninvasive device with a short cycling time is ideal, because it leaves the anesthesiologist's hands free to make interventions during the early stages of hypotension. A baseline blood pressure value should be established before performing any blocks that will produce sympathetic blockade.

The block level also should be monitored, especially when a sympathectomy is produced. Block level and blood pressure should be measured every 3 to 5 minutes for the first 15 minutes following the block to warn of unexpected high levels. Block level should be monitored during the course of epidural or spinal anesthesia, because both of these techniques may demonstrate a change of level over the first hour.

References

1. De Jong, R. H., Heavner, J. E. Local anesthetic seizure prevention: Diazepam versus pentobarbital. *Anesthesiology* 36: 449, 1972.
2. Moore, J. M., Liu, S. S., Neal, J. M. Premedication with fentanyl and midazolam decreases the reliability of intravenous lidocaine test dose. *Anesth. Analg.* 86: 1015, 1998.
3. Mulroy, M. F., Neal, J. M., Mackey, D. C., Harrington, B. E. 2-Chloroprocaine and bupivacaine are unreliable indicators of intravascular injection in the premedicated patient. *Reg. Anesth. Pain Med.* 23: 9, 1998.
4. Bernards, C. M., Carpenter, R. L., Rupp, S. M., Brown, D. L., Morse, B. V., Morell, R. C., Thompson, G. E. Effect of midazolam and diazepam premedication on central nervous system and cardiovascular toxicity of bupivacaine in pigs. *Anesthesiology* 70: 318, 1989.
5. Benumof, J. L. Permanent loss of cervical spinal cord function associated with interscalene block performed under general anesthesia. *Anesthesiology* 93: 1541, 2000.
6. Urquhart, M. L., White, P. F. Comparison of sedative infusions during regional anesthesia—methohexital, etomidate, and midazolam. *Anesth. Analg.* 68: 249, 1989.
7. Smith, I., Monk, T. G., White, P. F., Ding, Y. Propofol infusion during regional anesthesia: Sedative, amnestic, and anxiolytic properties. *Anesth. Analg.* 79: 313, 1994.
8. Smith, D. C., Crul, J. F. Oxygen desaturation following sedation for regional analgesia. *Br. J. Anaesth.* 62: 206, 1989.

5 Equipment

Regional techniques can be performed with almost any syringe and needle. Their success depends more on the skill of the operator than on the quality of the instrument. Nevertheless, there are differences in equipment that make some devices more effective than others and, in experienced hands, can optimize the performance of regional techniques.

General Principles

Equipment for regional blocks is usually stocked in prepared sterile trays. Trays should include skin-preparation swabs, drapes, needles, syringes, solution cups, and a sterility indicator. The choice of equipment will be dictated by the specific blocks attempted and by personal preference, but some general comments are warranted.

Disposable Versus Reusable Equipment

Reusable *block trays* allow maximum flexibility in choosing specific needles, syringes, and catheters. They allow for the purchase of products that are manufactured to more exact specifications than those usually found in disposable trays. However, reusable trays represent a significant initial capital investment and require additional technician time to maintain, as well as a perception of a greater risk of transmission of infectious diseases.

Concern about infectious diseases (1), especially newer ones that are resistant to conventional sterilization techniques, has created a greater reliance on disposable equipment. The quality of disposable trays has improved, and the willingness of the manufacturers to "customize" trays to the needs of individual institutions is widespread. They remove the burden of sterilization from the local department or hospital (although not the responsibility of checking for sterility).

Sterilization

If presterilized disposable trays are not used, reusable equipment must be both cleaned and sterilized between uses. Detergents are *not* desirable for cleaning reusable needles and syringes because of the chance of chemical contamination of local anesthetic solutions from residual cleansing agents left on the syringe or needle. Significant bacterial or viral contamination is removed by heat sterilization at 121°C or above for 20 minutes (steam under pressure). Appropriate indicators of adequate heat exposure must be placed both in the center of each sterilized packet and on the outside.

Plastic and rubber will not tolerate heat treatment and must be sterilized with ethylene oxide gas exposure. A long period of aeration is required to remove residual gas. A different indicator strip is used to document sterility. Disposable trays usually have such an indicator in their central compartment. This indicator must be checked before using the tray.

If local anesthetic drugs are added to trays after they are opened, they must be wrapped sterilely and handled in an aseptic manner.

Skin Preparation

Skin preparation (asepsis) also requires meticulous attention. The current standard solution is an iodophor preparation, also termed *povidone–iodine.* The activity of this solution is based on the release of free iodine, which is dependent on the water dilution of the solution. Careful adherence to the manufacturer's instructions for dilution and use is important. These are "contact" preparations; that is, they do not require scrubbing or prolonged contact to remove microorganisms. Unlike previous iodine–alcohol solutions, these preparations are not likely to burn tissues, although excessive quantities in body folds can cause irritation, and should be washed off after completion of the block. Single-use containers are preferable because of the potential of contamination of larger bottles (2).

A few patients are truly allergic to topical iodine preparations and require alternative solutions. Chlorhexidine is a detergent that requires scrubbing and longer contact time, and must be wiped from the skin before insertion of needles. Isopropyl alcohol (70%) is a third satisfactory alternative as a skin preparation, and it does not require scrubbing. Both of these carry a potential risk of unrecognized contamination of anesthetic solutions if used as colorless solutions.

Regardless of the agent used, total sterility of the skin is rarely achieved, and careful attention to aseptic technique is needed. A wide area should be prepped, and sterile towels or plastic drapes should be placed on the skin to extend the working field.

Syringes

Although syringes are generally considered only as carrying instruments for the local anesthetics, their features are important. The resistance between the barrel and the piston is critical when using the "loss of resistance" technique for identifying the epidural space. Here, glass syringes have been superior to most plastic material in allowing free movement. Some new lubrication techniques have produced plastic products with low friction, but generally the disposable products rely on a gasket to provide a seal, which gives firm resistance in the movement of the piston and will obscure changes in resistance to injection as the needle is advanced. Glass syringes have the disadvantage that a small amount of powder from sterile gloves can cause the piston to stick in the barrel, but generally these syringes provide better appreciation of resistance.

The size of the syringe also affects performance. The smallest syringes (1 mL) give the greatest accuracy in measurement, as is required in adding epinephrine to the anesthetic solution. A small-diameter (3 to 5 mL) syringe gives a better feel of resistance during epidural insertion but is impractical for injection of large volumes. For injection, a 10-mL syringe is most comfortably held in the hand; larger syringes are heavy and bulky and usually require two hands for good control. They do not allow the fine control needed for localizing nerves. Disconnecting and reconnecting the needle also can be awkward with large syringes if one hand is occupied in fixing the needle in place on the nerve. Larger syringes also add more weight and are more likely to cause an unwanted advancement of the needle. A 10-mL syringe appears to be a practical compromise. It is inconvenient to refill frequently, but use of a 10-mL syringe limits the quantity injected at any one time and thus serves to encourage incremental injection of large volumes of local anesthetic. If a larger syringe (20 or 30 mL) is used, it is desirable to avoid direct connection to the needle by using a short length of flexible intravenous tubing as a connector. This allows for finer control of the needle, but may require an assistant to handle aspiration and injection with the syringe.

A *three-ring adapter* is useful on the 10-mL syringe (*control syringe*, Fig. 5.1). It allows greater control in injecting solution and

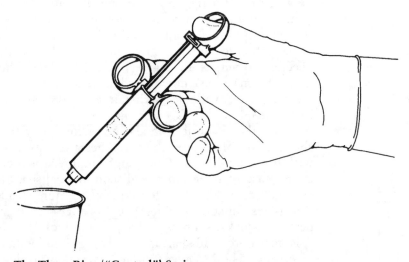

Figure 5.1   **The Three-Ring ("Control") Syringe**
This adaptation to the plunger of a standard 10-mL syringe allows greater control of injection, easier aspiration, and the opportunity to refill the syringe with one hand.

also allows the solo operator to refill the syringe with one hand while holding the needle in place in the patient with the other. These adapters are available on plastic as well as glass syringes.

The connection to the hub of the needle can affect the ease of fixation of the needle. The Luer-Lok adapter, which screws tightly onto the matching needle hub, does not require forceful friction to provide a seal and thus is less likely to cause unwanted movement of the needle when attaching the syringe. This coupling also provides a connection less likely to leak on injection. A tight seal is critical when using resistance to identify the epidural space.

Thus, an ideal tray would have Luer-Lok syringes in 1-, 3-, and 10-mL sizes with a three-ring adapter on the latter, plus a glass syringe for epidural localization.

Needles

Although local infiltration can be performed with almost any needle, special adaptations can facilitate success with regional techniques.

Regional-Block Needles

Peripheral nerve blocks are most commonly performed with special needles adapted for use with nerve stimulators (see below). These needles are usually around 22 gauge in size; with a specially adapted Luer-Lok hub or side-arm extension that includes an 8-to16-in. wire connection for attachment to the negative lead of the nerve stimulator (Fig. 5.2). The needles are also sheathed with a nonconducting cover to concentrate the electrical current at the tip, which is most commonly a short-beveled design. The incidence of nerve injury is presumed to be less with shorter-bevel needles (16 versus 12 degrees) (Fig. 5.2). The short-bevel needle may offer more resistance to advancement. Larger (19 gauge) needles are also available with curved tips that allow passage of catheters (3).

Regional anesthetics can also be performed with traditional unsheathed needles using the paresthesia technique or localization with other landmarks. The gauge employed is a compromise between ease of injection and discomfort caused. Smaller needles (25 to 32 gauge) are best for skin infiltration because their insertion is less uncomfortable. The 23-gauge size is suitable for superficial blocks, such as axillary or intercostals on thin patients. A larger, more rigid shaft is usually required for any deeper needle insertions. The 22-gauge 1.5- or 2-in. size is needed for the majority of regional techniques. A 5- or 6-in. 20-gauge needle is used for deep blocks, such as the celiac plexus, where free aspiration is desired.

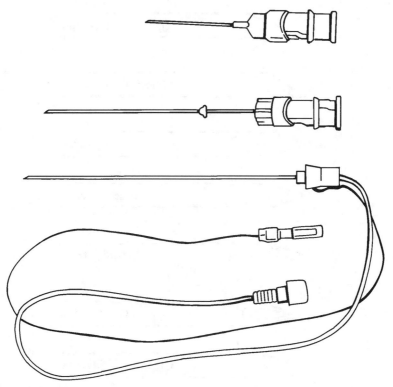

Figure 5.2   **Regional Anesthesia Needles**
For superficial blocks, such as the axillary, short 25-gauge needles (*top*) with a shorter bevel angle (compared to standard Quincke-type needle points) are very effective. For deeper injections, longer needles may be equipped with a "safety bead" on the upper shaft (*middle*) to prevent loss of the needle in the subcutaneous tissue if it separates from the hub. Needles used for peripheral nerve stimulator blocks (*bottom*) include the direct attachment for the nerve stimulator connection and the short tubing for the injection syringe. This tubing serves to remove the weight of the syringe from the needle hub, allowing finer control.

Spinal Needles

Spinal needles are necessarily longer (3.5 to 6 in.) and usually styletted to prevent occluding the lumen with a plug of skin or subcutaneous tissue before the dura is punctured. A number of bevel designs have been introduced since the original Quincke (sharp bevel) style was first used, and most are designated by the name of their inventor (Fig. 5.3). The rounded Greene and Whitacre points are designed to be less traumatic to the dura itself, apparently splitting or spreading rather than cutting the longitudinal fibers, and thus promoting more rapid sealing of the dural hole. Experience with the rounded-bevel design (especially the Whitacre and the Sprotte derivation of it) has shown an impressive reduction in the incidence of postdural puncture headache.

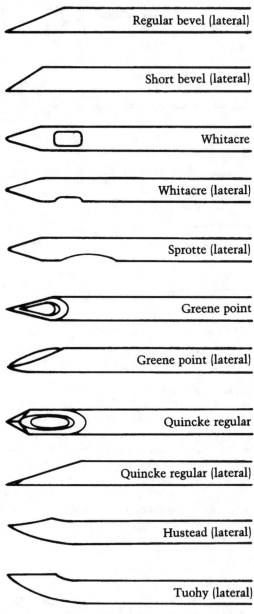

Figure 5.3   **Standard Regional Anesthesia Needle Bevels**

The gauge of spinal needles is also important in terms of the probability of a headache, although it is apparently not as important as the needle type (see Chapter 6). Smaller needles create smaller holes and less transdural leak, but they are more difficult to insert and to aspirate. The 25-gauge rounded-bevel needle is the size most frequently chosen as a reasonable compromise.

Epidural Needles

Epidural needles are of a larger gauge, both to permit better assessment of loss of resistance and to allow the passage of catheters. An 18-gauge thin-walled needle is the smallest that will pass a 20-gauge catheter, and 16- or 17-gauge needles are commonly used for catheters. A 19-gauge needle is satisfactory for single injections. A 22-gauge needle has been used, but the perception of resistance is more challenging through the narrower opening.

A conventional Quincke-point needle can be used for a single-injection technique, although some practitioners prefer the blunter, short-beveled Crawford needle for epidural or caudal insertion. The Tuohy needle with a curved point was first introduced to facilitate the passage of catheters. Hustead modified this needle to reduce the bevel angle slightly in the hope of reducing the chance of shearing the catheter during passage (Fig. 5.3). The angle of both of these bevels may allow better direction of the catheter into the main axis of the epidural canal, but the greater curvature and the offset of the point of the needle from the midaxis of the shaft also make them more likely to deviate from the intended path during advancement. The longer bevel also creates the possibility that the tip of the needle may communicate a loss of resistance before the full opening of the bevel is completely through the ligamentum flavum. These needles may need to be advanced another 2 to 3 mm beyond their initial penetration of the ligament before a catheter will pass. Most of these needles are manufactured with 1-cm markings along the shaft to allow better appreciation of the needle depth or movement. Tuohy needles have also been manufactured with additional channels and end holes to facilitate simultaneous insertion of spinal needles for combined spinal–epidural anesthesia (CSE) (4).

The hubs of epidural needles also have been adapted in some cases with "wings" to allow better control of the depth of advancement, particularly in the thoracic region (Fig. 5.4).

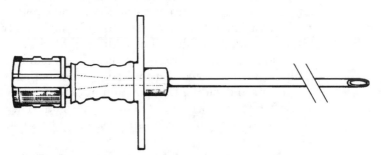

Figure 5.4   **Wing Adapters on Needle Hub**
The flanges attached to the hub of a standard epidural needle allow greater control of the advancement of the tip when the flanges are grasped between the thumb and forefinger while the other fingers rest on the skin and control the depth of insertion. These flanges come in several modifications.

Introducers

Introducers are useful in spinal and epidural anesthesia. These are short, large-bore, sharp-pointed needles. For spinal anesthesia, these can be inserted through the skin and into the interspinous ligament. They create a rigid path to guide the more flexible small-gauge spinal needles. They offer the added advantage of allowing the tip of the spinal needle to bypass the skin and thus avoid contamination with prep solution or residual skin bacteria. For epidural use, a skin hole made with these needles reduces the resistance to insertion of the epidural needle and allows more sensitive appreciation of the ligaments themselves.

Catheters

A multitude of catheters is available for insertion through epidural or peripheral nerve block needles. The primary difference among them is the construction material, which gives different performance characteristics. Newer catheters of nylon, polyamide, or polyvinyl offer compromises between flexibility (increased risk of kinking) and rigidity (risk of puncturing dura or veins), and the appropriate balance is a matter of personal choice among the wide selection available. A spring-wire reinforced flexible catheter is available which combines the ideal features of easy passage, minimal trauma, and low risk of occlusion or migration. If the catheter is to remain in place for several days for postoperative analgesia, these devices allow adaptation of the catheter to patient movement, and may reduce the frequency of catheter migration.

Another feature offered in epidural catheters is the presence of lateral injection ports proximal to a closed, soft-tip end. This may reduce the chance of dural puncture, and the presence of multiple holes reduces the chance of occlusion of the catheter by tissue or blood clot blocking a single hole. However, multiple holes may also allow unrecognized dural or venous puncture, because a test dose may not give a reliable response if only one hole is in a vessel or into the dura. Many practitioners prefer a single-port catheter for this reason. On the other hand, aspiration is more likely to be an effective test with multiple-orifice catheters. Marks at 1- or 5-cm intervals along the first 20 cm are useful in guiding insertion of the catheter to the correct depth. Radiopaque markers on the catheter are useful in documenting position of chronic indwelling catheters or catheters for injection of neurolytic agents. The selection of any or all of these features is again a matter of personal experience and choice.

Adapters are needed to allow injection from a syringe into a catheter. These are usually of the Tuohy-Borst type, where screwing one fitting onto another tightens a rubber sleeve around the catheter and holds it in place. There are as many connectors available as there are catheters, and the selection is again a personal choice based on reliability and ease of use. All connectors should have a Luer-Lok adapter for fitting a syringe and a cap to provide sterility of the fitting between injections. All catheters used for repeated injections on surgical wards should be clearly labeled as epidural catheters to prevent unintentional injection of intravenous drugs.

Epidural catheters can also be inserted into the subarachnoid space, although the larger needles used for the standard catheters may increase the risk of headache. At one point, smaller micro-catheters (27 gauge or smaller) were employed through smaller needles to reduce this problem. Unfortunately, problems with neurotoxicity (see Chapter 3) led to their withdrawal from the market.

Infusion Devices

In the last 10 years, anesthesiologists have become more actively involved in the continuation of regional techniques in the postoperative period for pain relief (see Chapter 24). There are several continuous-infusion devices available to assist in the delivery of local anesthetics or local anesthetic–opioid mixtures for postoperative pain relief (Fig. 5.5). For inpatient use, there are small electrically driven pumps that provide not only the ability to deliver continuous infusion, but also a patient-controlled option that allows supplemental doses at times of increased need. These devices are individually programmable and demonstrate a high degree of flexibility. They usually contain a locked chamber for the infusion itself, because opioids are used commonly in this setting. It is important that such devices have the potential for a continuous infusion, as well as a lockout interval to prevent excessive dosage by the patients. Mechanical failures with such devices are extremely rare, and they are highly effective for inpatient postoperative analgesia.

The use of continuous catheters for peripheral nerve blocks also benefits from the attachment of a continuous-infusion pump. Several modalities are available. The simplest are elastomeric bulbs that contain a fixed amount of local anesthetic under a constant pressure, which is then delivered at a fixed rate through a flow valve connected to the catheter. These pumps can provide continuous infusions for 24 to 48 hours for brachial plexus and lower extremity analgesia. The limitation of the elastomeric pumps is the fixed delivery volume. Alternatively, there are small battery-operated, programmable, mechanical pumps available, which have the same options as the inpatient infusion devices; that is, they can deliver both continuous infusion and incremental additional boluses on patient demand. Again, mechanical problems with these pumps are very rare and they appear to provide a useful option for prolonging postoperative analgesia in both inpatients and outpatients.

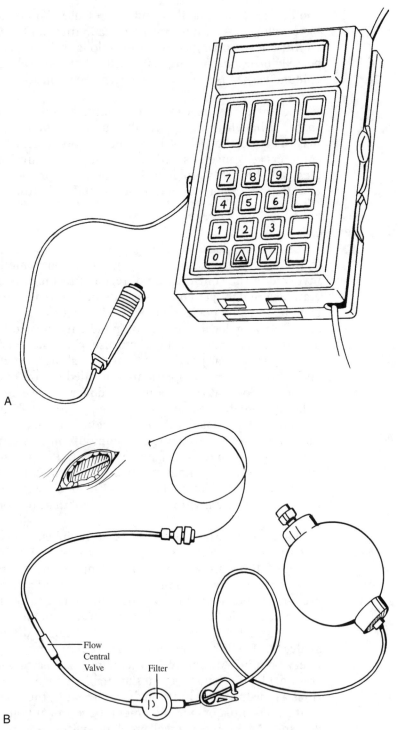

A

B

Flow
Central
Valve   Filter

Figure 5.5   Samples of infusion pumps for inpatient use (**A**), outpatient fixed infusions (**B**) and outpatient patient-controlled analgesia (PCA) infusions (**C**).

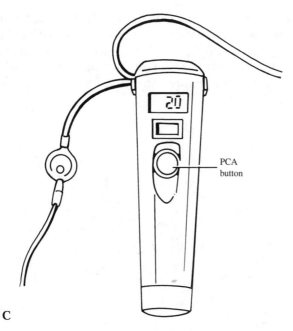

C

Figure 5.5 *(continued)*

Nerve Stimulators

The *peripheral nerve stimulator* delivers a pulsed electric current to the tip of an exploring needle. As the needle approaches a nerve, depolarization is produced. Efferent motor nerves (A alpha fibers) are most easily depolarized, so these devices have the advantage of identifying mixed peripheral nerves by producing a muscle twitch rather than eliciting uncomfortable sensory paresthesias. This also offers the anesthesiologist a method of confirming nerve localization in the obtunded or uncooperative patient.

The degree of stimulation is dependent on the total current (amperage) and the distance between the current source and the nerve. This principle led to the development of nerve stimulators with variable outputs. A high current (approximately 1 to 2 mA) can be used to identify the approach to a nerve. A progressively lower current will document increasing proximity of needle to nerve. In practice, 2 mA will produce depolarization of a motor nerve at a distance of about 1 cm. As the needle is moved closer to the nerve, a smaller current (0.5 to 0.6 mA) suggests adequate proximity to the nerve (5). This is confirmed if 2 mL of local anesthetic injected at this point abolishes the twitch response.

The ideal nerve stimulator has a variable linear output with a clear display of current delivered. The positive (red, ground) lead of the stimulator is connected to an electrocardiogram (ECG) skin electrode near the site of the block. The negative (black, cathode) lead is attached to the exploring needle. The connection can be made with an "alligator"-type clamp, but commercial sheathed needles with electrical connectors incorporated in their design are more commonly used (Fig. 5.6).

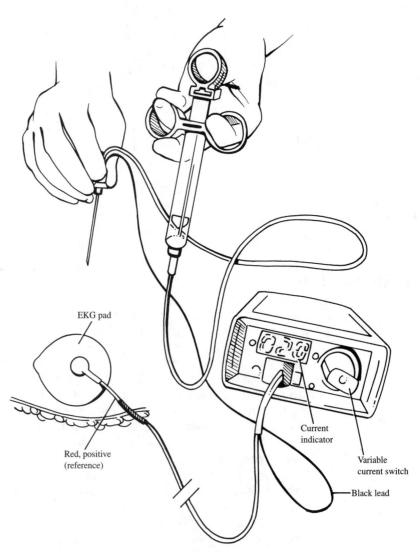

Figure 5.6

Nerve Stimulator Attached to Regional Block Needle
The negative (*black*) lead is attached to the exploring needle, while the positive (*red*) is connected to a reference electrocardiogram (EKG) pad used as a "ground." The stimulator is set to deliver 1 to 2 mA of current to detect the nerve. The current is reduced further as the needle is advanced closer to the nerve. Motor stimulation at a current of 0.5 mA or less suggests that the needle is adjacent to the nerve.

Electrically insulated (sheathed, Teflon-coated) needles concentrate more current at the needle tip and will increase the accuracy of nerve localization. The electrical isolation of the needle shaft causes the depolarization to decrease after the needle point passes the nerve, which is not the case with unsheathed needles. Sheathed needles are more expensive, but are the best choice.

Nerve stimulators are not a substitute for knowledge of anatomy and proper initial needle placement. They will only help document the proximity of the needle to the nerve once it is already near. The stimulator cannot find the nerve for the novice who has not reviewed anatomy. Although it is speculated that their use may reduce the potential for nerve damage, no study has shown an increased safety margin when nerve stimulators are used, and nerve injuries occur despite its use (6). Stimulators are particularly useful in the obtunded or uncooperative patient, however, in whom motor stimulation may be a needed substitute for identification of a paresthesia. Stimulators are also useful for teaching residents in a heavily premedicated patient, and they are particularly useful in pediatric practice, where blocks are usually performed on a sedated or anesthetized patient. Again, even the use of a nerve stimulator does not eliminate the risk of nerve injury when blocks are performed on unconscious adults (7). One challenge is that the use of a stimulator may require two individuals—one sterilely gloved for the procedure and the other operating the device, although there are new foot control pedals available that will obviate this obstacle.

References

1. Tait, A. R., Tuttle, D. B. Prevention of occupational transmission of human immunodeficiency virus and hepatitis B virus among anesthesiologists: A survey of anesthesiology practice. *Anesth. Analg.* 79: 623, 1994.
2. Birnbach, D. J., Stein, D. J., Murray, O., Thys, D. M., Sordillo, E. M. Povidone iodine and skin disinfection before initiation of epidural anesthesia. *Anesthesiology* 88: 668, 1998.
3. Steele, S. M., Klein, S. M., D'Ercole, F. J., Greengrass, R. A., Gleason, D. A new continuous catheter delivery system. *Anesth. Analg.* 87: 228, 1998.
4. Rawal, N., Van Zundert, A., Holmstrom, B., Crowhurst, J. A. Combined spinal-epidural technique. *Reg. Anesth.* 22: 406, 1997.
5. Choyce, A., Chan, V. W., Middleton, W. J., Knight, P. R., Peng, P., McCartney, C. J. What is the relationship between paresthesia and nerve stimulation for axillary brachial plexus block? *Reg. Anesth. Pain Med.* 26: 100, 2001.
6. Borgeat, A., Ekatodramis, G., Kalberer, F., Benz, C. Acute and nonacute complications associated with interscalene block and shoulder surgery: A prospective study. *Anesthesiology* 95: 875, 2001.
7. Benumof, J. L. Permanent loss of cervical spinal cord function associated with interscalene block performed under general anesthesia. *Anesthesiology* 93: 1541, 2000.

6 Spinal Anesthesia

Spinal anesthesia is the simplest and most effective technique available to the anesthesiologist. Injection of local anesthetic into the easily identified dural sac provides ready access to the exposed spinal nerves, resulting in anesthesia that is rapid, dense, and predictable.

Anatomy

The peripheral nerve tracts enter and depart the skull as a single cord (i.e., the spinal cord) and traverse the spinal canal enclosed in a protective sheath in which they are bathed in cerebrospinal fluid (CSF). The dura is the outermost layer of this sheath, and it is closely applied to the underlying arachnoid. Although a potential (subdural) space exists between them, the major space is the subarachnoid area between the arachnoid and the pia, which overlies the cord itself. Spinal CSF is in continuity with the intraventricular and intracranial fluid and identical in composition and pressure.

The cord itself usually terminates at the level of the L-1 vertebral body in the adult, whereas the dural sac generally continues caudad to the second sacral vertebra. The efferent fibers leave the cord from the ventral horn, whereas the afferent sensory fibers enter through the dorsal horns (Fig. 6.1). The dorsal and ventral fibers on each side of the cord join to form the segmental nerve for each dermatomal level. These nerves descend a variable distance in the canal before exiting the intravertebral foramina of their respective levels. The most distal fibers of the lower lumbar and sacral roots have the greatest distance between their level of origin and their exit, and they form the extensive filaments of the cauda equina as they traverse the lower regions of the canal.

As the fibers leave the dural sac, they draw with them dural sleeves that extend their protective bath of CSF. These sleeves extend to the foramina in the cervical region, but they are more likely to end in the canal itself in the lumbar area. While still within the dural sac, the nerves are devoid of the extensive perineural tissue that impedes the diffusion of local anesthetics into peripheral nerves. They are also deprived of the buffering capacity of the extracellular fluid. Local anesthetics injected into this milieu find little resistance to their action on nerve membranes and thus produce rapid anesthesia.

The spinal column provides the supporting and protective conduit for the cord. Each vertebra surrounds and protects the cord on all four sides, yet the openings between the pedicles allow the roots to exit on each side. There is also a posterior opening in the spinal canal between the laminae of each vertebra (Fig. 6.1). It is through this opening that spinal anesthesia is delivered. Entry into this

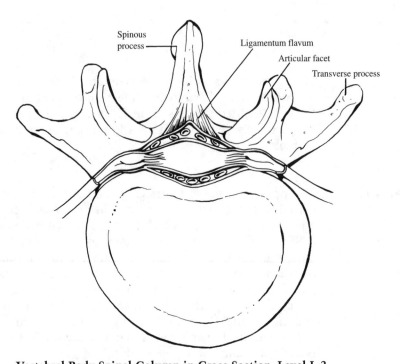

Spinous
process

Ligamentum flavum

Articular facet

Transverse process

Figure 6.1   **Vertebral Body Spinal Column in Cross Section, Level L-3**
The dura extends laterally to envelop the emerging nerve roots. In the
thoracic region, these dural "sleeves" can extend through the lateral
foramina. The epidural space is generously endowed with veins. The
posterior epidural space is 3 to 5 mm in depth in the lumbar area at its
widest point, just under the triangular ligamentum flavum.

space is protected by the dense ligamentum flavum and by the spinous process of the cephalad vertebra at each level, which angles
downward to protect the space below. The spinous processes maintain their alignment by the dense interspinous ligament that attaches between them (see Fig. 6.6).

The spinal column has characteristic curves in the lumbar and
thoracic regions that influence the spread of injected drugs. The
lumbar anterior convexity affects the cephalad spread of solutions
injected below the second lumbar vertebra. The thoracic concavity
encourages the pooling of hyperbaric solutions in the thoracic region when the patient is turned supine.

Indications   Local anesthetics in the subarachnoid space generally produce total
neural blockade caudad to the site of injection; anesthesia cephalad
to the site of injection is produced to a variable extent dependent on
patient position, total dose of drug, and baricity of the local anesthetic solution. There is a gradually decreasing concentration of lo-

cal anesthetic at the cephalad extent of blockade, which causes a gradient of anesthesia due to differential sensitivities of the spinal nerves. Sympathetic fibers are blocked by lower concentrations of drug and thus (depending on the drug used) may be anesthetized two to six segments higher than sensory fibers. Likewise, the level of sensory anesthesia may be two dermatomes higher than that of motor blockade, which requires the highest concentration of local anesthetic.

A low-level spinal (L-1, or saddle block) is useful for perineal or perianal surgery. A moderate-level block (T-10 sensory dermatome) is adequate for hip pinning or lower-extremity and foot surgery, although a slightly higher level may be required to prevent tourniquet discomfort. It is ideal for transurethral prostatectomy because it provides good anesthesia while preserving sensation in the abdomen and dome of the bladder, giving early warning of extravasation of irrigation fluid into the abdominal cavity. Higher levels of spinal anesthesia (T4-6 block) are suitable for lower abdominal surgery, such as inguinal herniorrhaphy, appendectomy, cesarean delivery, and abdominal hysterectomy. In such procedures, however, the patient may perceive an unpleasant discomfort associated with traction on the peritoneum or abdominal contents, and higher levels of block or supplemental sedation is required.

These higher levels of spinal anesthesia are associated with changes in cardiovascular and respiratory function. Thoracic sympathetic block will produce hypotension, which may be exacerbated in the patient who is hypovolemic as a result of blood loss, dehydration, diuretic therapy, or overvigorous catharsis (1,2).

Ventilation is usually adequate despite a high spinal block because the phrenic nerve is not blocked. Spinal anesthesia itself does not alter ventilatory response to carbon dioxide. The obese patient in the head-down position, however, may have difficulty with ventilation, especially with a large lower abdominal incision and extensive "packing" of the bowel. The expiratory reserve volume and the force of a cough decline progressively as the level of spinal anesthesia increases (1), and thus high spinal anesthesia may not be desirable in the patient with respiratory disease. A block above T-10 without ventilatory assistance is unwise in the patient who is dependent on abdominal muscles for normal respiration.

Higher levels (T-1) of block have been advocated for upper abdominal surgery because of the excellent muscle relaxation provided for cholecystectomy, pyloroplasty, bowel resection, and abdominal exploration. Spinal block offers the surgeon a contracted bowel because of blockade of the sympathetic innervation. Upper-abdominal procedures usually require supplementation with a light general endotracheal anesthetic to ensure adequate ventilation, protection of the airway, and blunting of residual visceral and diaphragmatic sensation. If a high spinal technique is used, the cardiovascular changes are more profound, and severe bradycardia may occur with total sympathetic blockade unless anticholinergic vagal blockade is added.

Certain patients are not candidates for spinal anesthesia. The presence of infection at the site of injection, untreated sepsis, severe hypovolemia, or coagulopathy are considered contraindications to the technique. Patients dependent on high venous filling pressures (such as in aortic stenosis) are poor candidates for extensive sympathetic blockade. Fever alone is not a contraindication if appropriate therapy is instituted (3).

Drugs   Lidocaine has been the most extensively used local anesthetic for spinal anesthesia: 50 mg will produce a T6-10 level of block for approximately 45 to 60 minutes, and as long as 120 minutes in the leg. Lower doses, such as 20 to 25 mg, will produce a T-10 block with a shorter duration, and may be better suited to outpatient anesthesia for knee arthroscopy. These lower doses also may produce less transient neurologic symptoms (TNS, see Chapter 3). The commercial 5% solution contains 7.5% dextrose and thus is already hyperbaric. The 2% commercial solution gives essentially isobaric anesthesia and can be diluted with an equal volume of sterile water to produce hypobaric anesthesia.

Procaine is also available for short-duration procedures, but it is not as reliable an anesthetic and is not significantly shorter in duration than lidocaine. The 10% solution should be diluted to 5% concentration by addition of an equal volume of CSF (isobaric) or glucose (hyperbaric). Mepivacaine has been used for spinal anesthesia in doses and duration slightly more potent than lidocaine.

Bupivacaine is the desired alternative for longer duration blockade. The extent and duration are dose related (4). Doses of 5 mg will give a T-10 block for about 90 minutes, and may be acceptable for some outpatient procedures. A 10-mg dose produces midabdominal anesthesia for 2 to 3 hours, but the more extensive anesthesia associated with doses above 10 mg will frequently cause urinary retention. The standard commercial preparation is hyperbaric, but the 0.5% solution is essentially isobaric. Levobupivacaine will produce a similar pattern of spinal blockade, whereas ropivacaine appears to be slightly shorter in duration and extent of anesthesia (5). Tetracaine is now used almost exclusively for spinal anesthesia also, and has the advantage that the crystalline preparation can be diluted to any baricity desired. It is slightly more potent than bupivacaine, so the dose can be reduced by 30% for equivalent blockade.

Any of these drugs can be employed for a continuous technique, but should be used in a dilute concentration to improve accuracy of dosing. The 5% lidocaine preparation has been associated with neurotoxicity when injected through microcatheters, and should be used with caution.

Epinephrine (0.2 mg) has been traditionally added to spinal anesthetic solutions to prolong blockade and improves the quality of anesthesia (see Table 6.1). It also prolongs the time to voiding (6). Phenylephrine is slightly more effective in prolonging duration than epinephrine, but both drugs prolong the ultimate resolution of blockade more than the regression, and thus are most useful for prolonging lower abdominal anesthesia. Increased milligram dosage of the local anesthetic is another alternative. Clonidine can also prolong spinal anesthesia when given orally or with the local anesthetic, but may be associated with sedation or cardiovascular side effects. Intrathecal neostigmine also prolongs anesthesia, but at the price of unacceptable nausea. Fentanyl, in doses of 10 to 25 µg will produce sensory prolongation equivalent to epinephrine, but without prolongation of voiding (Table 6.1). Because it potentiates the local anesthetic, it allows use of lower milligram doses, and may be the preferred additive, especially in the outpatient setting (7). In these doses it may also provide some analgesia, and has not been associated with a high frequency of respiratory depression, although itching may occur.

Although total dose appears to be the major factor in determining final extent of spinal anesthesia, multiple other factors affect the extent of spread (Tables 6.2 and 6.3). The most important factor appears to be one that is not easily measured, the CSF volume of the patient (8). Among the factors that we can control, baricity and position are major factors determining spread of spinal anesthesia. If a hyperbaric injection is made in the sitting position, this can produce sacral anesthesia ("saddle block"), whereas the same injection in the standard supine position usually includes the midthoracic nerves, which lie in the most dependent portion of the spine in this position (Fig. 6.2) (9). An isobaric solution (without dextrose) is less influenced by gravity and will generally resist extensive spread from the site of injection despite manipulations of patient position,

Table 6.1 Duration of 50-mg Lidocaine Spinal Anesthesia

Solution	Height of Block	Duration (minutes) ± SD				
		Two-Segment Regression	T-12 Surgical Anesthesia	Motor Block	L-1 Regression	S-2 Regression
1.5% Plain (isobaric)	T-6 (T3-L2)	56 ± 5	20 ± 13	71 ± 8	104 ± 5	130 ± 18
1.5% Dextrose	T-3 (T7-L1)	39 ± 5	29 ± 10	30 ± 8	73 ± 10	99 ± 11
5% with dextrose only	T-3 (C8-T5)	50 ± 16	49 ± 30	88 ± 20	109 ± 6	150 ± 8
5% with epinephrine	T-4	56 ± 11	45 ± 30	108 ± 30	96 ± 42	156 ± 43
5% with fentanyl	T-3	70	75 ± 32	89 ± 31	100 ± 31	157 ± 11
25 µg with fentanyl	T10 (T5-12)					

SD, standard deviation.
Data from Chiu et al. (8) and Liu et al. (18).

Table 6.2   **Factors Affecting Subarachnoid Local Anesthetic Injections**

Determinants of spread
  Major factors
    Baricity of solution
    Position of patient (except isobaric solution)
    Dose and volume of drug injected (except isobaric)
  Minor factors
    Level of injection
    Speed of injection/barbotage
    Size of needle
    Physical status of patient
    Intraabdominal pressure
Determinants of duration
  Drug employed
  Dose injected
  Presence of vasoconstrictors
  Total spread of blockade

Adapted from Wildsmith, J. A. W., Rocco, A. G. Current concepts in spinal anesthesia. *Reg. Anesth.* 10: 119, 1985.

Table 6.3   **Spinal Anesthesia Doses**

Local Anesthetic	Dose (mg)			Duration (T-10 regression) (h)	
	Saddle	T-10 Level	T2-4	Plain	With Epinephrine
Procaine	50	75	100	1.5	2
Lidocaine	40	50	75	1.5	2
Tetracaine	4	6	8–12	1.5	3–4
Bupivacaine	5	10	12	0.5	3–4

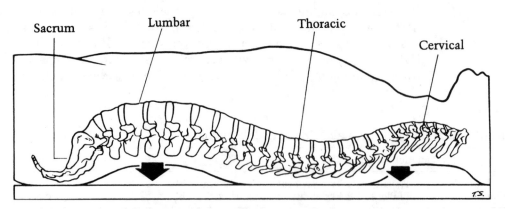

Sacrum   Lumbar   Thoracic   Cervical

Figure 6.2   **Normal Curvature of the Spinal Column**
Hyperbaric solutions injected at the L-2 interspace will gravitate to the lower sacral levels and to the most dependent midthoracic levels. The lumbar lordosis is often reduced in the supine position under anesthesia (*arrow*), but the spread of anesthetic solution usually precedes this flattening. Placing the legs in lithotomy stirrups will also reverse this curvature, but it has little effect on the spread of solution. (From Raj, P. P. *Handbook of Regional Anesthesia.* New York: Churchill Livingstone, 1985. P. 225, with permission.)

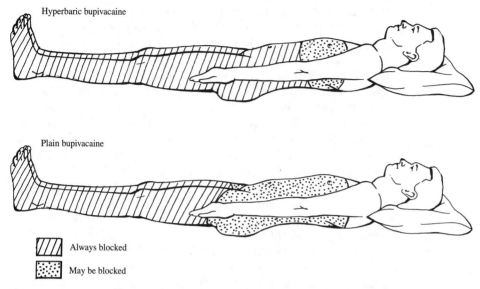

Hyperbaric bupivacaine

Plain bupivacaine

▨ Always blocked

▦ May be blocked

Figure 6.3 **Extent of Spinal Anesthesia**
The probable spread of anesthesia using two different preparations of bupivacaine, each injected slowly at the L3-4 interspace in the classic lateral midline position.

although the ultimate spread is less predictable (Fig. 6.3). A hypobaric solution will tend to rise away from the site of injection. This is useful for perineal anesthesia in the jackknife position.

These major factors are also influenced by several minor variables, such as the volume and force of injection, the level of injection, and patient status (Table 6.2). Although patient height does not correlate well with spread of anesthetic, obese and elderly patients will have higher than expected levels. The multitude of factors makes the prediction of final anesthetic level difficult.

Technique

Hyperbaric, Lateral Position, Midline Approach

The lateral position, midline approach, using a hyperbaric solution is the most common technique for spinal anesthesia. This technique is usually performed in the operating room, because the onset of anesthesia is rapid and surgical preparation is rarely delayed. Also, movement or transferring of the patient within 30 minutes after injection may produce an undesirable increase in the anesthetic level and decrease in blood pressure. The block can be performed on a stretcher or bed if movement of the unanesthetized patient is painful.

1. After appropriate monitors and supplemental oxygen are applied, the patient is turned to the lateral position. The operative side is generally placed down in order to provide the earliest and most dense anesthesia at the surgical site (with hyperbaric solution). A pillow or folded towel is placed under the head, both for patient comfort and to maintain the neutral alignment of the spinal column (Fig. 6.4).

2. The patient's back is moved to the edge of the operating table, and the shoulders are adjusted so that they are perpendicular to the floor. The knees and hips are flexed and then also the head so that the patient assumes the maximum anterior flexion of the spinal column. The hips and the back are then adjusted so that they also are perpendicular to the floor. A warm blanket and light sedation will enhance patient cooperation. The use of an assistant to remind the patient of the correct position is helpful.

3. The spinous processes and iliac crests are identified and marked. A line between the iliac crests passes through the L4-5 interspace or the L-4 spinous process itself. The processes are thus identified and numbered, with the widest interspace noted. The L2-3 interspace is usually preferred because injection at this

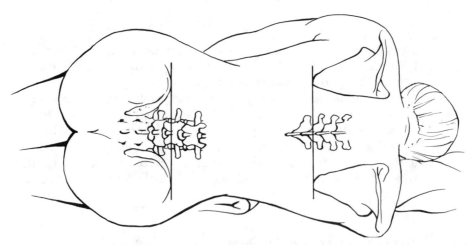

Figure 6.4   **Patient Position for Spinal or Epidural Blockade**
The patient's knees are drawn up toward the chest and the head flexed downward to provide the maximum anterior flexion of the vertebral column. The pillow should be placed under the head but not under the shoulders to avoid rotation of the spine. The hips and shoulders should be perpendicular to the surface of the bed, resisting the usual inclination of the patient to roll the superior shoulder forward. A line drawn between the posterior iliac crests usually crosses the spinal column at the L4-5 interspace or L-4 spinous process. Similarly, for thoracic epidural injection, a line between the inferior tips of the scapulae crosses the T-9 spinous process.

level will take maximum advantage of the lumbar spinal curvature to encourage spread of the solution both cephalad and caudad. Injections at L-1 or above are avoided because of the possibility of injury to the underlying cord itself. An "X" is marked on the skin at the anticipated site of the needle entry.

4. After the skin is marked, patient position is rechecked to ensure that the back is in full flexion and perpendicular to the floor. Then the regional tray is opened and the prep solution and drapes are applied.

5. After the prep, the patient is warned and a skin wheal of local anesthetic is raised at the "X" with a small-gauge needle. A longer (1.5 in.) needle is then used to identify the interspace and inject more local anesthetic along the intended needle track, which is in the midline but angled 10 to 15 degrees cephalad. Some of the local anesthetic solution is held in reserve in case further anesthesia is required or another interspace is attempted later.

6. After local infiltration, patient position is once again checked, because the patient will frequently pull away from the burning sensation of the local anesthetic and reduce the flexion of the back.

7. An introducer needle is inserted at the "X" in the direction of the local infiltration with a slight cephalad angulation. An introducer needle reduces contamination of the spinal needle with prep solution, epidermis, and skin bacteria, but it is most useful in guiding thinner needles. Its use will reduce the deflection of the needle point by the bevel. If properly positioned, the introducer will seat firmly into the dense fibers of the interspinous ligament. A rounded-bevel spinal needle is inserted through the introducer following the cephalad angulation but otherwise perpendicular to the back in order to remain in the patient's midline during its course (Fig. 6.5).

8. If bone is encountered, a mental note of the depth is made, and the needle is partially withdrawn and readvanced in a more cephalad direction. If bone is encountered again, the depth is compared to the first encounter (Fig. 6.6). If the bone is deeper than previously noted, the needle is probably advancing along the superior crest of the spinous process below the interspace, and it should be angled more cephalad and advanced further. If the bone is shallower than previously noted, it is most likely the inferior surface of the spinous process above the interspace, and less cephalad angulation is indicated. If bone is repeatedly encountered at the same depth, it is most likely the flat lamina of the vertebral body, and the needle point is not in the midline. The direction of the needle and introducer is reevaluated to ensure that they are perpendicular to the back, and then they are readvanced. This type of logical analysis will produce a minimum number of readjustments.

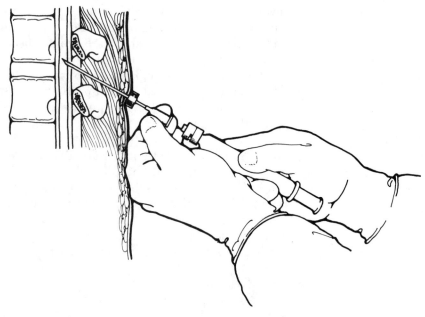

Figure 6.5   **Spinal Needle and Introducer**
The spinal needle is inserted through a larger-gauge introducer. The use of
the introducer avoids the problem of contamination of the tip of the
spinal needle with prep solution, epidermis, or skin bacteria, and allows a
rigid channel for the smaller-gauge needles frequently used to reduce the
incidence of headaches. Whenever the syringe is attached or removed
from the needle hub, the opposite hand rests firmly against the back and
grasps the hub firmly, preventing unintentional advancement or
withdrawal.

The most frequent misdirection occurs when the patient rolls
slightly away from the anesthesiologist in an attempt to flex the
spine, and the needle may be advanced parallel to the floor, but
not perpendicular to the back (Fig. 6.7). In general, the needle
will need to be oriented slightly toward the floor to compensate
for this rotation of the spine.

9. If the needle is on the correct course, two changes in resistance
to advancement will be perceived. The firm ligamentum flavum
will be encountered, followed by the dura. After this second
change in resistance (often perceived as a "pop"), the stylet is
withdrawn to check for fluid. If free flow does not occur, the hub
is rotated 90 degrees, in the event that a small flap of dura or
arachnoid is obstructing the orifice. With small-gauge needles,
gentle aspiration may be necessary to confirm the presence of
fluid. As a last resort, 0.1 mL air may be injected through the
needle to clear any obstruction. If no fluid is obtained, the stylet
is replaced and the needle is advanced further. The preceding
steps are repeated until fluid is identified. If the needle is ad-

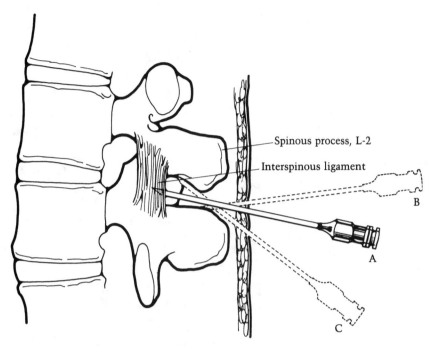

Spinous process, L-2

Interspinous ligament

B

A

C

Figure 6.6

Spinal Needle Insertion, Lateral View
For the classic midline approach, the needle is introduced in the middle of
the interspace and advanced with a slight cephalad angulation. If correctly
angled (A), it will enter the interspinous ligament, ligamentum flavum,
and epidural space. If bone is contacted, it may be the inferior spinous
process (B), and cephalad redirection will identify the correct path. If
angling cephalad causes contact with bone again at a shallower depth (C),
it is probably the superior spinous process. If bone is encountered at the
same depth after several attempts at redirection (not shown), the needle is
most likely on the lamina lateral to the interspace, and the position of the
true midline should be reassessed.

vanced to the hub without finding fluid, then the stylet is removed and the needle is withdrawn in 3-mm steps, with rotation of the hub 90 degrees and gentle aspiration at each increment of withdrawal until fluid is identified.

10. If a paresthesia is encountered at any time, the needle is immediately immobilized. Occasionally, the paresthesia is fleeting
and mild and serves as an indication that the subarachnoid
space has been reached. Injection may proceed as usual if fluid
is obtained and the paresthesia does not recur. More often, the
paresthesia indicates that the needle is in the spinal canal but
away from the midline, and the needle must be redirected ac-
cordingly. *Under no circumstance should an injection be made
if it produces a paresthesia at the time.*

11. Once fluid is obtained, the syringe with the anesthetic solution
is attached to the hub. The hub is fixed in position during this

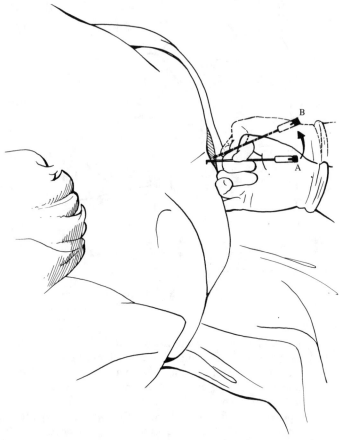

Figure 6.7   **Patient Position, Lateral View**
Most patients will rotate their body anteriorly in an attempt to flex their
back, and the spinal (or epidural) needle will thus need to be directed
slightly inferior (B) to be truly perpendicular to the midline.

maneuver by placing the hand firmly against the patient's back
and then grasping the hub between the thumb and forefinger
(Fig. 6.5). Gentle aspiration of 0.1 to 0.2 mL CSF confirms subarachnoid position before injection. The solution is injected
slowly (0.5 mL per second). To confirm that the needle did not
move during injection, CSF is again aspirated after the entire
dose is injected. The aspirated CSF is reinjected, and the syringe,
needle, and introducer are removed as a unit.

12. The patient is instructed to extend his or her legs at this point.
   If an isobaric solution is used, positioning can proceed for
   surgery with little effect on level of anesthesia. When hypobaric
   solutions are used, the patient is usually positioned for surgery
   before injection (jackknife or lateral position), and no further
   changes are made. With a hyperbaric solution, if a low "unilat-

eral" anesthesia is desired, the patient may be kept on his or her side for 5 minutes. (This will not produce total one-sided anesthesia, but it will give more dense and long-lasting anesthesia on the dependent side.) If the patient is turned immediately supine, the block will usually rise to the midthoracic level. When repositioned, the patient is given assistance. Excessive motion or straining may cause further spread of the block. The legs must be positioned carefully to avoid pressure on peripheral nerves or bony prominences, because the patient is no longer able to warn of uncomfortable pressure points.

13. The heart rate and blood pressure are checked immediately. The sympathetic fibers are anesthetized earliest, and venous pooling in the legs begins immediately. The loss of venous return can produce a decrease in blood pressure and heart rate, particularly in elderly or volume-depleted patients. A gradual increase of the anesthetic level also can produce a block of high sympathetic fibers 30 to 60 minutes after injection, often manifest as a profound bradycardia as the loss of venous return and block of cardioaccelerator sympathetic fibers combine to reduce the heart rate (see Complications, this chapter).

14. The level of temperature sensation is tested with an alcohol sponge 2 minutes after injection (temperature sensation is anesthetized as rapidly as pain). This early test will confirm the presence of anesthesia and suggest the ultimate height of the block. If it is lower than expected, the head of the bed can be lowered to encourage cephalad spread of a hyperbaric solution. Further spread will occur during the first 10 minutes and as long as 30 minutes after injection. If temperature sensation is difficult to assess, a pinch or pinprick can be employed.

15. Intraoperatively, supplemental oxygen is desirable, especially for elderly patients or those with high blocks or deep sedation. End-tidal carbon dioxide monitoring can be utilized with a probe inserted through either a facemask or nasal cannula, and is very useful in following respiratory rate. Sedation may be required during long procedures, and narcotics and systemic vagal blockade may be indicated if intraabdominal manipulation produces distress.

16. At the end of the procedure, the blood pressure may be unstable again and must be carefully monitored. Movement from the operating table to the stretcher and the recovery area is frequently associated with a redistribution of blood volume and transient hypotension. Sympathetic blockade may reliably be expected to have dissipated when all sensory and motor anesthesia has resolved (including return of proprioception in the big toe), but ambulation should still be done cautiously (10).

17. Bed rest for 24 hours has historically been recommended after a dural puncture to prevent spinal headache. There is no substantiation that this reduces the incidence of headache, although it

will obviously delay the appearance of symptoms. Heavy lifting and straining are best avoided, but spinal anesthesia is compatible with outpatient surgery and early ambulation of hospitalized patients.

Prone Position

When the jackknife position is selected for rectal or perineal surgery, the block can be performed after the patient is positioned (this may reduce the chance of injury in turning the anesthetized patient). Because the operative site is usually above the level of injection, the prone position is well suited to the use of hypobaric solutions.

1. The patient is placed prone on the operating table with a pillow or blanket under the hips to provide flexion of the lower spine. The arms are placed on arm boards for patient comfort (Fig. 6.8).

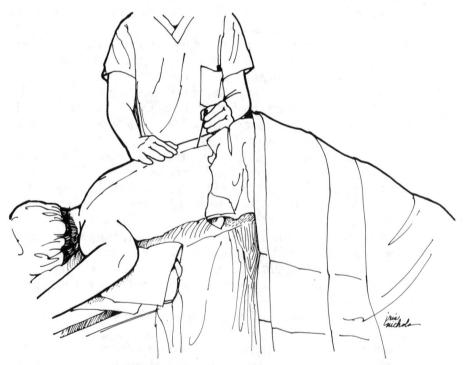

Figure 6.8   **Jackknife Position**
Hypobaric spinal anesthesia can be administered with the patient positioned on a flexed operating table, such as for rectal procedures. The flexion point of the table should be directly under the hip joint, and the use of a pillow under the hips will help accentuate the flexion needed to identify the lumbar spinous processes. Aspiration of the spinal needle is often necessary to confirm dural puncture, because the lower cerebrospinal fluid (CSF) pressure in this position will not necessarily generate a spontaneous flow of fluid.

Flexion of the operating table will help keep the hypobaric solution caudad.

2. The spinous processes and iliac crests are marked as in the lateral position, and skin analgesia and needle introduction are performed in the same manner. The guidelines for the adjustment of needle direction are the same as in the lateral position, and are easy to appreciate if a three-dimensional vision of the anatomy is maintained.

3. Aspiration is frequently required because of the relatively low CSF pressure in this position. Injection is made slowly, and the needle is left in place until anesthesia is established. Anesthesia is confirmed by gentle testing with pinprick or alcohol swab in the perianal area on both sides.

Sitting Position

In the obese patient or in anyone with whom the midline is difficult to discern, the sitting position is frequently helpful in identifying midline landmarks. If the patient is left in this position after injection of a hyperbaric anesthetic, sacral anesthesia is produced, creating the classic saddle block.

1. After monitors are placed, the patient is asked to sit up on the operating table and turn sideways so that the legs drop over the opposite side. Sedation should be minimal. If given, assistance in positioning is required. The feet are best supported on a stool, so that some flexion of the hips is maintained. The back is moved as close to the edge of the table as practical, and the patient is asked to "hunch over" so that the lower back is flexed (Fig. 6.9). Flexion is enhanced by allowing the patient to lean forward onto an over-bed table or Mayo stand.

2. The iliac crests and the spinous processes are identified and marked as in the lateral position. In the obese patient, the intercrest line is more likely to pass through the L3-4 space than the L4-5. An "X" is placed in the desired interspace.

3. The prep and drape are done, although the draping is limited to a single towel on the bed unless self-adherent drapes are used.

4. The local infiltration and needle advancement proceed as in the lateral position. If the midline is difficult to discern, the small-gauge infiltrating needle may be used as a gentle "seeker" to find the spinous processes, and thus confirm the midline. In the morbidly obese patient, a 3.5-in. 25-gauge spinal needle may also be used for this purpose.

5. Unless a true saddle block is desired, the needle is removed after injection and the patient is immediately assisted back into the supine position. The legs are positioned with care, because they may already be numb. If pure sacral anesthesia is desired, the patient may remain sitting for 5 minutes, but some cephalad spread will inevitably occur.

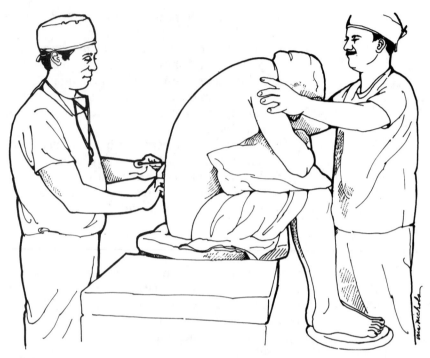

Figure 6.9   **Sitting Position for Spinal Anesthesia**
The patient's legs are allowed to hang over the edge of the bed, and the
feet are supported on a stool to encourage flexion of the lower spine. The
shoulders are hunched forward and the patient is encouraged to grasp
firmly onto a pillow held over the abdomen. If sedation is given, an
assistant should maintain the position and monitor the vital signs. This
position is optimal for identifying the midline in obese patients or those
with unusual spinal anatomy.

Paramedian (Lateral) Approach

The classic midline approach is adequate with most patients and
has the advantage of being simple to teach. In some elderly patients,
the interspinous ligament is heavily calcified, and, in some younger
patients, advancement of the needle through this dense structure is
uncomfortable. The ligament can be avoided by using other approaches.

One alternative, the lateral approach, simply moves one to one
and a half fingerbreadths off the midline while staying in the same
interspace. The needle is then introduced with a slight medial angle
as well as the usual cephalad angulation (Fig. 6.10). The anesthesiologist maintains a three-dimensional mental image of the tissues
as he or she advances the needle, so that the tip ends up in the midline as it reaches the depth of the ligamentum flavum. From here,
the advancement and injection proceed as before, but the interspinous ligament has been bypassed.

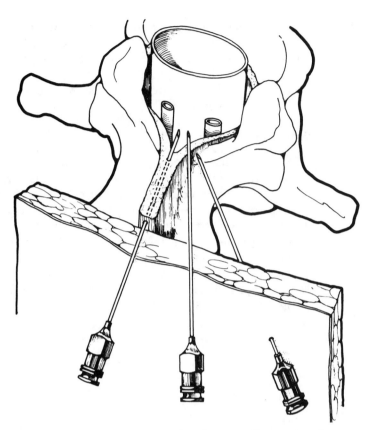

Figure 6.10   **Spinal Needle Insertion, Lateral and Paramedian Approach**
In the classic midline approach, the needle traverses the entire
interspinous ligament in a slight cephalad direction and exits through the
triangular ligamentum flavum into the epidural space before puncturing
the dura. In elderly patients with calcified interspinous ligaments, the
entry point can be moved one fingerbreadth lateral to the ligament, still
passing in the midline of the interspace, but approaching the ligamentum
flavum from a slightly oblique angle. A third alternative is to enter the
skin much further laterally and inferior to the interspace (a fingerbreadth
opposite the inferior spinous process) and pass the needle directly
perpendicular onto the lamina, and then "walk" superior and medially
until the ligament is contacted. All three of these approaches are suitable
for spinal or epidural blockade.

The paramedian or lateral oblique approach also starts lateral to
the midline, but from a level opposite the spinous process below
the interspace. From here, the needle must be advanced almost 45
degrees to the midline and 45 degrees cephalad to enter the ligamentum flavum in the midline (Fig. 6.10). A variation of this approach is to introduce the needle straight down onto the lamina of
the vertebra and then "walk" the needle up over the superior ridge

of the lamina into the ligamentum flavum. This gives the anesthesiologist an appreciation for the anticipated depth of the ligament, although it may cause the patient some discomfort. The oblique approach also provides an ideal angle for catheter insertion, because the exit angle at the skin is less likely to promote kinking of the catheter.

Taylor Approach

In an occasional patient, none of the approaches previously described allows entry to the spinal canal because of calcification or fusion of the intervertebral spaces or extensive scarring. In such a case, the lumbosacral (L5-S1) foramen may still be passable, because it is the largest of the openings into the canal. The lateral oblique approach to this space is referred to as the Taylor approach in recognition of the urologist who popularized it.

1. This approach can be used with the patient in the prone, lateral, or sitting position.

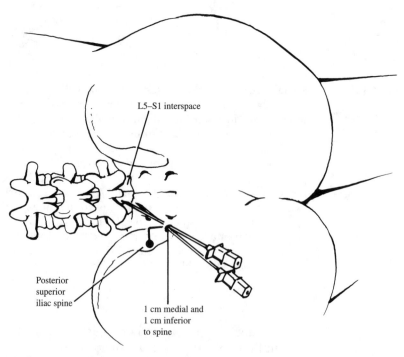

Figure 6.11   Taylor Approach for Spinal Anesthesia
The needle is introduced 1 cm medial to and 1 cm inferior to the posterior superior iliac spine and advanced at an angle 45 degrees to the midline and 45 degrees cephalad. On contacting the lamina, the needle is then walked upward and medially to enter the L5-S1 interspace.

2. The posterior superior iliac spine is identified, and a skin mark placed 1 cm medial and 1 cm inferior to this point. The L5-S1 interspace is also identified and marked.
3. After a skin wheal is placed, a 4- or 5-in. needle is introduced and directed approximately 45 degrees cephalad and 45 degrees medially, aiming at the fifth lumbar interspace in the midline (Fig. 6.11). A longer needle is usually required because the oblique angle creates a greater distance of travel at this level. The loss of resistance of the ligament and the dura is felt in the same manner as for the midline approach.
4. Aspiration may be needed to produce CSF flow in the prone position. In other positions, confirmation of the puncture and injection of drug proceed as described.

Continuous Technique

As in epidural anesthesia, a catheter can be passed into the subarachnoid space. The technique is identical to continuous epidural anesthesia (see Chapter 7), except that a needle that can accommodate a catheter is advanced until fluid is obtained; then the catheter is passed through the lumen. The bevel should be directed cephalad or caudad (depending on the direction of anesthesia desired); lateral direction will impede catheter placement. The same drugs are used as for an ordinary spinal. Extreme care should be taken to avoid injecting excessive doses because there is much greater potential for pooling of local anesthetic, which might be associated with local neurotoxicity (see Chapter 3). Sufficient time must be allowed for onset of anesthesia before additional injections are made, and testing for onset should be in sacral segments where a caudad catheter will produce earliest onset. After appropriate intervals (45 to 90 minutes, depending on the drug), supplemental injections can be given, starting with half the original dose. This is usually injected at a time equal to two-thirds the expected duration of the original dose. Because catheter and connector "dead space" account for a large volume relative to the volume of anesthetic injected, the catheter must be flushed with previously aspirated CSF after each injection. The drug and flush syringes can be arranged on a three-way stopcock to enhance the preservation of sterility. A more dilute local anesthetic solution may be desired for convenience of administration.

The continuous technique represents a theoretical risk of infection, because a foreign body is introduced into the subarachnoid space. This has not proven to cause a significant increase in risk. Nevertheless, sterility of the catheter, connector, and syringe must be maintained. The incidence of postspinal headache may increase because of the need for the large needle to accommodate the catheter. This technique is well suited to elderly patients, who have a low risk of postspinal headache.

Complications

Hypotension

Hypotension is the most frequent side effect of spinal anesthesia and is a direct result of the venous pooling and arteriolar dilation produced by sympathetic blockade. The extent of the decrease in blood pressure is dependent on the extent of sympathetic block, intravascular volume of the patient, and cardiovascular health (1,5) (Table 6.4). The decrease in pressure can be reduced by preloading with at least 250 to 500 mL of a crystalloid solution, but this is not reliable. If the decrease in pressure is abrupt, a mild vasopressor is appropriate to support the pressure temporarily until fluid replacement can be provided. Ephedrine in 5- to 10-mg increments intravenously is the drug of choice because it produces not only vasoconstriction but also increased cardiac output (11). The duration of this therapy is only 5 to 10 minutes, and an intramuscular dose of 25 mg may be needed if longer support is indicated. Phenylephrine is a reasonable second choice if tachycardia is present, but this drug will cause vasoconstriction with minimal increase (or a decrease) in cardiac output (12).

Elevation of the legs will help reverse the undesirable pooling, but lowering of the head during a hyperbaric spinal may drive the block to unwanted higher levels. Flexion of the operating table is an ideal compromise, because the feet can be raised while the head remains flat or elevated, thus increasing venous return while delaying further spread of the sympathetic block. A rapidly rising block occasionally prompts the novice to turn the operating table into the head-up, foot-down position to stop the cephalad spread. This is particularly dangerous because it exaggerates the venous pooling.

Although fluid loading is the treatment of choice to reverse spinal hypotension, this must be used cautiously in the elderly or those with limited cardiac reserve. A 1.5- or 2-L salt-containing solution load can precipitate congestive heart failure in the susceptible patient when the spinal anesthesia and associated sympathectomy resolve. In this situation, a vasopressor infusion may be more desirable if spinal anesthesia is the technique of choice. Another

Table 6.4   **Cardiovascular Response to Subarachnoid Blockade at 20 Minutes**

	T-10 Level	T-1 Level
Mean arterial pressure	−8%	−22%
Heart rate	Unchanged	−14%
Peripheral resistance	−10%	−7%
Cardiac output	Unchanged	−19%

Adapted from Sivarajan, M., Amory, D. W., Lindbloom, L. E., Schwettmann, R. S. Systemic and regional blood-flow changes during spinal anesthesia in the rhesus monkey. *Anesthesiology* 43:78,1975.

alternative in the high-risk group is the incremental injection of small doses of local anesthetic through a spinal catheter while monitoring blood pressure. This technique results in a lower requirement for supplemental fluid and vasopressors (13).

Bradycardia

Even in the absence of hypotension or hypoxia, bradycardia can occur independently (although rarely) during spinal anesthesia, even after 30 to 45 minutes (14). As the level of sympathetic anesthesia reaches T-2 and the cardioaccelerator fibers are blocked, the action of the vagus is unopposed. Bradycardia may be associated with a stimulus such as traction on the peritoneum or decreased venous return, or it may be unexplained. As the heart rate slows to 60, 50, or 45 beats per minute, cardiac output drops to the point where myocardial perfusion is inadequate, and a rapid deterioration occurs (Fig. 6.12). Bradycardia to a rate below 50 beats per minute occurs in 13% of normal patients (15) and may even progress rapidly to asystole and cardiac arrest (14). Early treatment with atropine (0.6 to 1.0 mg) and ephedrine may abort this downward spiral, but the drugs will be ineffective if circulation has already ceased. In this situation, external cardiac compression by the surgeon (or anyone else who is available) and intravenous epinephrine may be required to restore circulation. Again, sequelae are rare if rapid treatment is instituted.

Early recognition is essential, and prevention or early treatment is easier and less dramatic than chest compression in the operating room. The use of 0.4 to 0.6 mg atropine is appropriate whenever the pulse slows to below 60 beats per minute.

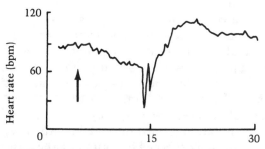

Figure 6.12

Sudden Bradycardia During Spinal Anesthesia
At the time indicated by the *arrow*, spinal anesthesia with 50 mg lidocaine was administered to an 85-year-old patient. Despite the use of 25 mg ephedrine prophylactically, the heart rate declined to 68 beats per minute, and 8 minutes after injection, she abruptly became asystolic while conversing with her anesthesiologist. The frequency of this phenomenon is not known. (From Mackey, D. C., Carpenter, R. C., Thompson, G. E., Brown, D. L., Bodily, M. N. Bradycardia and asystole during spinal anesthesia: A report of three cases without morbidity. *Anesthesiology* 70: 142, 1989, with permission.)

Total Spinal

Total spinal is the term used to describe a spinal anesthetic that rises above the cervical regions. This level of block is usually unintentional, resulting from unanticipated patient movement, inappropriate positioning, or inappropriate dosage. The major consequences are loss of consciousness, profound bradycardia, hypotension, and respiratory arrest. Although phrenic nerve paralysis may be involved, the respiratory arrest is usually due to hypoperfusion of the medullary respiratory control center. Fortunately, when the local anesthetic spreads this far cephalad, the concentration of drug is usually quite dilute—motor paralysis is limited and the duration is short. Prompt recognition is essential to prevent cardiac arrest and hypoxic organ damage.

Treatment of total spinal anesthesia is symptomatic. Ventilation is immediately supported. An endotracheal tube and mechanical ventilator may be necessary. Atropine, ephedrine, and fluids are given rapidly to support the cardiac output. The patient usually becomes unconscious, but verbal reassurance that he or she will recover is still appropriate. An amnesic agent may be desirable if a period of ventilatory support is needed. Sequelae do not occur if ventilation and perfusion are maintained.

Prevention is desirable. Vigorous motion and the head-down position (for hyperbaric solutions) after injection should be avoided.

Nausea

A frequent companion to high spinal and epidural anesthesia, nausea is a troublesome yet relatively benign side effect. Hypotension, bradycardia, or hypoxia must be excluded as the cause. The imbalance of sympathetic and parasympathetic tone on the viscera is often implicated. Atropine is again an appropriate initial step in treatment (11). If unsuccessful, an antiemetic can be employed, such as 2 mg of ondansetron or 0.625 mg droperidol. Compounds with vasodilating properties such as chlorpromazine are not suitable, but a number of antihistamines, phenothiazine derivatives, or serotonin antagonists have been recommended.

If a spinal has been given because of concern about a "full" stomach, the temptation to treat the nausea with heavy sedation must be avoided. This may succeed in obtunding the airway reflexes so that aspiration following vomiting is again a risk.

Postspinal Headache

This type of headache is due to a persistent leak of CSF through an unhealed dural puncture site. The consequent depletion of the fluid cushion for the cord and the brain is believed to allow a stretching of the meninges whenever the upright position is assumed. Thus, the characteristic spinal headache occurs when the patient is standing and is relieved when the patient lies down. This pathognomonic feature is often the only diagnostic clue available. The location and severity are variable, and the onset may even be delayed for days following dural puncture (5).

The incidence is higher in younger patients. Females have a slightly greater incidence than males, and pregnant women appear to be especially susceptible. The size of the needle is also important. Rounded-bevel and smaller-gauge needles will significantly reduce the incidence of headache (16), and these are the needles of choice (Fig. 6.13). Recumbency will delay the perception of symptoms, not reduce the incidence of headache. Air travel and heavy lifting and straining have been associated with the onset of symptoms, even after a previously successful epidural blood patch.

The headaches are benign in that they all resolve spontaneously without neurologic sequelae. Even the rare diplopia that results from abducens nerve stretching resolves completely. Two-thirds of the headaches resolve spontaneously within a week, but a rare few may persist for months. Standard therapy includes bed rest and analgesics, and the advice to increase fluid consumption (although the effectiveness of this step has not been documented). More specific therapy is available in the form of the epidural blood patch (see Chapter 7). The timing and use of this therapy depend on the severity of the headache and the social condition of the patient. A moderate headache in a hospitalized surgical patient requires less urgent treatment than the same headache in a postpartum patient anxious to go home and care for her new baby.

Prevention is the least expensive therapy. A lower incidence of headache may be achieved if epidural anesthesia is used in younger

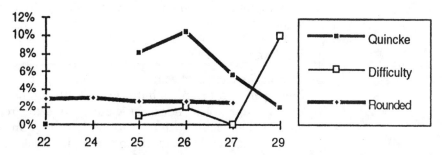

Figure 6.13   **Spinal Headache and Needles**
Although smaller-gauge Quincke needles will reduce the chance of postspinal headache, they are associated with a higher incidence of technical difficulty. Rounded-bevel needles significantly reduce the frequency of headache. (From Mulroy, M. F., Wills, R. P. Spinal anesthesia for outpatients: Appropriate agents and techniques. *J. Clin. Anesth.* 7: 622, 1995, with permission.)

patients. If a spinal is performed in young patients, the smallest practical round-beveled needle should be employed, usually 25- or 27-gauge Whitacre point. Patients should be cautioned about lifting heavy objects or planning air travel following dural puncture. Spinal anesthesia is not contraindicated in the outpatient setting, but other alternatives should be considered when a patient lives sufficiently far away from an ambulatory surgical center that returning for a blood patch would be a major inconvenience.

Neuropathy

Nerve damage due to the drug alone (in proper dose and concentration) is extremely rare (17,18) (see Chapter 3). Although laboratory studies confirm that nerve damage is possible with all of the local anesthetics, clinical experience suggests that it occurs infrequently. The major problem in this regard has been associated with the use of spinal microcatheters when repeated doses have been injected in a short period of time, apparently causing a pooling of a toxic concentration in the cauda equina region. These catheters should be used with caution, if at all (see Chapter 5).

Nerve damage may occur from a direct needle injury to a nerve root and is usually associated with a severe paresthesia at the time of performance of the block (19). Intraneural injection, signaled by a paresthesia on injection, has been implicated in nerve injury. Contamination of the anesthetic with prep solutions, detergents, and sterilizing chemicals also has been implicated.

The presence of a documented preexisting stable neurologic deficit is not a contraindication to spinal anesthesia. There is a general reluctance to use spinal anesthesia in the presence of demyelinating diseases, but there is no evidence to prove that it aggravates conditions such as multiple sclerosis.

Despite concerns about the possibility of neuropathy, large series of patients have shown the relative safety of correctly performed spinal anesthesia.

Backache

Pain in the back at the site of injection may be due to multiple, vigorous periosteal trauma, but backache after spinal or epidural anesthesia is more often nonspecific and related to stretching of the ligaments that occurs with relaxation of the back muscles. This is also seen after general anesthesia in the supine position, especially on a hard, flat operating table. In any case, heat, rest, and time usually provide relief within 1 or 2 days. As many as 40% of patients may complain of this annoying side effect.

Hearing Loss

Transient minor hearing loss has been described after spinal anesthesia. The mechanism is unclear and may be related to a temporary decrease in CSF pressure or traction on intracranial nerves. The frequency appears higher with larger-gauge needles (22 versus 26 gauge) (20,21). The problem is temporary and mild, but it is well documented with audiometry and can be a troublesome side effect for some patients.

Subdural Injection

The subdural space is essentially a potential space between the dural and the arachnoid membranes, and is usually passed through unnoticed in the performance of spinal anesthesia. On rare occasions, local anesthetic is injected through a needle or catheter tip while in this space, and the resulting drug injection is spread widely through this compartment. If the dose injected is intended as a subarachnoid anesthetic (a small dose), the resulting dispersion of the injection results in widespread but minimal and patchy anesthesia of nerves, and may explain many of the cases of failed spinal anesthesia. If an epidural dose is injected, the wider spread of anesthetic inside the dural sheath results in a surprisingly extensive block, described as massive extradural anesthesia. This situation is obviously more of a problem when epidural anesthesia or postoperative analgesia is being attempted. If it results in a failed spinal, a repeat injection is the simple solution (although care should be taken to avoid reinjection of spinal catheters, as described in Neuropathy, this chapter).

Epidural or Spinal Hematoma

Epidural or spinal hematoma is an extremely rare but potentially disastrous complication, because prolonged nerve compression can produce permanent nerve damage (see Chapter 3). Although these hematomas most often occur spontaneously, they can be precipitated by inserting a needle into the epidural venous plexus in a patient with a bleeding disorder or who is receiving anticoagulant therapy. A hematoma should be suspected when a spinal anesthetic is unusually long in duration, and computerized tomography (CT), or magnetic resonance imaging (MRI) of the spinal canal is indicated. Early surgical decompression (within 6 to 8 hours) is the only available therapy, and is only successful in 50% of cases.

Spinal Abscess or Meningitis

Abscess or meningitis from bacterial infection is rare. Contamination of the CSF by skin bacteria or from the anesthesia provider has been reported, but as isolated case reports (18). The use of indwelling catheters that create a track for contamination may increase this risk. The development of meningitis after lumber puncture in bacteremic patients has been a more frequent event, especially in pediatric patients. In animal models, it appears that treatment with antibiotics before the lumbar puncture eliminates this risk (3).

Diagnosis of abscess is best performed with MRI or CAT scan of the spine, whereas a lumbar puncture is needed to confirm the presence of meningitis and to identify antibiotic sensitivity.

The issue of lumbar puncture in patients already infected with human immunodeficiency virus is controversial. This virus infects the CSF early in the course of the disease, and 40% of patients with acquired immunodeficiency syndrome have clinical signs of neuropathy. Nevertheless, neuraxial techniques have been performed on these patients, including epidural blood patch. Individual patient evaluation and assessment of the risk–benefit situation are indicated.

References

1. Butterworth, J. Physiology of spinal anesthesia: What are the implications for management? *Reg. Anesth. Pain Med.* 23: 370, 1998.
2. Ward, R. J., Bonica, J. J., Freund, F. G., Akamatsu, T., Danziger, F., Englesson, S. Epidural and subarachnoid anesthesia. Cardiovascular and respiratory effects. *J.A.M.A.* 191: 275, 1965.
3. Carp, H., Bailey, S. The association between meningitis and dural puncture in bacteremic rats. *Anesthesiology* 76: 739, 1992.
4. Liu, S. S., Ware, P. D., Allen, H. W., Neal, J. M., Pollock, J. E. Dose-response characteristics of spinal bupivacaine in volunteers. Clinical implications for ambulatory anesthesia. *Anesthesiology* 85: 729, 1996.
5. Liu, S. S., McDonald, S. B. Current issues in spinal anesthesia. *Anesthesiology* 94: 888, 2001.
6. Chiu, A. A., Liu, S., Carpenter, R. L., Kasman, G. S., Pollock, J. E., Neal, J. M. The effects of epinephrine on lidocaine spinal anesthesia: A crossover study. *Anesth. Analg.* 80: 735, 1995.
7. Liu, S., Chiu, A. A., Carpenter, R. L., Mulroy, M. F., Allen, H. W., Neal, J. M., Pollock, J. E. Fentanyl prolongs lidocaine spinal anesthesia without prolonging recovery. *Anesth. Analg.* 80: 730, 1995.
8. Carpenter, R. L., Hogan, Q. H., Liu, S. S., Crane, B., Moore, J. Lumbosacral cerebrospinal fluid volume is the primary determinant of sensory block extent and duration during spinal anesthesia. *Anesthesiology* 89: 24, 1998.
9. Wildsmith, J. A. Predicting the spread of spinal anaesthesia. *Br. J. Anaesth.* 62: 353, 1989.
10. Pflug, A. E., Aasheim, G. M., Foster, C. Sequence of return of neurological function and criteria for safe ambulation following subarachnoid block (spinal anaesthetic). *Can. Anaesth. Soc. J.* 25: 133, 1978.
11. Ward, R. J., Kennedy, W. F., Bonica, J. J., Martin, W. E., Tolas, A. G., Akamatsu, T. Experimental evaluation of atropine and vasopressors for the treatment of hypotension of high subarachnoid anesthesia. *Anesth. Analg.* 45: 621, 1966.
12. Brooker, R., Butterworth, J., Kitzman, D., Berman, J., Kashtan, H., McKinley, A. Treatment of hypotension after hyperbaric tetracaine spinal anesthesia. A randomized, double-blind, cross-over comparison of phenylephrine and epinephrine. *Anesthesiology* 86: 797, 1997.
13. Schnider, T. W., Mueller-Duysing, S., Johr, M., Gerber, H. Incremental dosing versus single-dose spinal anesthesia and hemodynamic stability. *Anesth. Analg.* 77: 1174, 1993.

14. Caplan, R. A., Ward, R. J., Posner, K., Cheney, F. W. Unexpected cardiac arrest during spinal anesthesia: A closed claims analysis of predisposing factors. *Anesthesiology* 68: 5, 1988.
15. Carpenter, R. L., Caplan, R. A., Brown, D. L., Stephenson, C., Wu, R. Incidence and risk factors for side effects of spinal anesthesia. *Anesthesiology* 76: 906, 1992.
16. Mulroy, M. F., Wills, R. P. Spinal anesthesia for outpatients: Appropriate agents and techniques. *J. Clin. Anesth.* 7: 622, 1995.
17. Hodgson, P. S., Neal, J. M., Pollock, J. E., Liu, S. S. The neurotoxicity of drugs given intrathecally (spinal). *Anesth. Analg.* 88: 797, 1999.
18. Horlocker, T., Wedel, D. Neurologic complications of spinal and epidural anesthesia. *Reg. Anesth. Pain Med.* 25: 83, 2000.
19. Auroy, Y., Narchi, P., Messiah, A., Litt, L., Rouvier, B., Samii, K. Serious complications related to regional anesthesia: Results of a prospective survey in France. *Anesthesiology* 87: 479, 1997.
20. Schaffartzik, W., Hirsch, J., Frickmann, F., Kuhly, P., Ernst, A. Hearing loss after spinal and general anesthesia: A comparative study. *Anesth. Analg.* 91: 1466, 2000.
21. Wang, L. P., Magnusson, M., Lundberg, J., Tornebrandt, K. Auditory function after spinal anesthesia. *Reg. Anesth.* 18: 162, 1993.

7 Epidural Anesthesia

In contrast to spinal anesthesia, epidural anesthesia is technically more difficult to perform, but it offers greater flexibility in the extent, density, and duration of anesthesia. The technique has been favored over spinal anesthesia because of the segmental and graded anesthesia and the lower incidence of headaches in young patients. The potential for continuation of postoperative analgesia with narcotics or local anesthetics with a continuous (catheter) technique has dramatically increased its popularity (1).

Anatomy

Epidural blockade anesthetizes the emerging nerve roots of the spinal cord in the central peridural space of the spinal canal (see Chapter 6). This spinal epidural space is bounded anteriorly by the vertebral bodies and posteriorly by the laminae and the ligamenta flava that join these bony arches. This dense ligament creates a continuous posterior border to the space. It is 3 to 5 mm thick and is "tented" to form an acutely angled arch in the midline (see Fig. 6.10). Here the two lateral portions join and meet the anterior extension of the interspinous ligament, which lies between the spinous processes. The ligamentum flavum lies from 3.5 to 5 cm deep to the skin in patients of average build. Laterally, the boundary formed by the pedicles is interrupted by the intervertebral foramina, which allow the lateral exit of the nerve roots from the epidural space. These openings vary in size with the level of the spine and the age of the patient. At the caudal end of the spinal canal, the sacral vertebral bodies become fused and the foramina become anterior and posterior structures. The terminal point of the canal is the channel lying under the midline sacral–coccygeal membrane.

The center of the canal is occupied by the dural sac, which is suspended in position by thin lateral ligaments. A variable dorsal midline band of connective tissue holds the dura in close approximation to the ligamentum flavum and may rarely interfere with the passage of a catheter or the spread of local anesthetic. Generally, however, these septae do not interfere with the spread of solutions in the epidural space. The epidural space is widest in the posterior midline. The dural sac tapers and ends near the fifth lumbar vertebra, making the caudal end of the canal the most spacious. In the cervical region, the epidural space is smaller and the dura extends a sleeve to the foraminal openings along each exiting nerve. This sleeve ends inside the canal in the lumbar region. At the cephalad end of the canal, the space ends where the dura is attached to the borders of the foramen magnum.

The peridural space is not empty, but is filled with loose areolar tissue and fat. It is generously endowed with veins, particularly in

93

the pregnant patient (see Fig. 6.1). In the thoracic region, the space shares a negative pressure with the intrapleural space. In the lumbar region, this pressure may be equal to atmospheric pressure or slightly less. The posterior depth of the space varies from 3 to 4 mm in the thoracic region to 5 or 6 mm in the lumbar region. The greatest depth is at the second lumbar interspace. The brachial plexus and the lumbar plexus enlargements of the spinal cord distort the canal space at their corresponding levels (C-3 through T-2 and T-9 through T-12).

A larger volume of local anesthetic is required to produce epidural anesthesia than for equivalent subarachnoid blockade. A 10-fold in-

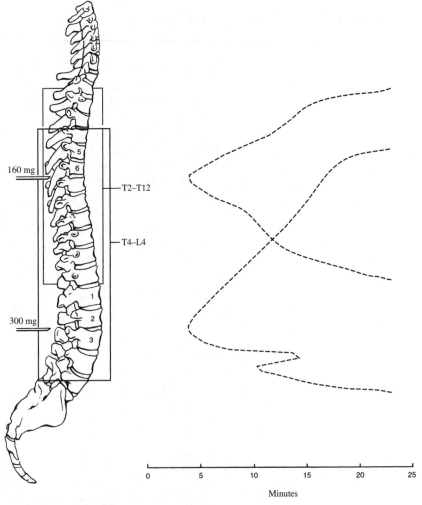

Figure 7.1   **Diagram of Spread of Local Anesthetic in the Epidural Space**
The onset of epidural anesthesia is noted first in the segments nearest the site of injection, and spreads over the next 20 minutes both cephalad and caudad from this point.

crease in volume over spinal anesthesia is usually required in the lumbar area, although smaller volumes are sufficient to fill the thoracic space. The larger volume of local anesthetic must fill a larger potential space and penetrate the protective layers surrounding the nerves. Higher concentrations are required, and slower onset is characteristic. Spread of the anesthetic solution is influenced by the contents of the space. Anesthesia extends both cephalad and caudad from the point of injection (Fig. 7.1), but upward spread above the cervical portion of the canal is limited by the dural attachment. This prevents the high brainstem levels of anesthesia that are possible with unintentionally high spinal anesthesia.

Indications

Epidural injection of anesthetic produces a regional dermatomal "band" of anesthesia spreading cephalad and caudad from the site of injection. The height of the band will vary depending on the mass and volume of drug injected, and the level of injection. Lumbar segmental epidural anesthesia is particularly suited for lower abdominal surgery or hip or knee surgery. Generous lumbar dosages or thoracic injections also can be used for upper abdominal surgery but will usually require light general anesthesia supplementation to provide control of diaphragmatic motion and ventilation. Combination of general anesthesia with epidural anesthesia is associated with a reduction in the general anesthetic requirement (2). Thoracic epidural anesthesia can be used for thoracic and breast surgery. Peridural anesthesia at the lower end of the spinal canal is produced with caudal injections (see Chapter 8) and is more appropriate for surgery in the sacral nerve distributions.

Epidural anesthesia provides the advantages of muscle relaxation and decreased bowel distension, as with spinal anesthesia. In contrast to spinal anesthesia, epidural blockade is segmental and can produce a variable number of anesthetized dermatomes, which is ideal for such situations as labor pains or thoracotomy surgery. In addition, it gives added flexibility in depth and duration. The ability to insert a catheter into the epidural space provides flexibility in duration regardless of the drug chosen. It is ideal for long surgical procedures or where duration may vary unpredictably, and may provide an ideal alternative in ambulatory surgery where adjustment of duration to the surgical procedure allows earlier discharge (3). It also is an optimal anesthetic for labor and delivery, where duration is unknown and the requirements for level and density of anesthesia vary. Continuous epidural catheter analgesia is also the optimal postoperative treatment for thoracic and upper abdominal surgery (see Chapter 24). Segmental thoracic blockade has also been used to relieve chest pain due to coronary ischemia (4).

The avoidance of postdural puncture headache makes the epidural technique particularly appropriate in the young patient. This should never be stated as a guarantee to a patient, because the possibility of a headache after a large-gauge needle puncture of the dura still exists and is significant. Contraindications to epidural blockade, as with spinal anesthesia, include patient refusal or the presence of local infection, hypovolemia, or coagulopathy.

Drugs

Almost all of the local anesthetics have been employed for epidural anesthesia. Higher concentrations are required to penetrate the protective dural layers and produce adequate sensory and motor blockade. Lower concentrations can (unlike with spinal anesthesia) produce sympathetic or sensory analgesia without total motor paralysis.

For short procedures, 2-chloroprocaine produces excellent block in a 2% or 3% concentration and will give 45 to 60 minutes of surgical anesthesia with a rapid recovery (5). It may be ideal for selected outpatient surgeries (3). If used with a catheter technique, repeat injections should be made at 45- to 60-minute intervals or at the earliest sign of regression. Intraoperative dissipation of chloroprocaine anesthesia can be distressingly rapid. Procaine is not a reliable epidural anesthetic drug.

Lidocaine (1.5% or 2%) will produce 60 to 90 minutes of abdominal anesthesia. Mepivacaine (1% or 1.5%) may last 90 to 120 minutes (Fig. 7.2). If a catheter technique is used with these intermediate-duration amides, reinjection should be planned at 75 to 90 minutes into the procedure. For upper abdominal and thoracic procedures, these intermediate drugs are ideal to confirm the function of the epidural catheter, yet allow dissipation of the block at the end of the surgery to allow transition to an analgesic infusion.

Bupivacaine provides longer-acting anesthesia. A 0.5% solution will give adequate blockade, but the addition of epinephrine or the use of the 0.75% concentration gives a more profound motor block. Levobupivacaine appears to be equal in potency and duration to the racemic mixture. Ropivacaine performs in a similar fashion, but it is slightly less potent and of slightly shorter duration so that concentrations of 1% and 0.75% may be required for similar effects. Etidocaine 1.5% also will give 3 to 5 hours of abdominal anesthesia and may provide better apparent caudal spread of anesthesia than bupivacaine, although it is not as popular because of the more profound motor block.

Epinephrine is generally used to prolong the effect of these anesthetic drugs, but it is also indicated for other reasons in epidural anesthesia. Because of the plethora of vessels in the space, a test dose to rule out intravenous injection is appropriate (see Chapter 3). Epinephrine is usually an essential component of this test (6). Epinephrine also will reduce peak systemic blood levels and intensify the block (7). This intensification may allow lower concentrations of the local anesthetic to be used and thus further reduce the chance

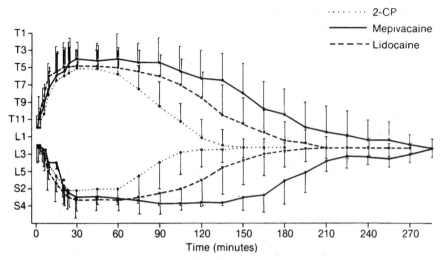

Figure 7.2   **Duration of Epidural Anesthesia**
Sensory dermatomal blockade level (with standard deviations) versus time following injection of 20 mL of 3% 2-chloroprocaine, 1.5% lidocaine, or 1.5% mepivacaine with 1:200,000 epinephrine at the L-2 interspace. Average total durations were 133, 182, and 247 minutes, respectively. (From Kopacz, D. J., Mulroy, M. F. Chloroprocaine and lidocaine decrease hospital stay and admission rate after outpatient epidural anesthesia. *Reg. Anesth.* 15: 19, 1990, with permission.)

of systemic toxicity. Epinephrine also may reduce the phenomenon of tachyphylaxis sometimes seen with continuous techniques.

In epidural anesthesia, addition of epinephrine helps preserve cardiovascular stability. The amount that is absorbed systemically has positive inotropic effects on the myocardium that tend to offset the hypotension produced by vasodilatation in the lower extremities. Although epidural anesthesia to thoracic dermatomal levels lowers the blood pressure, cardiac output actually increases if epinephrine is added to the local anesthetic. This effect is not sufficient to maintain perfusion in the presence of hypovolemia.

Other adjuvants have been recommended in epidural anesthesia in the past. Hyaluronidase has been used to increase the onset and spread. It produces unreliable anesthesia, however, and is not recommended. The use of bicarbonate to alkalinize the solutions and the use of carbonated salts are discussed in Chapter 2. Clonidine has been added to enhance analgesia, but has hemodynamic side effects and sedation that may limit its use (8,9). Opioids are the most effective additives for postoperative synergism with local anesthetics (1,10), but their intraoperative advantages in the epidural space have not been studied as widely as their intrathecal use.

Table 7.1   **Factors Affecting Epidural Dosage**

Major factors
    Patient age
    Site of injection
Minor factors
    Patient weight
    Patient height
    Position
    Pregnancy
Minimally relevant
    Speed of injection/incremental injection
    Direction of needle bevel
    Presence of atherosclerosis

Dosage

Calculating dosage for epidural anesthesia is more complex than for any other regional blockade. A greater number of factors influence the spread of drug in the epidural space (Table 7.1). Both the total drug dose and the volume affect the extent of anesthesia, but several patient and technique factors also modify the result.

Drug Mass

The total milligram dose and the volume injected both affect the height of block. When equal volumes are injected, the solution with the higher concentration (greater milligram dose) will produce greater spread. A more dilute solution (larger volume) of equal milligram dose will spread farther than a lower volume at higher concentration. In general, a more dilute solution may be advantageous in providing spread while reducing the total milligram dosage (and thus the chance for systemic toxicity).

The effect of increasing the volume of injectate is not linear and seems to have an upper limit of usefulness at approximately 20 mL for lumbar injections. At this point, further volume increases the spread of solution out of the epidural space through the intervertebral foramina (especially in younger patients).

Patient Factors (Age, Height, Weight)

Patient factors are more important in determining epidural dose requirements than in spinal anesthesia. *Age* is the major factor in the spread of epidural anesthesia (Fig. 7.3). Smaller volumes produce higher spread in older patients (11). This may be due to narrowing of the intervertebral foramina with age. In young patients, these openings allow dissipation of the injected solutions and increase the apparent dose of local anesthetic required to anesthetize a given number of segments. The relationship is not linear. *Body weight* is a second factor. Heavy patients have a reduced requirement. *Height* is a third factor influencing dose, with taller patients requiring more solution, but this, like weight, seems less of a factor than age.

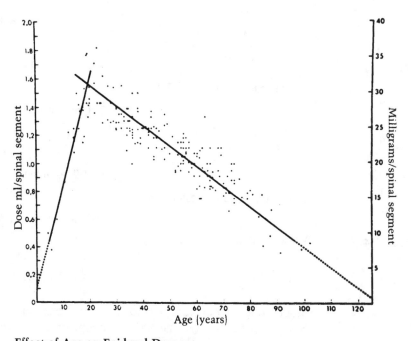

Age (years)

Figure 7.3

Effect of Age on Epidural Dosage
The dose requirement for epidural anesthesia declines with age, as
illustrated here using 2% lidocaine over a wide range of patient ages.
Despite this general trend, there is a wide scatter of patient variability,
which makes specific prediction extremely difficult based on age alone.
(From Bromage, P. R. *Epidural Analgesia.* Philadelphia: Saunders, 1978. P.
138, with permission.)

Technical Factors

Gravity has a minimal clinical effect, but there is reasonable justification for performing the block with the operative side dependent.
Unfortunately, the sitting position does not appear to enhance
sacral spread. The *site of injection* influences spread. Caudal anesthesia requires larger volumes, with 25 mL usually required to produce a T-10 level of block. Thoracic anesthesia can be attained with
6 or 8 mL of solution injected at the thoracic levels because of the
smaller volume of the epidural space there. The direction of the
needle bevel and the speed of injection have a small influence on
spread. If a catheter is advanced more than 5 cm into the space, it
will likely lie off the midline, and often is positioned near an intervertebral foramen, allowing passage of much of the injectate out of
the canal (12). Fortunately, there is a relatively homogenous spread
of anesthetic despite these aberrations.

The calculation of an epidural drug dose is highly empirical. Although each of the mentioned factors has some mathematical correlation to the height of block in a given population, the variability

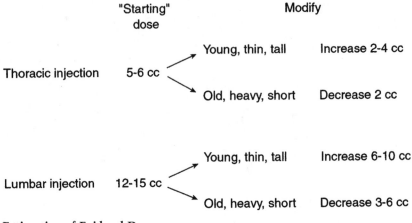

Figure 7.4 **Estimation of Epidural Dose**

associated with each is so wide as to make exact dosing impossible. Several authors have used the concept of a milliliter per segment dose, but all agree that there is a wide range for every formula and that age and total dose can alter the relation. A reasonable approach is to estimate an approximate volume or milligram dosage for the desired spread in a given patient and then adjust the volume higher or lower according to the most important individual patient factors, specifically, age, height, and weight (Fig. 7.4). Starting with a small estimate and adding incrementally through a catheter is prudent, especially in the elderly or obese patient.

Technique

The technical procedure of epidural blockade is similar to that for spinal anesthesia. As with subarachnoid blockade, several positions can be employed and several approaches to the epidural space can be used. The classic midline approach in the lateral position will be described, but the alternatives discussed in Chapter 6 are all applicable here also, including the prone position.

1. The patient is placed in the lateral position, with a pillow under the head to maintain the spine in a straight plane parallel to the bed surface. The shoulders as well as the hips are kept perpendicular to the surface of the bed. The knees are drawn up toward the head and the head is bent down toward the knees to attain a fetal position with maximal flexion of the lumbar spine.
2. The iliac crest and spinous processes are marked as for spinal anesthesia. An "X" is placed over the desired interspace.
3. Prep, drape, and local infiltration are carried out as for spinal anesthesia. A wider draping area may be needed if a catheter is

to be passed, in order to avoid contamination of the free end during passage. The infiltrating needle can serve as a "seeker" to identify the depth of the ligamentum flavum in the thin patient, as well as the cephalad–caudad orientation of the interspinous space.

4. The epidural needle is inserted through the skin wheal with the bevel directed cephalad. Lateral direction of the bevel, especially of a Tuohy or Hustead type, will encourage lateral deviation of the needle point. The needle is advanced into and slowly through the interspinous ligament, stopping at the point of increased resistance, which represents the ligamentum flavum (Fig. 7.5). If the midline is correctly identified, the needle will meet steady, consistent resistance up to contact with the ligament. This depth of the ligament will vary from 3.5 to 5 cm from the skin in the normal adult and is most closely related to patient weight.

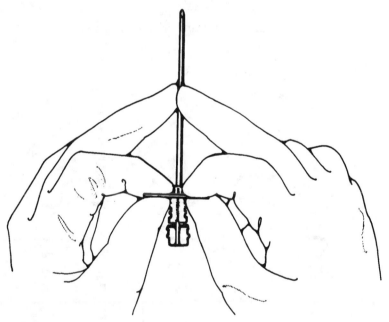

Figure 7.5   **Hand Position for Epidural Needle**
The epidural needle is introduced into the skin at the same point and direction as the spinal needle. During passage through the interspinous ligament, firm, sensitive control is needed to allow identification of the subtle increase in resistance that represents the entry into the ligamentum flavum. Although many approaches are used, a common technique is to grasp the hub of the needle firmly using the flanges present on many epidural needles, and to brace the other fingers of the hands against the back, either along the shaft of the needle itself (as shown) or slightly away from it on the back. This bracing prevents unintentional advancement of the needle due to either patient or operator motion.

The ability to perceive the increase in resistance is an acquired skill. Novices must have—literally—a helping hand. A number of unintentional dural punctures may occur before this crucial step is mastered. The pregnant patient is notorious for ligamentous softening at term and is the most challenging in whom to demonstrate this subtle increase in resistance.

5. When the resistance of the ligament is perceived, the stylet is withdrawn, and a 3- to 5-mL glass syringe with 1 to 3 mL of local anesthetic or saline solution is attached to the hub. A small air bubble (0.1 to 0.2 mL) is introduced into the syringe before attachment.

   The syringe is carefully tested beforehand to ensure that the plunger moves freely. Care is taken in handling the plunger so that powder-covered gloves do not come in contact with its shaft. A sticky syringe will frustrate attempts to identify a loss of resistance.

   At all times, the hub of the needle is controlled by the thumb and forefinger of the nondominant hand, the back of which is resting solidly against the patient's back (Fig. 7.6).

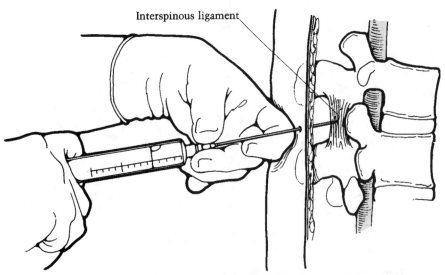

Interspinous ligament

Figure 7.6   **Advancement of the Epidural Needle into the Space**
Once the ligamentum flavum is identified, a syringe with 1 mL of fluid and a 0.1-cm³ bubble of air is attached to the hub of the needle. The dominant hand rests firmly against the back while grasping the hub of the needle between thumb and one finger. The opposite hand exerts pressure on the plunger of the syringe so that the bubble is compressed to one-half its normal size. If the needle is in the true ligament, compression is possible without injecting any fluid. The dominant hand then "rotates" slightly to advance the needle slowly while constant pressure is held on the plunger. Entry to the epidural space is heralded by the dramatic release of resistance, allowing all of the fluid in the syringe to be injected easily.

Moderate pressure is exerted on the plunger of the syringe with the thumb of the dominant hand. If the needle tip is fully in the ligamentum flavum, injection of solution will not be possible, but the force exerted will compress the air bubble in the syringe.

6. If adequate compression is not obtained, the needle is advanced slightly and the test is repeated until compression is established. If there is uncertainty about the location of the tip, or if there is no resistance at all, the needle is withdrawn and redirected after the landmarks are reassessed.

7. If the bubble is compressed to half its original size without injection of fluid, the tip lies in the ligamentum flavum. The needle is advanced through the ligament slowly by the nondominant hand, with constant pressure on the plunger of the syringe exerted by the opposite thumb. The nondominant hand holding the hub of the needle performs all the advancing. The dominant hand maintains constant unremitting pressure on the plunger but does not advance the syringe–needle combination. As the advance begins, the patient is warned that he or she may feel a "splash" or "squirt" sensation in the back, but this sensation will not be painful and he or she must not move.

8. As soon as the tip of the bevel penetrates the inner surface of the ligament, there is a dramatic loss of resistance. The contents of the syringe empty rapidly into the epidural space. The sudden discharge of fluid into the back may cause some patients to move; the nondominant hand must maintain firm control of the depth of the needle, and the needle must remain fixed at this depth.

9. The syringe is removed carefully, allowing no change in needle depth. If a catheter is to be inserted, the hub is grasped firmly between thumb and forefinger and advanced 1 to 2 mm while the heel of the hand rests on the patient's back to control depth. This ensures that the entire opening of the bevel passes into the epidural space.

10. Then 0.5 mL air is drawn into the syringe, which is carefully reattached to the hub. Gentle aspiration is performed to detect blood or cerebrospinal fluid (CSF). If no fluid returns, the air in the syringe is forcefully injected. The epidural space will offer no resistance to injection, although a small amount of the air may "rebound" back into the syringe. If there is any resistance to air injection, the needle is repositioned and the epidural space is sought again. If there is no resistance, the depth of needle insertion is noted.

A false release (loss of resistance) may occur if the needle was seated only in the interspinous ligament and passed laterally out of this ligament before reaching the ligamentum flavum. This air test usually will detect the situation where the needle tip still lies in connective tissue outside the epidural space, because there will be residual resistance. This air test may be omitted if injection of air is undesirable, as in lithotripsy or pediatric anesthesia (13).

11. Once placement of the needle is reasonably certain, a test dose is injected and appropriate observations are made to exclude intravascular or subarachnoid injection (see Chapter 3). Although a catheter can be inserted at this point, the potential for intravascular placement appears higher if the passage is made into the space before the injection of the local anesthetic rather than after (14,15). The chosen therapeutic dose is injected in 5-mL increments at 30-second intervals. If a catheter is to be inserted, 2 to 3 mL of the local anesthetic solution is reserved for a test dose through the catheter.

12. If a catheter is used, it is inserted with the dominant hand while the nondominant hand continues to fix the needle in position (Fig. 7.7). As the catheter is inserted, resistance will be felt as it passes the angle at the end of the needle. If the tip does not exit

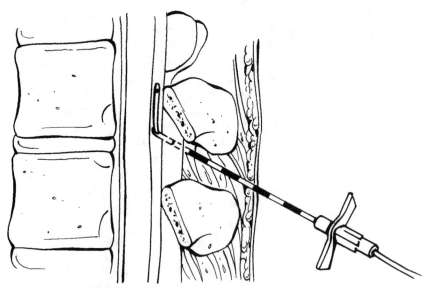

Figure 7.7   **Insertion of an Epidural Catheter**
The needle is again secured by resting one hand on the back and grasping the hub firmly (not shown) while the other hand inserts the catheter into the hub and gently advances it beyond the tip of the needle. The bevel is usually directed cephalad, which produces the most reliable insertion; caudad orientation may allow the catheter to exit one of the intervertebral foramina. Ideally, the catheter is advanced only 3 to 4 cm beyond the needle tip; further placement increases the potential for lateral misdirection or foraminal exit.

the end of the needle freely, the catheter is removed and the needle is advanced another millimeter; the confirmatory tests are then repeated.

After the catheter passes the needle tip, it is advanced no more than 5 cm beyond the needle tip. Further insertion increases the chance of coiling or misdirection into a foramen or elsewhere off the midline. If resistance is felt, it is a hint that the needle may not be in the epidural space. The catheter should not be withdrawn once it has passed the needle tip. This maneuver may shred the catheter or cut it completely on the sharp leading edge of the angled needle tip. If difficulty is encountered, the entire needle and catheter combination should be withdrawn as a unit and the procedure started anew.

13. When the catheter is in place, it is held firmly and advanced through the needle as the latter is withdrawn from the skin, so that the length of catheter in the epidural space remains constant. The needle is withdrawn with a slight curving motion in the direction of the arc of its bevel so that the sharp edge of the bevel is less likely to drag alongside or shear the catheter. Once out of the skin, the needle is carefully removed over the end of the catheter and an appropriate connector is attached in a sterile manner to the free end of the catheter.

    The length of catheter in the epidural space is then confirmed by assessing the total length at the skin and subtracting the previously noted depth of the epidural space. If more than 4 cm has been introduced, the excess is withdrawn before securing the catheter and injecting the dose. The patient can be instructed to extend the legs at this point, and the catheter is carefully aspirated for blood or CSF.

14. In a single-injection technique, the needle is then removed and the patient may be asked to move to the supine position. In a catheter technique, the legs are fully extended and the catheter is securely taped to the back before the patient turns. Care is taken to avoid a sharp angle or kink at the point where the catheter exits the skin. A gentle loop at the skin exit site is usually required to avoid kinking. If the catheter is to remain in place for several days for postoperative analgesia, a sterile adhesive dressing should be placed over the skin entry site. The free end is brought over the patient's shoulder and secured there so that neither the free loops nor the adapter is accidentally dislodged.

15. Onset of epidural anesthesia is slower than that of spinal anesthesia. Testing for a level may be deferred for several minutes, especially with the longer-acting drugs. Sacral anesthesia is the last to evolve, and it cannot be assumed to have occurred when abdominal anesthesia is present. Its presence should be confirmed if it is required for the procedure.

16. Each reinjection of the catheter must be preceded by the same safety steps performed with the initial dose, recognizing that the response to a test dose may be altered if general anesthesia is present (6).
17. Unless it is to remain in place for postoperative anesthesia or narcotic analgesia, the catheter should be removed at the completion of the procedure. The integrity of the tip should be noted.

Paramedian (Lateral) Approach

In addition to the traditional midline approach, the ligament can be entered from the lateral aspect. As in a spinal, the needle can be directed to the ligament at an angle by entering the skin a few centimeters lateral to the midline while still in the center of the interspace. This avoids calcified interspinous ligaments, but loses the advantage of using the interspinous ligament to identify the midline as the needle is advanced.

A popular approach with epidurals is the *paramedian approach*, where the needle is introduced through the skin opposite the spinous process below the interspace and is advanced into the ligament from a lateral and inferior direction, as described in Chapter 6. The advantage of this technique is that the bony lamina opposite the spinous process is identified first, giving a clear indication of the anticipated depth of the ligament. The needle can then be redirected medially and superiorly to "walk over the top" of the lamina and enter the ligament. This approach also offers the advantage of a more oblique entry to the epidural space. This obliquity may facilitate catheter advancement, and the less acute angle at the skin also may reduce the chance of catheter kinking at that point. Despite these theoretical advantages, there is no substantial difference in success with this approach compared to the midline approach (14).

Thoracic Epidural

Segmental anesthesia of the upper abdomen or chest can be obtained by injecting the local anesthetic in the thoracic epidural space. This technique reduces the total dose requirement and greatly improves the postthoracotomy analgesia with lipid-soluble opioid infusions, but the anatomy presents a technically greater challenge. First, the spinous processes (particularly T4-10) are longer and more steeply angled, so that the midline approach is more difficult. More significantly, the dural sac lies closer to the ligamentum flavum, and in this region the spinal cord is in closer proximity to the dura. A dural puncture here carries the risk of direct spinal cord damage. For these reasons, the paramedian approach (see Chapter 6) may be preferred, both because of its lateral approach to the interspace and because of its early identification of the safe depth of the lamina and ligament.

1. The patient is placed in the lateral or sitting position with the neck and upper back flexed as much as possible. The spinous processes are identified and marked. The process of C-7 is usually the most prominent in the neck and serves to identify this level. The tip of the scapula will identify the T-9 level (see Fig. 6.4). An "X" is marked on the skin 1 to 1.5 cm lateral to the spinous process at the level desired, usually the dermatomal level below the center of the intended surgical incision. In the thorax, the spinous processes lie over the vertebral bodies and laminae of the segment below. A catheter should be inserted one to two levels below the desired center of the block area, because it will advance up the canal as it is introduced.

2. Local infiltration with anesthetic solution is performed with a 1.5-in. 22-gauge needle. The tip of this needle may be used to identify the lamina of the vertebral body. In the obese patient, a 3.5-in. spinal needle may be needed to identify the bone and provide adequate analgesia. Infiltration of the periosteum is also performed. The exploring needle should "walk up" the lamina and identify the upper border where the ligamentum flavum has its insertion.

3. With a mental note of this anatomy, the Tuohy needle with stylet is advanced onto the lamina with the bevel directed cephalad. The needle is advanced upward and medially at a 45- to 50-degree angle and "walked off" the lamina until the ligament is reached (Fig. 7.8). The epidural space is identified by the loss of resistance technique or the "hanging drop" technique (see "Hanging Drop" and Other Adjuncts, this chapter).

4. Once through the ligament, the needle is advanced only a millimeter before the catheter is threaded. The same procedure and cautions are followed as in the lumbar region. Again, only 3 to 4 cm of catheter is inserted at this level.

5. For pure thoracic anesthesia, more dilute solutions of local anesthetics can be used (1% lidocaine, 0.25% to 0.5% bupivacaine). Dosages again depend on patient age and weight, but are generally 30% to 50% of the lumbar doses, because the epidural space is smaller in this region. As in the lumbar region, a segmental block will spread several dermatomes above and below the site of injection. Sympathectomy may include the cardioaccelerator fibers, but it does not produce the same degree of peripheral vasodilatation and hypotension as lumbar blockade.

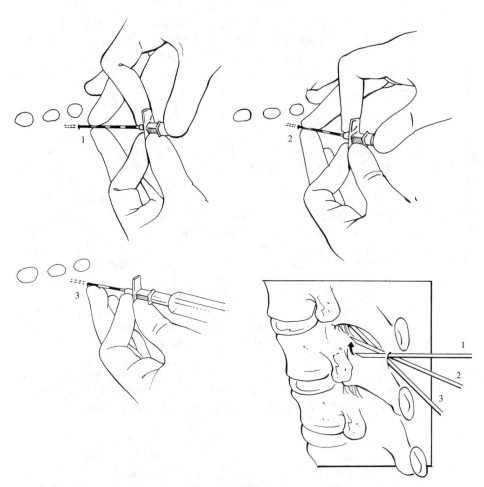

Figure 7.8　　　**Thoracic Epidural Approach**
The needle is introduced one fingerbreadth lateral to the inferior tip of the spinous process overlying the desired interspace. The needle is introduced directly perpendicular to the skin, and will contact the lamina. The needle is then gently repositioned, angling both 45 degrees medially and 45 degrees cephalad to walk up and in over the lamina to the ligamentum flavum and enter the epidural space with the loss of resistance technique or the hanging drop technique once the needle is seated in the ligament.

"Hanging Drop" and Other Adjuncts

The loss of resistance technique described earlier is a modification of the original (classic) method of identification of the lumbar epidural space. In addition to the fluid and bubble method described, identification also can be performed with an air-filled syringe with intermittent ballottement of the plunger. This technique appears to be simpler, but it involves intermittent advancement between evaluations of resistance rather than the constant appreciation provided by the compressed bubble. In addition, concern about the introduction of air into the epidural space may make this technique less desirable (13). Another alternative is the use of saline alone, although the use of a noncompressible medium carries the risk of failing to recognize a sticky plunger as the source of resistance. Neither of these alternatives is as smooth or as dramatic as the combination of air and fluid.

In the thoracic region, the epidural space shares the negative pressure with the chest cavity. In this area, a drop of solution on the hub of the advancing needle will be dramatically sucked into the epidural space by the negative pressure as soon as the ligamentum flavum is pierced. This alternative "hanging drop" technique is acceptable in the thorax, but it is not as reliable in the lumbar region, where the pressure may be equal to atmospheric pressure.

Several mechanical devices, such as balloons or manometers, have been devised in the past to aid in identification of the epidural space. Although their reliability may be satisfactory, the practiced hand will usually find no need of mechanical assistance in locating the ligament and the epidural space with the simple techniques already described. Likewise, the use of ultrasound and fluoroscopy to facilitate identification of the space has been described, but these are generally unnecessary. They may be helpful in rare cases of extreme obesity or anatomic deformity.

Other Positions

Epidural anesthesia also can be performed with the patient in the sitting and prone positions, as previously described for spinal anesthesia (see Chapter 6). As with spinals, the sitting position is useful in the obese patient. This position allows the easiest identification of the bony landmarks and the midline.

Epidural anesthesia in the prone position is less common, but it is practical. The technique and approach are the same as described earlier. Avoidance of repositioning the patient after a block may be an indication for the prone position, but epidural blockade will provide 5 to 10 minutes of adequate residual sensory and motor function to allow prone positioning with safety after injection of the anesthetic. Prone positioning may allow greater separation of spinous processes and a wider separation of the dura from the ligament, but these minor advantages may not merit the additional effort required.

Combined Spinal–Epidural Technique

The advantages of both spinal and epidural anesthesia can be obtained with the combination technique—the rapid onset and sacral spread of subarachnoid injection, plus the potential to provide ongoing anesthesia or analgesia with an epidural catheter (16). This is particularly useful in obstetrics, but also applicable for surgeries such as abdominal–perineal resections and total knee replacements, where sacral anesthesia is needed at the onset, and postoperative analgesia is a challenge. The technique is usually limited to lumbar insertion, where subarachnoid injection is safer.

1. The patient is prepared for lumbar epidural anesthesia as with any of the approaches described. A designated epidural needle is introduced in the epidural space in the standard fashion.
2. After entering the epidural space, the syringe is removed from the epidural needle and an appropriate 25- or 27-gauge spinal needle is inserted through it a sufficient distance to puncture the dura (see Fig. 22.1). These needles are provided as a "pair" in the commercial packets, so that the length of the spinal needle (11 to 12 cm) allows it to protrude a full 5 to 10 mm beyond the tip of the epidural needle, either by exiting along its normal shaft, or through a specifically designed hole in the outer curvature of the bevel of the epidural needle.
3. Once free flow of CSF is obtained, the spinal needle is fixed in place, or locked into the hub of the epidural needle (in some kits). The chosen dose of subarachnoid local anesthetic or opioid is injected in the standard fashion for spinal anesthesia or obstetrical analgesia. The spinal needle is then withdrawn, and an epidural catheter is threaded through the epidural needle and secured in the standard fashion.
4. If the spinal needle fails to penetrate the dura, the epidural needle might be directed off the midline, or not sufficiently advanced into the epidural space. Repositioning should be attempted to correct the error.
5. When the spinal anesthesia begins to recede (or the opioid effect dissipates), local anesthetic is injected in the epidural catheter, with a 10% to 20% reduction in dosage from the normal. (The epidural injection may "raise" the level of spinal anesthesia, creating the potential for unintended high block.) From this point, the epidural catheter is managed in a standard fashion.

Epidural Blood Patch

This technique is the definitive treatment for postdural puncture headache. The symptoms, indications, and associated treatment are all discussed in Chapter 6. The simple technique is described here.

1. The patient is placed in the lateral position, and the landmarks are identified as indicated earlier for a routine epidural. If possible, the injection is made at the same interspace as the original dural puncture.
2. The back is prepped and draped with careful aseptic technique.
3. Local infiltration and needle placement proceed as with a routine epidural. As soon as the epidural space is identified by loss

of resistance, the needle is left in place and the patient is instructed to hold this position.

4. The anesthesiologist or an assistant then uses aseptic technique to draw blood from one of the patient's veins. If the anesthesiologist is working alone, the arm can be positioned, the tourniquet applied, and the prep performed before the rest of the procedure is started. Blood must be drawn *after* identification of the epidural space to avoid premature clotting. Once the blood is drawn, it is injected slowly through the epidural needle, with a warning to the patient that some cramping or pressure may be felt. The injection should be terminated if the patient perceives pain in the back or leg. The epidural needle is then removed.

   Controversy exists over the optimal volume of blood to be injected. A higher success rate with 20 mL of blood has been reported, although most series have reported 90% to 95% success with the "standard" 10-mL injection. A 10-mL injection spreads six segments above and three segments below the site of injection. Further injection (up to an average volume of 14 mL) will produce radicular pain attributed to nerve compression (17). It would appear that 10 to 15 mL is a reasonable volume and that if the patient perceives pain before that point, the injection has probably filled the space sufficiently and can be discontinued.

5. Onset of relief varies following injection. Some patients can rise up and walk away immediately, cured in a biblical fashion. Others, particularly those suffering CSF volume depletion, may profit from additional bed rest and may not perceive a cure for several hours. The need for fluid administration at the time of patch has not been documented, but the intravenous administration of a liter of balanced salt solution may be helpful in the dehydrated or vomiting patient. All patients should be advised to avoid lifting, straining, or air travel for a period of time after a blood patch—the desired duration is unclear. A second patch can be performed within 24 hours if symptoms persist or recur. Although the success rate of performing the patch within 24 hours of the puncture is reported to be lower than if the procedure is delayed, this may simply reflect that those patients with more severe headaches respond less well.

Complications

Sympathetic Blockade

As with spinal anesthesia, the sympathectomy produced by epidural blockade will usually produce a decrease in the systolic blood pressure, with the degree of hypotension roughly related to the extent of sympathetic blockade. In contrast to spinal block, the onset of hypotension is usually slow enough to allow compensation

Table 7.2   **Cardiovascular Changes with Epidural Anesthesia**

	Epidural Block with Lidocaine		
	Plain	Epinephrine 1:200,000	Spinal Block
Heart rate	7%	16%	4%
Mean arterial pressure	–9%	–22%	–21%
Peripheral resistance	–3%	–40%	–5%
Cardiac output	–5%	30%	–18%

Data from Ward, R. J., et al. Epidural and subarachnoid anesthesia: Cardiovascular and respiratory effects. *J.A.M.A.* 191:275,1965.

by fluid infusion alone. If not, intravenous or intramuscular ephedrine is the drug of choice, as with spinal anesthesia. As with spinal blockade, the hypotension is more profound in the presence of preexisting volume depletion or hemorrhage, and these are relative contraindications to epidural block.

Epinephrine added to epidural anesthetics has a dual effect. The sympathetic block produced by plain lidocaine solutions produces minimal decreases in blood pressure, whereas addition of epinephrine 1:200,000 is associated with a more dramatic decrease (Table 7.2). This phenomenon is attributed to the vasodilatory (peripheral beta) effects of the low dose of epinephrine absorbed systemically. Fortunately, it is associated with increased cardiac output and blood flow to the lower extremities.

Sympathectomy also produces other side effects. Urination is often inhibited, and the frequency of required bladder catheterization (as with spinal anesthesia) is roughly related to the duration of action of the local anesthetic. Concern has been expressed that sympathetic blockade might precipitate intestinal perforation due to increased peristaltic tone if an obstruction is present. This does not appear to be a clinically significant problem.

Intravascular Injection

Intravascular injection is the most serious threat during epidural anesthesia, particularly because of the large volumes of concentrated local anesthetic solution employed. The hazard is increased by the generous venous plexus in the epidural space. This is further complicated by the low or negative pressure in these veins, which may frustrate attempts to identify intravascular placement by aspiration of blood. The vessels may simply collapse when aspiration is attempted with a syringe. The problem is not avoided by the use of a catheter, because even these soft plastics can penetrate the vessels and appear to do so in the range of 1% to 8% of epidurals (5,14,15). It appears that vessel entry is less likely if the epidural space is dis-

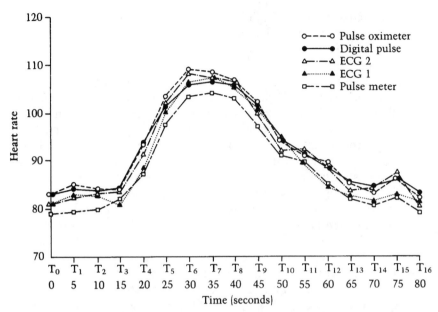

Figure 7.9   **Cardiovascular Response to an Epinephrine Test Dose**
Intravascular injection of 15 μg of epinephrine will cause a 30% increase
in heart rate within 30 seconds in a normal patient, which is easily
detected by a pulse oximeter, electrocardiogram (ECG), or other electronic
pulse counter. This figure illustrates the average heart rates in six subjects
monitored with five devices after injection of epinephrine. This is the
typical pulse rate change and duration.

tended by injection of the local anesthetic solution before insertion
of the catheter. Catheters also have been known to migrate into a
vessel between intermittent injections. Prevention and treatment
are discussed at length elsewhere; careful test dosing and incremental injection are the mainstays of prevention. Careful monitoring of
the cardiovascular response to an epinephrine test dose (Fig. 7.9) is
the current standard, although there are many clinical situations
that interfere with this test (6). Resuscitation equipment is mandatory, even in the family-centered birthing suite. Monitoring and precautions are mandatory every time a catheter is reinjected with a
large volume of concentrated solution.

Total Spinal Anesthesia

Total spinal anesthesia can occur when the local anesthetic solution is unintentionally injected into the subarachnoid space. As
with intravascular injection, the large volumes used for epidural
anesthesia lead to dramatic complications. Treatment is identical to
that for an unintentionally high spinal (see Chapter 6), but the onset, severity, and duration are far more rapid, extensive, and pro-

longed. Unanticipated high blocks also can result from *subdural injection* (see Subdural Injection, this chapter).

Again, prevention is more rewarding. Test doses and incremental injection with the initial and all subsequent injections are indicated. Two full minutes may be required to detect the onset of sensory anesthesia in the sacral segments following lidocaine injection (18), and actual pinprick sensation in sacral dermatomes should be tested at this time rather than mere subjective signs or ability to "wiggle the toes." Detection of dural puncture by the catheter is difficult once the initial injection has been made. All supplemental injections should be in increments, with careful monitoring of sensory anesthesia levels and systolic blood pressure.

If a dural puncture is detected before injection, several courses of action are available. A spinal anesthetic may be substituted, if appropriate, and alternate drugs or reduced dosage should be used. An epidural can be performed at an adjacent interspace, or the needle can be withdrawn back into the epidural space at the same level and a catheter inserted. If an epidural dose is injected at the same level (or even at a different level), a 15% to 25% reduction in dosage appears to be appropriate, along with careful monitoring to ensure that diffusion of the anesthetic through the dural rent does not precipitate high spinal blockade (19).

Unilateral or "Patchy" Blocks

Rarely, an epidural anesthetic will fail to produce the expected segmental anesthesia. Unilateral block has been described, most often when a catheter is advanced more than 5 cm and its tip lies well to one side of the midline (12). "Patchy" block, with a lack of anesthesia in a few isolated segments, also has been reported. Most often, the sacral segments are not anesthetized because of the mechanical block to spread produced by the S-1 root or by a stenosis of the spinal canal.

Rarely, air bubbles in the epidural space may interfere with spread of solution and produce scattered patches of missed anesthesia. The use of significant volumes of air also has been reported to produce venous air embolization and supraclavicular emphysema (13). Although air has been advocated to distend the epidural space to facilitate passage of catheters, it would appear wise to use a minimum volume, or saline instead.

Neuropathy and Cord Damage

Nerve-root damage may occur with lumbar epidural anesthesia, as with spinals, although it is rare here also. Thoracic or cervical attempts carry the added risk of damage to the cord itself. This is signaled by an abrupt complaint of severe radiating pain by the patient during needle advancement. Because of the large gauge of the needles used and the nonregenerating nature of cord fibers, the result can be permanent and significant motor or sensory deficit below the level of injury. Although there is no treatment for these injuries, they are fortunately rare.

Prevention is critical. Care should always be taken when advancing any needle near the neuraxis. Attempts at epidurals above the L-2 level should not be performed without premedication and adequate training. Meticulous technique is essential, and the practitioner who is unsure of himself or herself should use alternate methods for anesthesia. Performance of such blocks in the presence of a general anesthetic may increase the risk of unrecognized nerve contact (20).

Headache

Dural puncture can occur with attempts at epidural anesthesia. The larger needle employed will lead to a higher frequency of headaches (as high as 50% in young patients, particularly in obstetrics). These headaches are evaluated and treated the same as those following spinals. Prophylactic blood patching does not appear to decrease the incidence of headache.

Retained Catheter

As mentioned earlier, an attempt to withdraw a catheter through a needle with an angled bevel may produce shearing or complete transection. No direct harm results from this, because the materials used are nonirritating and "tissue-implantable." The patient should be informed of the foreign body present, but surgical removal is usually not indicated. The patient must be aware of this, lest a subsequent abdominal x-ray detect an opaque fragment that a zealous surgeon may offer to remove.

Of more concern is the catheter that has been excessively advanced and allowed to curl sufficiently to produce a knot in the epidural space. This rare condition is best avoided by limiting catheter advancement to less than 5 cm in the epidural space. If knotting occurs, some catheters can be retrieved by gentle traction alone. Surgical removal may be indicated if the catheter breaks at the skin and creates a tract for potential contamination of the epidural space.

Subdural Injection

As mentioned in Chapter 6, the subdural space is a potential space between the dural and the arachnoid membranes, and may be entered with a Tuohy needle or catheter. The resulting drug injection is spread widely through this compartment, resulting in a surprisingly extensive block, described as massive extradural anesthesia. This situation can be a problem when epidural anesthesia or postoperative analgesia is being attempted, and it should be suspected whenever an epidural dose produces a more extensive spread than expected.

Epidural Hematoma

Epidural hematoma is rare and is associated usually with preexisting coagulopathy if it occurs during anesthesia (20,21). In the unanesthetized patient, pain may be the first complaint, followed by weakness in the legs. Under epidural anesthesia, any block that fails to resolve in the expected time must be suspected of representing spinal cord compression from bleeding and hematoma formation. This is more likely if a coagulopathy is present. Magnetic resonance imaging (MRI) or computerized axial tomography (CAT scan) is an appropriate diagnostic test. Recovery is rare if decompressive laminectomy is not performed early.

The role of epidural anesthesia in the face of anticoagulant therapy is discussed in Chapter 3.

Epidural Abscess

Infection is rare in the epidural space, but in immunocompromised patients it is a potential risk, which may be increased by the injection of steroids. An abscess may present as pain and neurologic changes several days after epidural injection, and may be associated with localized tenderness, fever, and leukocytosis. MRI is the best diagnostic tool, and early surgical decompression is indicated if neurologic symptoms exist. Superficial inflammation or infections at the site of catheter insertion are more common and usually resolve with removal of the catheter.

Wrong Solution

Injection of the wrong solution into the epidural space occurs more often than officially reported. Solutions of potassium chloride, thiopental sodium, antibiotics, and many other drugs intended for intravenous use have been inadvertently administered through poorly labeled injection ports by those not familiar with the use of these catheters. This is more likely as epidural narcotic analgesia gains further popularity for postoperative pain control on hospital wards. Fortunately, there is buffering capacity in the epidural space, and the dural layers appear to protect the nerves to some extent from chemical injury. Consequently, serious sequelae have not been reported. Careful labeling of catheters and (ideally) the use of special color-coded injection ports may reduce this problem.

References

1. Liu, S., Carpenter, R. L., Neal, J. M. Epidural anesthesia and analgesia. Their role in postoperative outcome. *Anesthesiology* 82: 1474, 1995.
2. Hodgson, P. S., Liu, S. S. Epidural lidocaine decreases sevoflurane re-

quirement for adequate depth of anesthesia as measured by the Bispectral Index monitor. *Anesthesiology* 94: 799, 2001.

3. Mulroy, M. F., Larkin, K. L., Hodgson, P. S., Helman, J. D., Pollock, J. E., Liu, S. S. A comparison of spinal, epidural, and general anesthesia for outpatient knee arthroscopy. *Anesth. Analg.* 91: 860, 2000.
4. Meissner, A., Rolf, N., Van Aken, H. Thoracic epidural anesthesia and the patient with heart disease: Benefits, risks, and controversies. *Anesth. Analg.* 85: 517, 1997.
5. Kopacz, D. J., Mulroy, M. F. Chloroprocaine and lidocaine decrease hospital stay and admission rate after outpatient epidural anesthesia. *Reg. Anesth.* 15: 19, 1990.
6. Mulroy, M. F., Norris, M. C., Liu, S. S. Safety steps for epidural injection of local anesthetics: Review of the literature and recommendations. *Anesth. Analg.* 85: 1346, 1997.
7. Burm, A. G., van Kleef, J. W., Gladines, M. P., Olthof, G., Spierdijk, J. Epidural anesthesia with lidocaine and bupivacaine: Effects of epinephrine on the plasma concentration profiles. *Anesth. Analg.* 65: 1281, 1986.
8. Milligan, K. R., Convery, P. N., Weir, P., Quinn, P., Connolly, D. The efficacy and safety of epidural infusions of levobupivacaine with and without clonidine for postoperative pain relief in patients undergoing total hip replacement. *Anesth. Analg.* 91: 393, 2000.
9. Paech, M. J., Pavy, T. J., Orlikowski, C. E., Lim, W., Evans, S. F. Postoperative epidural infusion: A randomized, double-blind, dose-finding trial of clonidine in combination with bupivacaine and fentanyl. *Anesth. Analg.* 84: 1323, 1997.
10. Curatolo, M., Petersen-Felix, S., Scaramozzino, P., Zbinden, A. M. Epidural fentanyl, adrenaline and clonidine as adjuvants to local anaesthetics for surgical analgesia: Meta-analyses of analgesia and side-effects. *Acta. Anaesthesiol. Scand.* 42: 910, 1998.
11. Bromage, P. R. Ageing and epidural dose requirements: Segmental spread and predictability of epidural analgesia in youth and extreme age. *Br. J. Anaesth.* 41: 1016, 1969.
12. Hogan, Q. Epidural catheter tip position and distribution of injectate evaluated by computed tomography. *Anesthesiology* 90: 964, 1999.
13. Saberski, L. R., Kondamuri, S., Osinubi, O. Y. Identification of the epidural space: Is loss of resistance to air a safe technique? A review of the complications related to the use of air. *Reg. Anesth.* 22: 3, 1997.
14. Griffin, R. M., Scott, R. P. Forum. A comparison between the midline and paramedian approaches to the extradural space. *Anaesthesia* 39: 584, 1984.
15. Verniquet, A. J. Vessel puncture with epidural catheters. Experience in obstetric patients. *Anaesthesia* 35: 660, 1980.
16. Rawal, N., Van Zundert, A., Holmstrom, B., Crowhurst, J. A. Combined spinal-epidural technique. *Reg. Anesth.* 22: 406, 1997.
17. Szeinfeld, M., Ihmeidan, I. H., Moser, M. M., Machado, R., Klose, K. J., Serafini, A. N. Epidural blood patch: Evaluation of the volume and spread of blood injected into the epidural space. *Anesthesiology* 64: 820, 1986.
18. Abraham, R. A., Harris, A. P., Maxwell, L. G., Kaplow, S. The efficacy of 1.5% lidocaine with 7.5% dextrose and epinephrine as an epidural test dose for obstetrics. *Anesthesiology* 64: 116, 1986.

19. Hodgkinson, R. Total spinal block after epidural injection into an inter-space adjacent to an inadvertent dural perforation. *Anesthesiology* 55: 593, 1981.
20. Horlocker, T. T., Wedel, D. J. Neurologic complications of spinal and epidural anesthesia. *Reg. Anesth. Pain Med.* 25: 83, 2000.
21. Vandermeulen, E. P., Van Aken, H., Vermylen, J. Anticoagulants and spinal-epidural anesthesia. *Anesth. Analg.* 79: 1165, 1994.

8 Caudal Anesthesia

An alternative approach to the peridural space is through the base of the spine at the sacral hiatus. Injection into the sacral canal produces an epidural block but requires a higher volume of solution to reach abdominal levels. The caudal approach is handicapped by a greater variability of the anatomy and a higher potential for venous injection.

Anatomy

The caudal canal is the lowermost extension of the spinal canal. The dorsal roof is the fused posterior laminae of the sacral vertebral bodies. The only direct opening into the canal normally occurs at the level of the fifth sacral vertebra, where the failure of development of the spinous process and the laminae leaves a hiatus in the bony roof of the canal. This opening is bounded laterally by the prominent cornu (the incompletely developed articular processes) and covered by the thick sacral–coccygeal ligament. Along the lateral border of the canal itself are openings both anterior and posterior in the sacral bone at the levels of S-1 through S-4. The sacral nerve roots emerge both posteriorly and anteriorly through these modified intervertebral foramina.

The canal is concave anteriorly but basically flat at the point of entry from the sacral hiatus (see Fig. 8.1). The angle of the canal to the skin surface varies with sex and race. In whites, the canal is angled approximately 35 degrees to the skin surface, whereas in blacks, the angle may be 45 degrees. In women of each race, the angle is slightly less steep than in their male counterparts. The degree of fusion of the bones is variable; the canal may be absent in 5% to 10% of the population (1).

Within the canal, the dural sac normally can be expected to terminate above the level of the second sacral vertebra. It may extend into the sacral portion of the canal and be as close as 3.5 cm from the hiatus. Areolar tissue, nerve roots, and a generous venous plexus are the other occupants of the space.

Indications

Local anesthetics injected into the sacral canal produce dense sacral root anesthesia. This is an ideal technique for perineal and perianal surgery, such as hemorrhoidectomy or rectal tumor fulguration. With adequate lumbar levels of block, foot or leg procedures are possible. If larger volumes are used, anesthesia to the lower thoracic dermatomes can be obtained, and transurethral prostatectomy or vaginal hysterectomy is possible. The advantages of a continuous technique can be obtained by inserting a catheter in the canal.

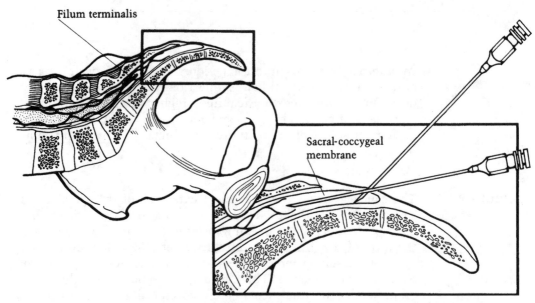

Filum terminalis

Sacral-coccygeal
membrane

Figure 8.1 **Sacral Anatomy, Lateral View**
A needle directed through the sacral–coccygeal membrane at a 45-degree
angle will usually "pop" through the ligament and contact the anterior
bone of the sacral canal. The needle needs to be rotated so that the bevel
does not scrape the periosteum of this layer, and the angle of
advancement changed to allow passage directly 2 to 3 cm up the canal
without contacting bone again. This space is generously endowed with
blood vessels, and the terminal point of the dural sac extends a variable
distance into the sacral canal, but usually lies at the S-2 level.

Caudal anesthesia offers an advantage over lumbar epidural anesthesia in that anesthesia for lower-extremity surgery is limited to
lumbar and sacral roots. When compared to spinal anesthesia, caudal anesthesia offers less chance of postdural puncture headache
than spinal anesthesia, but this complication is still possible. With
the lower incidence of headache with rounded-bevel spinal needles,
this advantage is less significant. These potential comparative advantages must be weighed against the slower onset, higher drug
dose, and anatomic difficulties of caudals.

The major application of the caudal approach is in pediatric anesthesia, where the anatomy is more superficial and reliable, and excellent postoperative analgesia can be offered. Obstetric practice has
seen a decline in the use of continuous caudals, related to the high
volume of anesthetic solution required and the greater interference
with the "pushing" reflex. Caudal anesthesia is available for the
rare patient who cannot be offered the advantages of lumbar
epidural anesthesia, such as the mother with a previous Harrington
rod spinal fusion.

Drugs   The drugs used for caudal anesthesia are the same as those used for lumbar epidural anesthesia. The same considerations apply when choosing desired density (motor versus sensory) and duration of anesthesia.

Because of leakage through the lateral sacral foramina and the greater space in the canal, the volume of solution required is greater for caudal than for epidural anesthesia. A dose of 15 mL of solution may produce only sacral (perineal) anesthesia, whereas 25 mL is required to obtain a T10-12 level of block. This is an average of 2 to 3 mL per segment, in contrast to the requirement for half this amount with lumbar injections. Age and weight are not predictable determinants of extent of anesthesia, as they are in adult lumbar epidural anesthesia. The dose requirement does appear to be slightly reduced in pregnancy—16 to 18 mL will give a T-10 level of block.

The same additives can be used as in epidural injection. Epinephrine prolongs duration. Clonidine and opioids will enhance degree and duration of analgesia (2,3).

Technique   Caudal anesthesia may be performed with the patient in the prone, lateral, or knee–chest position. The latter is preferred in obstetrics, where the uterus makes lying prone unsuitable. For that position, the patient is instructed to turn prone but with the knees brought up into a kneeling position. It is the least "glamorous" position, but it is also the most effective in causing the gluteal muscles to "fall away" from the sacral hiatus.

In the lateral position, the upper leg is flexed at the hip and knee, again to help spread the gluteal muscles away from the hiatus. In the prone patient, a pillow is placed under the hips to flex the hip joint and spread the muscles, and the patient is also asked to spread the legs and internally rotate the feet.

1. Once the patient is in the appropriate position, the landmarks are identified. The sacral cornu may be easily palpated on the thin patient, lying just above the intergluteal crease. The sacral coccygeal membrane forms a soft valley between and just below these peaks. The position is confirmed by drawing the triangle formed by the hiatus and the posterior superior iliac spines; it should be equilateral. The membrane also should be 4 to 5 cm above the palpable tip of the coccyx. The sacral foramina also may be drawn (Fig. 8.2).

2. Before skin preparation in the prone position, a small sponge is placed in the gluteal skin crease to prevent solution dripping into the perineal area. Following aseptic preparation and draping, a small skin wheal is raised with a small-gauge needle over the membrane. Generous infiltration will obscure the landmarks.

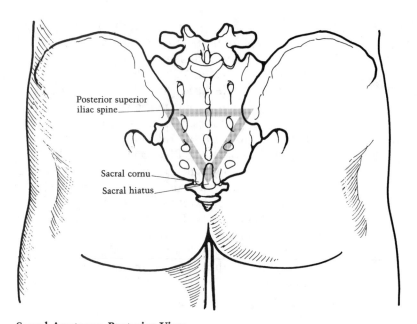

Figure 8.2   **Sacral Anatomy, Posterior View**
The sacral hiatus is covered by a thick ligament that lies between and slightly inferior to the two prominent sacral cornua. A triangle drawn between the posterior superior iliac spines and this foramen is usually equilateral in shape.

3. Deeper infiltration is done with a 22-gauge needle, again avoiding excessive distortion of the tissues. If a catheter is not used, the entire single-injection block can be performed with the 22-gauge needle, keeping in mind that the loss of resistance in the peridural space will be harder to appreciate with the smaller needle than with the traditional 17- to 19-gauge needle. Even when a large needle is used, the preliminary approach with the 22-gauge needle helps identify the membrane and canal so that the larger needle can be placed in a single attempt.

4. The needle is introduced through the anesthetized tissue to the membrane at about a 70-degree angle to the skin (perpendicular to the membrane [Fig. 8.1]). Firm pressure will allow the needle to penetrate the fibrous band and "drop" into the caudal canal. The canal here is shallow, however, and vigorous advancement will produce a painful laceration of the periosteum of the anterior wall of the canal. If multiple attempts do not produce a penetration of the membrane within a few minutes, the landmarks are reassessed. Six percent to 10% of patients will have a fusion of the structures that prevents entry (1), and alternative techniques may have to be considered.

5. Once in the canal, the hub of the needle is dropped downward toward the gluteal crease so the tip now advances no more than 4 cm up the center of the canal, almost parallel to the axis of the back itself. The bevel should be rotated to face downward to reduce the chance of the sharp point lacerating the tender periosteum as it advances. The angle of the canal can normally be expected to be almost flat in relation to the skin in females, but somewhat steeper in males or African-Americans (the hub will drop less from the perpendicular). If the angle is 50 degrees or greater, intraosseous or transsacral placement should be suspected. The path of advancement should be directly up the caudal canal following the midline course of the spine; if lateral deviation occurs, the needle is withdrawn and the landmarks are reassessed.

6. With 2 to 4 cm of needle within the canal, a small syringe with 1.5 mL of air is attached to the hub, and gentle aspiration is performed. If no blood or cerebrospinal fluid (CSF) is obtained, the air is injected forcefully to gauge the resistance. There should be no resistance to injection other than the caliber of the needle itself, just as in the epidural space. Sharp pain on injection indicates subperiosteal placement and requires reinsertion.

7. If no pain or resistance is felt, an additional 5 mL of air is injected forcefully while the fingers rest lightly on the area of skin over the tip of the needle. If crepitance is felt, the needle is probably in the subcutaneous tissue and needs to be reinserted. Air may emerge laterally through the sacral foramina (Fig. 8.2); this is acceptable. The patient may confirm proper needle placement by describing cramping discomfort in the posterior thighs with injection.

8. An alternative confirmation of proper entry is the use of the nerve stimulator, which will produce perirectal contractions if the needle is in the caudal canal (4).

9. If a catheter is used, it is inserted after these confirmatory tests. A longer length of insertion (12 to 13 cm) into the canal may be required here than in the lumbar area, especially if lower abdominal (thoracic root) anesthesia is desired.

10. A test dose of 3 mL of local anesthetic with 1:200,000 epinephrine is injected through the catheter or needle (single-injection technique), and the heart rate or blood pressure is monitored appropriately.

11. If no intravascular or subarachnoid injection is demonstrated, the anesthetic dose may be injected and the catheter secured. Twenty minutes are usually required before adequate surgical anesthesia is obtained.

12. As with all continuous techniques, the test dose is repeated before each injection.

Complications

Intravascular Injection

Intravascular injection is the most common serious problem, and is more likely here than with epidural anesthesia (5). The canal is highly vascular, but the veins have a low pressure that frustrates detection of vascular entry by aspiration of blood. Careful test doses are mandatory, along with frequent monitoring of the patient's mental status. Incremental injection is appropriate.

Periosteal Damage

Periosteal damage is infrequent but may be a painful disability for the patient for several weeks. Vigorous treatment with heat and antiinflammatory drugs, along with concerned support, is needed.

Dural Puncture

Dural puncture is rare and carries the same risks of total spinal anesthesia and postspinal headache as epidural anesthesia.

Intraosseous Injection

Intraosseous injection is rare, but it can produce systemic toxicity similar to that of intravenous injection. Aspiration of the thick marrow is usually not possible, and absorption is slow enough that a test dose may not clearly reveal improper needle placement. Systemic symptoms may not occur for several minutes following injection of a therapeutic dose.

Presacral Injection

Presacral injection is also rare, but rectal injection and injection into the fetal scalp have occurred. Careful attention to landmarks and angles will reduce this possibility, and the needle need not be advanced its entire length into the tissues. Some authors suggest that obstetric caudal anesthesia is contraindicated once the fetal head has descended into the pelvis (and lies just anterior to the sacrum).

Hypertension

Hypertension also has been described on rapid injection. This may be due to a response to compression of the cord or spinal nerves. It is usually transient and can be avoided with slow injection.

References

1. Crighton, I. M., Barry, B. P., Hobbs, G. J. A study of the anatomy of the caudal space using magnetic resonance imaging. *Br. J. Anaesth.* 78: 391, 1997.

2. Constant, I., Gall, O., Gouyet, L., Chauvin, M., Murat, I. Addition of clonidine or fentanyl to local anaesthetics prolongs the duration of surgical analgesia after single shot caudal block in children. *Br. J. Anaesth.* 80: 294, 1998.
3. Van Elstraete, A. C., Pastureau, F., Lebrun, T., Mehdaoui, H. Caudal clonidine for postoperative analgesia in adults. *Br. J. Anaesth.* 84: 401, 2000.
4. Tsui, B. C., Tarkkila, P., Gupta, S., Kearney, R. Confirmation of caudal needle placement using nerve stimulation. *Anesthesiology* 91: 374, 1999.
5. Brown, D. L., Ransom, D. M., Hall, J. A., Leicht, C. H., Schroeder, D. R., Offord, K. P. Regional anesthesia and local anesthetic-induced systemic toxicity: Seizure frequency and accompanying cardiovascular changes. *Anesth. Analg.* 81: 321, 1995.

9 Intercostal Anesthesia

Intercostal nerve block provides an alternative to spinal or epidural anesthesia for abdominal and chest-wall procedures. This technique provides intraoperative and postoperative analgesia for up to 12 hours without the price of the sympathectomy associated with the axial blocks, and is a useful alternative if neuraxial blockade is contraindicated. It is more tedious, because multiple injections must be made and one missed nerve can reduce the analgesia provided.

Anatomy

The peripheral somatic nerves of the thorax depart the spinal column and immediately form a small dorsal and a major ventral branch. These ventral somatic branches travel laterally under their respective ribs. The interior lower edge of each rib provides a channel for the nerve and its companion artery and vein, leaving an overhanging external edge that protects these fellow travelers from direct external assault. This intercostal groove is further enclosed by the fascia of the internal and external intercostal muscles. Beneath the internal intercostal muscle lies the parietal pleura. Near the midaxillary line the groove becomes less well defined, and the nerve migrates away from the rib and gives off a lateral cutaneous branch as it moves anteriorly. Because of these two factors, reliable anesthesia is more difficult beyond the anterior axillary line. The main trunk continues anteriorly to provide sensory and motor innervation to the muscles and skin of the anterior chest (T2-6) and abdomen (T7-11).

The 12th intercostal nerve is unique in that it is not closely associated with its rib. Branches from the 12th nerve depart early to join the ilioinguinal nerve, and the standard subcostal injection is less likely to produce anesthesia of this nerve. The first and second intercostal nerves also differ in that their primary branches join with the lower nerves of the brachial plexus or extend onto the arm itself as the intercostobrachial nerve to provide sensation to the medial aspect of the upper arm.

The ribs themselves vary. In the posterior midline, all of them are well protected medially by the thick paravertebral muscle. The lower six are easily palpated lateral to this muscle and are broad, flat, and relatively superficial. The upper ribs are more protected by the scapula and its associated muscles, appear narrower and deeper, and are technically more difficult to reach, making the paravertebral approach more practical in this region.

Indications

Bilateral blockade of the 6th through 12th intercostal nerves provides sensory anesthesia of the abdominal wall in these respective dermatomes, i.e., from the xiphoid to the pubis. The abdominal muscles

127

in this distribution are also relaxed. There is no anesthesia of the visceral peritoneum. Anesthesia of these nerves will thus produce sufficient analgesia and relaxation for an anterior abdominal incision. Bilateral blockade is needed for any midline incision because there is some lateral overlap of innervation such that sensory dermatomes for each side cross over the midline. Supplemental anesthesia of the celiac plexus or general anesthesia is necessary for intraabdominal procedures. This combined technique is ideally suited for upper abdominal surgery, such as cholecystectomy, splenectomy, or gastrectomy. Even with visceral anesthesia, endotracheal intubation, controlled ventilation, and light supplemental general anesthesia are usually required in all but the more debilitated patients. For midabdominal surgery (abdominal aortic aneurysm repair, colectomy, etc.), this technique can be further supplemented with paravertebral block of the first and second lumbar nerve roots.

Unilateral blockade of the intercostal nerves is also useful in reducing the anesthetic requirement during thoracotomy. It will reduce postoperative analgesia requirements, although not as successfully as for abdominal surgery. A paravertebral approach may be needed for the upper ribs (see Chapter 10). Intercostals are rarely useful as the sole anesthetic for superficial operations of the chest wall. They are applicable, however, for insertion of chest tubes or for providing analgesia for percutaneous biliary drainage. Unilateral blockade of three or more ribs is useful in relieving the pain of fractured ribs. The segments above and below the injury also must be blocked because of sensory dermatome overlap.

This technique is also useful for acute postthoracotomy pain or for subcostal incisional pain, as well as midline abdominal pain. Intercostal block in this setting has been shown to improve ventilatory function and reduce narcotic requirements in healthy patients. The relief is not as effective as with epidural infusions, and the intercostal blocks need to be repeated frequently to preserve the gains.

Drugs

Prolonged duration is usually a primary goal of this technique, and the longer-acting amino-amides are ideal. Bupivacaine or levobupivacaine 0.5% with 1:200,000 epinephrine in a dose of 3 to 5 mL per rib will give 9 to 14 hours of analgesia as well as adequate intraoperative muscle relaxation for a shorter time. Ropivacaine is equally effective, but the duration is shorter by a third [1]. The lower concentration of 0.25% is more appropriate for postoperative analgesia when motor relaxation is not needed. The total dose is thus reduced. This is an important consideration, because the highly vascular area of injection produces the highest blood levels of any of the peripheral nerve injections.

Technique

Posterior Approach
This classical approach can be performed with the patient in the traditional prone position (Fig. 9.1) or in the sitting or lateral positions

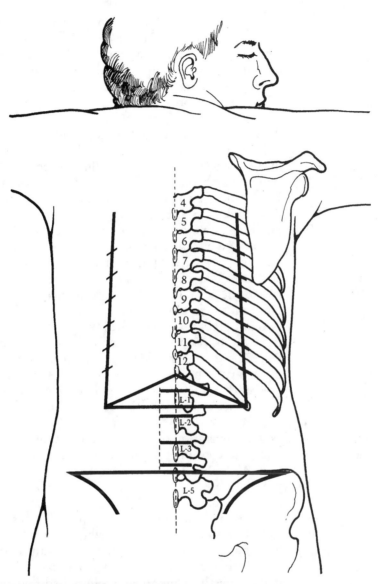

Figure 9.1 **Landmarks for Intercostal Block**
The inferior borders of the ribs are identified at their most prominent
point on the back. The marks usually lie along a line that angles slightly
medially from the 12th to the 6th rib. The marks for the 12th rib usually
lie approximately 7 cm from the midline. For a celiac plexus block (see
Chapter 11), a triangle is drawn between the 12th rib marks and the
inferior border of the 12th spinous process, with the base formed by
joining the two rib marks with a straight line. For lumbar somatic (see
Chapter 10) or lumbar sympathetic blocks (see Chapter 11), the transverse
processes of the lumbar vertebrae are identified by drawing a line across
the superior border of the lumbar spinous processes; the transverse
process for each vertebra usually lies along this line in the lumbar area.

for patients with abdominal pain or tenderness. The lateral position allows the greatest lateral displacement of the scapula, but it allows only one side to be blocked at a time. The major risk of the prone position is respiratory depression or airway obstruction from the sedation that is normally required for the patient to tolerate 14 injections. Close monitoring is needed.

1. The patient is positioned prone with the arms hanging over the sides of the stretcher or bed so that the scapulae fall laterally away from the midline. A pillow placed under the abdomen helps to arch the back and facilitate palpation of the ribs. The head is turned to one side, and an adequate airway is ensured.
2. The landmarks are drawn. The spinous processes are marked, and then a mark is drawn on the lower border of the 12th rib at a point 7 cm from the midline (Fig. 9.1). This usually marks the point of the sharpest posterior angulation of the rib. The sixth or seventh rib is then marked where it can be most easily felt between the scapula and the paraspinous muscles, usually 4 to 5 cm from the midline. A line is drawn on each side joining these two initial rib markings. The lower borders of the rest of the ribs from the 6th to the 11th are marked along these lines on each side. These lines should fall along the prominent posterior angle of each rib. The distance between the 11th and 12th rib will be greater than that between the other ribs. If a celiac plexus block is to be performed also, skin markings are made at this time (see Chapter 11).
3. While preparation of the back and equipment is proceeding, an assistant continues monitoring and begins intravenous sedation. A combination of analgesic and amnestic drugs is most appropriate.
4. After skin preparation and draping, a skin wheal is made at each mark with a small needle. The patient's reaction to these 14 injections will usually indicate whether sedation is adequate.
5. Starting at the lowest rib, the intercostal nerves are blocked. The 12th nerve may be skipped because its variable course makes anesthesia unreliable. The anesthesiologist stands at the patient's side with the syringe in his or her caudad hand (right hand if he or she is on the patient's left). The index finger of the cephalad hand is placed on the skin just above the lowest skin mark and should lie on the body of the rib. The skin wheal is retracted cephalad so that it lies over the midpoint of the rib. The 22-gauge needle is inserted through the wheal to rest on the rib (Fig. 9.2). The periosteum is contacted gently, both to avoid patient discomfort and to avoid barbing the point of the needle.
6. With the needle resting safely on the rib, the cephalad hand now assumes control of the needle and syringe. The hub of the needle is grasped between the thumb and forefinger while the middle finger rests along the needle shaft (Fig. 9.3). The ulnar border

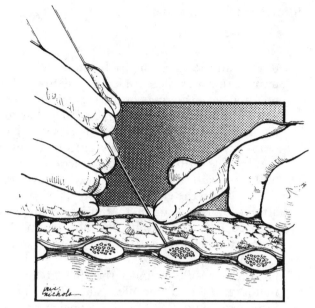

Figure 9.2

Hand and Needle Position for Intercostal Block; Needle on Rib
The index finger of the cephalad hand identifies the lower margin of the
rib and the needle is gently inserted onto the bone. The cephalad hand
then is used to grasp the hub of the needle and control the movement of
the syringe.

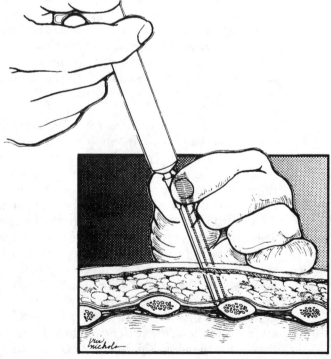

Figure 9.3

Hand and Needle Position for Intercostal Block; Needle Under Rib
The depth of the needle is controlled by the hand resting on the back. The
other hand injects solution when the needle is under the rib, but that is
the only function performed while the needle is near the pleura.

of the palm rests on the back and steadies the hand to prevent unintentional changes in depth. The fingers of the caudad hand now move to the rings of the syringe and prepare for injection. While maintaining a 20-degree cephalad angulation of the needle and syringe, the needle tip is raised slightly off the periosteum and "walked" inferiorly until it passes under the inferior border of the rib. The natural traction of the skin (previously pulled upward to move the skin wheal over the rib) helps move the needle to the correct position. The syringe and needle must always remain parallel to their original cephalad angulation with each "step" toward the rib margin. The most frequent cause of inadequate analgesia is allowing the syringe to pivot to a caudad angle.

7. Once the needle is under the rib, the cephalad angulation is maintained and the needle is advanced 2 to 3 mm to lie in the intercostal groove. While the cephalad hand continues to control the syringe, 3 to 4 mL of anesthetic solution is injected. Intravascular injection should be prevented by careful aspiration. A deliberate infinitesimal "jiggling" of the needle tip may help prevent intravenous injection. If the needle lies within a vessel, the jiggling makes the intravascular presence temporary. Paresthesias are not necessary unless a neurolytic block is sought.

During the injection, the upper hand rests on the chest wall, providing firm control of the syringe. The fingers of the caudad hand are used only to inject, not to advance the syringe or needle.

8. After injection, the needle and syringe are immediately moved back to the safe dorsal surface of the rib. The fingers of the caudad hand are removed from the rings of the syringe, and the barrel is cradled between the thumb and forefinger to allow control of the syringe. Now the upper hand relinquishes control to the caudad hand and is again employed to seek the next rib while the needle remains "parked" on the rib just blocked.

9. By alternating control of the syringe between the hands, the syringe and needle are moved from one rib to the next. If the syringe is to be refilled, it is detached from the needle, and the needle is left in the skin as a marker of the last nerve injected.

10. The ribs of the opposite side may be injected by reaching across the midline or by moving to the opposite side of the stretcher. If the anesthesiologist moves to the opposite side, the syringe is best held in the caudad hand again. This is now an opposite arrangement, and appears awkward to the beginner when the nondominant hand is caudad. If a right-handed anesthesiologist attempts to block the patient's right side with the syringe in his or her right hand, it is difficult to maintain the necessary cephalad angle. The needle often pivots and points caudad when "walked off" the rib, and the local anesthetic solution is injected away from rather than toward the nerve.

11. If a celiac plexus or lumbar somatic block is to be added, it is performed at this point.
12. After completion of the block, the stretcher can be taken to the operating room and the patient simply rolled over onto the operating table, where the block can be tested and further anesthesia and surgery can begin.

Midaxillary Approach

When the patient's abdomen is distended or pain prevents the prone or lateral approach, the intercostal nerves can be reached in the mid- or posterior axillary line while the patient lies supine. This is also a good approach for postoperative pain relief at the conclusion of surgery if intercostal blocks were not performed at the beginning of the procedure. It is more awkward, but it is not difficult technically.

1. With the patient in the supine position, both of the patient's arms are extended laterally on arm rests. The ribs are palpated and marked as far posteriorly as practical, usually in the posterior axillary line.
2. Skin preparation and draping are done on both sides, and skin wheals are raised if the patient is alert. (This can be performed at the start or end of a general anesthetic with no need for local anesthesia.)
3. The anesthesiologist may stand either at the head of the bed or at the side. The technique of injection is the same as that in the prone position, with the syringe held in the caudad hand and control alternating between the upper and lower hands as the needle is "walked off" the rib, injection is made, and the syringe is advanced to the next rib.

Continuous Technique

A continuous technique also has been described, using insertion of a standard epidural catheter in the intercostal space by means of a Tuohy needle. This may produce anesthesia of several levels because of medial spread of injected solutions to the peridural or paravertebral levels. This usually provides anesthesia for three or four segments. This technique of intrapleural injection may be useful for postoperative analgesia (see Chapter 10).

Complications

Pneumothorax

Pneumothorax is the most commonly feared complication of the technique, but it is rare in experienced hands. The key to prevention is rigid control of the depth of penetration of the needle by the upper hand resting solidly on the back during the time of injection. In addition, the needle remains safely on top of the rib for every part of the block except the injection itself. The lower hand, which exerts poorer control because of its lack of fixation and longer "lever arm," does nothing except inject while the needle is below the rib. The fingers of this hand are not moved in and out of the rings except when the needle is "parked" on the top of the rib.

With these precautions, the technique is quite safe, and pneumothorax will occur in less than 1% of patients. It should be suspected if the patient experiences coughing or chest pain during injection or if localization of the ribs is difficult and associated with frequent deep, blind probings (an undesirable variant of the technique). If pneumothorax is suspected clinically, a chest x-ray should be ordered and the air leak treated appropriately if confirmed.

Airway Obstruction and Respiratory Depression

Airway obstruction and respiratory depression are the more frequent complications, related to generous sedation in the prone position during performance of the block. Ventilation and resuscitation equipment, including naloxone, should be available. Supplemental nasal oxygen and pulse oximetry are indicated.

Respiratory Inadequacy

Respiratory inadequacy can occur after intercostal block if motor blockade of the intercostal and upper abdominal muscles is produced in a patient whose diaphragm is ineffective and who depends on intercostal muscles for tidal ventilation.

Systemic Toxicity

Systemic toxicity is also possible. Owing to the large volume of solution injected into a highly vascular space, systemic absorption is significant. Even with epinephrine added to 0.5% bupivacaine, blood levels of bupivacaine may reach 2 μg/mL, the highest for any of the peripheral nerve blocks. A lower concentration of either bupivacaine or ropivacaine (0.25%) will reduce the blood levels to approximately 1 μg/mL (1).

Hypotension

Hypotension occurs rarely and may be the result of subarachnoid injection into a dural sleeve if the injection is made too far medially. More commonly, it is produced by epidural or paravertebral spread of local anesthetic to the sympathetic chain. Drugs injected in the intercostal space can easily track medially and spread to several dermatomes above and below the injection.

Reference

1. Kopacz, D. J., Emanuelsson, B. M., Thompson, G. E., Carpenter, R. L., Stephenson, C. A. Pharmacokinetics of ropivacaine and bupivacaine for bilateral intercostal blockade in healthy male volunteers. *Anesthesiology* 81: 1139, 1994.

10 Paravertebral Blocks

In addition to blocking the peripheral nerves of the trunk along the ribs, the anesthesiologist also may approach these nerves near their exit from the intervertebral foramina. This is particularly useful for the lumbar roots, which do not have a convenient rib to mark their peripheral course, and for the upper thoracic nerves, where the ribs are more difficult to reach.

Anatomy

The thoracic and lumbar nerve roots emerge from the spinal canal through their respective intervertebral foramina at the lateral border of the canal. These foramina lie anterior to the level of the transverse processes and are positioned midway between these processes. The spinal nerves thus emerge from the canal just caudad to and 2 cm anterior to their respective transverse processes. In the thoracic area, the transverse processes, vertebral bodies, and overlying pleura form a triangular space between each pair of ribs (1). In this area, a small posterior branch departs each spinal nerve to innervate the muscles and skin along the middle of the back. The majority of the nerve fibers continue as the primary anterior root to their respective dermatomes and myotomes (Fig. 10.1).

The transverse processes cannot be identified directly, but must be located in relation to their respective spinous processes. In the thoracic area, the long spinous processes extend caudally to overlie the transverse process of the vertebra below them. The 11th and 12th vertebrae constitute a transitional zone where the spinous process lies opposite the intervertebral space. In the lumbar region, the straighter spinous processes overlie their own transverse processes. With the exception of the transition zone at T11-12, a transverse process can usually be located 3 to 4 cm lateral to a spinous process and slightly cephalad to it.

Indications

Thoracic paravertebral blocks may be used as an alternative to epidural or intercostal anesthesia (2), but the accuracy of location of the nerve is not as great, with a 10% failure rate reported in several series (3,4). Identification of paresthesias may improve success, but the standard technique relies on large volume and bony anatomy. This reliance creates two problems. First, blind advancement of the needle beyond the transverse process increases the possibility that the needle will unintentionally puncture the closely underlying pleura. Second, the larger volumes required limit the number of levels that can be blocked before the maximal recommended dose of local anesthetic is exceeded. Thus, this technique is limited to situations where segmental anesthesia of only a few dermatomes may

137

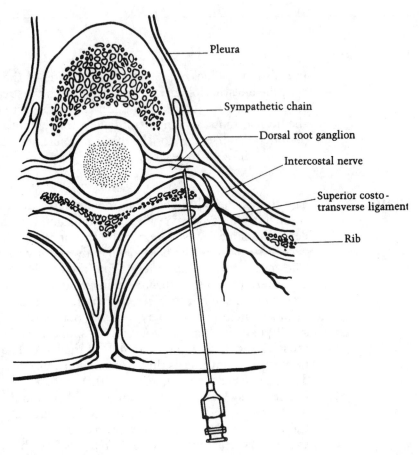

Figure 10.1   **Paravertebral Block**
As it exits the intervertebral foramen, the thoracic somatic nerve enters a small triangular space formed by the vertebral body, the plane of the transverse process, and the pleura. The needle is advanced over the superior border of the transverse process through the ligament into this space. Medial direction of the needle is obviously important in reducing the chance of a pneumothorax. (From Barash, P. G., Cullen, B. F., Stoelting, R. K., Eds. *Clinical Anesthesia*. Philadelphia: Lippincott, 2001, with permission.)

be needed, and especially where more proximal blockade of the intercostal nerve may be desired. Pain relief for acute herpes zoster infections of the thorax is a classic application, as well as attempts to relieve postthoracotomy neuralgia that is believed to be related to injury to the intercostal nerve distally. Relief of pain due to rib fractures is another potential use. Thoracic blockade has been used for breast surgery (5,6), including cancer procedures performed on an outpatient basis (7). For most applications, several roots (at least one above and one below the desired segment) must be blocked because of the extensive overlap of sensory innervation. The use of an indwelling continuous catheter at a single level may overcome this problem by allowing spread of a larger volume of anesthetic to two or three adjacent segments on either side.

Lumbar paravertebral blocks also can be used for pain problems, but additionally can supplement intercostal blocks in providing surgical anesthesia for the lower abdomen and upper leg. This technique does not carry the risk of pneumothorax as does thoracic paravertebral block, but high volumes are again required. Anesthesia for aortobifemoral bypass grafting is a procedure in which this combined technique is useful. Lumbar blockade alone is very effective for inguinal hernia repair, and allows pain-free discharge after ambulatory surgery (3), in contrast to neuraxial blockade alone. This technique can provide postoperative analgesia for 10 hours.

Drugs

As with intercostal blocks, intermediate-duration amino-amides (1% or 1.5% lidocaine, 1% mepivacaine) can be used for 3 to 5 hours of anesthesia, but generally the longer-duration amino-amides are employed. Sensory anesthesia can be obtained with 0.25% bupivacaine or ropivacaine, whereas somewhat longer and denser anesthesia and motor blockade can be obtained with 0.5% concentration. These drugs with 1:200,000 epinephrine may produce 8 to 14 hours of anesthesia.

Because of the less exact relationship of the nerve to the bony landmarks, larger volumes (5 to 10 mL versus 3 to 4 mL for intercostal blocks) are injected for each nerve. Attention needs to be focused on the total milligram dose to avoid systemic toxicity. If several nerves are blocked, a more dilute solution may be required to keep the total dose within acceptable limits.

Neurolytic agents may be employed (see Chapter 23). Smaller volumes are used, and a paresthesia or x-ray confirmation should be used to ensure identification of the nerve.

Techniques

Lumbar Technique

1. The patient is turned prone, and a pillow is placed under the abdomen to exaggerate the spinal curve. The spinous processes are identified. The seventh cervical process is identified by its prominence in the upper spine, whereas the fourth lumbar process lies on or slightly above the intercristal line.
2. The spinous processes associated with the nerves to be blocked are marked over their entire length. In the lumbar region, the superior border of the processes will correspond to the transverse process and nerve to be blocked, whereas in the thoracic region, the spinous process will be associated with the next lower transverse process and nerve.

3. Transverse lines are drawn across the top of the spinous processes desired, and then these lines are connected by vertical lines running parallel to the spinal column and 3 to 4 cm lateral to the midline (see Fig. 9.1).
4. Following aseptic skin preparation, a skin wheal is raised at each intersection of the horizontal and vertical lines.
5. A 3- or 4-in. 22-gauge needle is introduced through the wheal and directed 10 to 30 degrees cephalad. The greater angle will be re-

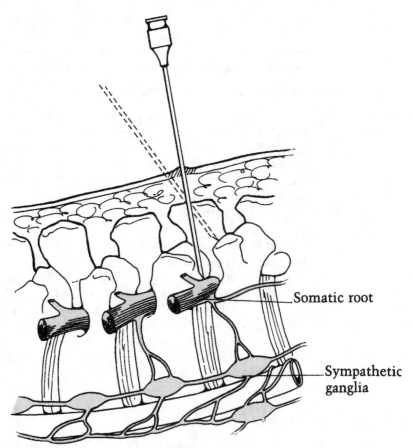

Somatic root

Sympathetic ganglia

Figure 10.2   **Lumbar Paravertebral Block, Lateral View**
The needle is introduced through the skin wheal at the lower border of the transverse process and angled 30 to 45 degrees cephalad to contact the bone at 3.5 to 5 cm depth. Once the process is identified, the angle of insertion is reduced to allow the needle to pass below the bone. The somatic nerve will be found approximately 2 cm below the transverse process. Paresthesias are not necessary, and injection of 10 mL of anesthetic will produce somatic nerve anesthesia. The needle can be advanced an additional 3 to 4 cm and angled slightly medially to contact the body of the vertebra if sympathetic blockade is desired (see Fig. 11.4); the sympathetic chain lies along the anterior margin of these bodies.

quired in the lumbar region. The needle should come in contact with the transverse process at 2.5 to 5 cm depending on the girth of the patient. If the bone is not contacted at the expected depth, gentle exploration is performed caudad and cephalad. Once the bone is found, the depth of the transverse process is noted.

6. The needle is withdrawn to the skin, redirected caudally (more perpendicular to the skin) and slightly medially, and reinserted to pass 2 cm beyond the lower edge of the transverse process (Fig. 10.2). The body of the vertebra may be contacted, and this serves as a useful landmark. No paresthesias are sought unless a neurolytic agent is used.

7. With the needle fixed in position 2 cm below the inferior border of the transverse process, 5 to 10 mL of solution is injected after careful aspiration.

8. When paravertebral anesthesia of T-12 and L-1 is desired to supplement intercostal nerve blocks, a single-needle insertion on each side is possible. The spinous process of L-1 is identified, and an "X" is marked 3 cm lateral to its superior border on each side. A 3-in. needle is inserted perpendicularly through each "X" and the transverse process is identified. The needle is then "walked off" the process cephalad, and 5 to 10 mL of anesthetic is injected in the area of the T-12 root. Next, the needle is "walked off" the caudad edge, and the injection is repeated for the L-1 root.

Thoracic Paravertebral Technique

Although the lumbar technique described can be used in the thoracic region, there is need for greater accuracy. The nerve tends to lie more superiorly under its transverse process. A modified approach can bring better identification of the paravertebral triangle (1).

1. The thoracic approach can be performed with the patient in the sitting or lateral position as well as prone.

2. The surface landmarks and skin wheal at the thoracic levels are the same as for the lumbar approach (Fig. 10.3), entering the skin 3 cm lateral to the superior margin of the spinous process of the level above the nerve to be blocked.

3. A 4-in. 22-gauge needle (or a Tuohy needle if a catheter is to be inserted) is introduced perpendicular to the skin and advanced onto the rib or transverse process, at a depth of approximately 2.5 to 3.5 cm.

4. After the bone is contacted, the needle is redirected cephalad to "walk over" the upper margin of the process. An air-filled syringe is attached and pressure maintained as the needle is advanced. A loss of resistance (as with epidural injection) marks the entry through the ligament into the paravertebral space.

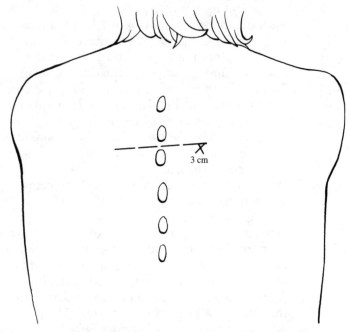

Figure 10.3.   **Surface Landmarks for Thoracic Paravertebral Injection**
The needle insertion point is 3 cm lateral to the upper edge of the spinous process, which overlies the segment to be blocked.

5. Careful aspiration is performed to exclude subarachnoid, intravascular, or intrapleural placement. Five mL of anesthetic solution is then injected for each segment to be blocked, or a bolus of 15 mL if a catheter is inserted.
6. A catheter will provide anesthesia for several segments above and below the site of injection. The catheter should not be advanced more than 2 cm beyond the needle tip.

Intrapleural Catheter

A modification of paravertebral–intercostal blockade is the use of intrapleural catheters to provide injection of local anesthetic solutions into the pleural space. The intrapleural anesthetic solution blocks several levels of thoracic nerves, either by diffusion across the parietal pleural into the intercostal space or into the paravertebral space. This block is successful with unilateral injections for cholecystectomy and nephrectomy surgery (8), but it is less effective for thoracotomy because of the loss of anesthetic solution through the chest drainage tubes. The large volumes required make bilateral blockade impractical. Although higher concentrations of local anesthetic will prolong duration, the resultant blood levels increase risk. The technique is comparable in pain relief to intercostal blocks, but the risks (especially of pneumothorax and high blood levels of local anesthetic) are significant (8,9), especially compared to the alternative of epidural opioids.

1. Catheter insertion can be performed with the patient in the lateral, sitting, or prone position.
2. An appropriate intercostal interspace is identified (usually the eighth for abdominal anesthesia) and marked 8 to 10 cm lateral to the midline along the upper margin of the rib below the space.
3. After aseptic preparation, a skin wheal is raised and local anesthesia infiltrated down to the level of the rib.
4. A Tuohy needle is introduced onto the superior margin of the rib and then angled 30 to 40 degrees superiorly and "walked off" the rib. A small, well-lubricated, air-filled syringe is attached, and entry to the pleural space is identified by the negative pressure, which aspirates the contents of the syringe.
5. A catheter is advanced 5 to 6 cm into the space, and 20 mL of anesthetic solution (0.25% to 0.5% bupivacaine) is injected. This will provide 6 to 8 hours of analgesia on the injected side.

Complications

Pneumothorax

Pneumothorax is the most serious complication of the thoracic approach, reported in approximately 0.5% to 1% of cases (2,6), and it should be handled appropriately if encountered. The pleura is quite close to the transverse process anteriorly, and the needle should not be advanced more than 2 cm beyond the posterior border of the process. Attempts at thoracic paravertebral sympathetic block require deeper insertion and involve greater potential risk. Pneumothorax is also a 2% risk with intrapleural catheter insertion (9).

Subarachnoid Injection

Subarachnoid injection is more likely with thoracic paravertebral blocks than with intercostal blocks because a dural sleeve is more likely to extend beyond the intravertebral foramen at this level. Total spinal anesthesia may result from thoracic injections and should be managed as previously discussed (see Chapter 6).

Systemic Toxicity

Systemic toxicity is possible because of the volumes of solution used and the proximity of blood vessels. Careful aspiration, incremental injection, and constant monitoring of the mental status are essential not only during injection but for a 30-minute period thereafter. When lumbar paravertebral injections are combined with intercostals, the concentration and total volume may both need adjustment to avoid toxic levels. Intrapleural injection with 0.5% bupivacaine produces significant systemic blood levels (8).

Spread of Solution

Spread of solution also may occur and is likely to cause a dermatomal sympathetic block if the rami communicantes are affected. An epidural band of anesthesia also may be obtained by diffusion of the local anesthetic into the intervertebral foramina, but neither of these events constitutes a problem unless a neurolytic agent is used.

References

1. Eason, M. J., Wyatt, R. Paravertebral thoracic block—a reappraisal. *Anaesthesia* 34: 638, 1979.
2. Karmakar, M. K. Thoracic paravertebral block. *Anesthesiology* 95: 771, 2001.
3. Klein, S. M., Greengrass, R. A., Weltz, C., Warner, D. S. Paravertebral somatic nerve block for outpatient inguinal herniorrhaphy: An expanded case report of 22 patients. *Reg. Anesth. Pain Med.* 23: 306, 1998.
4. Lonnqvist, P. A., MacKenzie, J., Soni, A. K., Conacher, I. D. Paravertebral blockade. Failure rate and complications. *Anaesthesia* 50: 813, 1995.
5. Klein, S. M., Bergh, A., Steele, S. M., Georgiade, G. S., Greengrass, R. A. Thoracic paravertebral block for breast surgery. *Anesth. Analg.* 90: 1402, 2000.
6. Pusch, F., Freitag, H., Weinstabl, C., Obwegeser, R., Huber, E., Wildling, E. Single-injection paravertebral block compared to general anaesthesia in breast surgery. *Acta Anaesthesiol. Scand.* 43: 770, 1999.
7. Greengrass, R., O'Brien, F., Lyerly, K., Hardman, D., Gleason, D., D'Ercole, F., Steele, S. Paravertebral block for breast cancer surgery. *Can. J. Anaesth.* 43: 858, 1996.
8. Scott, N. B., Mogensen, T., Bigler, D., Kehlet, H. Comparison of the effects of continuous intrapleural vs epidural administration of 0.5% bupivacaine on pain, metabolic response and pulmonary function following cholecystectomy. *Acta Anaesthesiol. Scand.* 33: 535, 1989.
9. Stromskag, K. E., Minor, B., Steen, P. A. Side effects and complications related to interpleural analgesia: An update. *Acta Anaesthesiol. Scand.* 34: 473, 1990.

11 Sympathetic Blocks

The peripheral sympathetic division of the autonomic nervous system is formed by the branches from the thoracic and upper lumbar spinal segments. The roots include efferent fibers that regulate vasoconstriction and afferent fibers responsible for intraabdominal and intrathoracic "visceral" sensation. Separate selective anesthesia of these paths may be particularly useful in some acute and chronic pain situations, and may provide useful supplemental surgical analgesia when combined with other regional or general techniques. Fortunately, many of the sympathetic fibers are grouped in separate nerves, ganglia, and plexuses and do not follow the regular somatic nerve pathways. Thus, they are susceptible to individual blockade in many situations without motor or sensory anesthesia.

Anatomy

The preganglionic sympathetic efferent nerve cell bodies lie in the sympathetic centers of the brain stem. The axons travel in the spinal cord to one of the thoracic or lumbar segments, where they emerge from the lateral column of gray matter. These peripheral fibers pass through the intervertebral foramina and immediately leave the somatic nerves by means of the white rami communicantes to join the sympathetic ganglia lying anteriorly along each side of the vertebral bodies. Although the preganglionic fibers emerge only from T-1 to L-2, the chains of ganglia form trunks that extend on each side upward into the neck and downward into the pelvis so that each area of the body receives its segmental share of sympathetic innervation. In the neck, the chains of sympathetic ganglia lie along the lateral border of the relatively flat vertebral bodies; in the chest, they lie more posteriorly near the head of each rib (see Fig. 10.1). In the abdomen and pelvis, they lie more anteriorly on the vertebral bodies and are more widely separated from the somatic nerves (see Fig. 10.2). In the ganglia, the preganglionic fibers can synapse with their postganglionic counterparts, travel up or down several segments until they synapse, or pass through the ganglia to a synapse in distal supplemental ganglia such as the celiac plexus or in a target organ such as the adrenal medulla. The postganglionic fibers to the somatic dermatomes leave the sympathetic trunks as the gray rami and travel back dorsally to rejoin the appropriate segmental somatic nerves. The exception is in the head, where these postganglionic fibers travel with the arterial blood vessels.

The ganglia of the head and neck organize themselves into three groups on each side by joining several of the expected segmental ganglia. The superior cervical ganglion lying along the first three cervical vertebrae is the largest of the three. All of the fibers to it and to the middle cervical ganglion must pass through the inferior cervical, or stellate, ganglion. The stellate ganglion is the fusion of the first thoracic segmental ganglion with the lower cervical segments. It lies along the lateral aspect of the seventh vertebra just anterior to its transverse process. This places it behind the carotid sheath and the vertebral artery, just above the pleura, and in close proximity to the recurrent laryngeal nerve.

The thoracic ganglia send extensive branches, in the form of the greater and lesser splanchnic nerves, to a subsidiary intraabdominal ganglion, the celiac plexus. This extensive network of autonomic nerves lies in the retroperitoneal space along the aorta at the origin of the celiac artery, at approximately the level of the L-1 vertebra. The abdominal organs receive their postganglionic innervation from this plexus and from the superior and inferior mesenteric ganglia, which lie caudad to it.

Below the L-2 vertebral body, the sympathetic ganglia continue to lie astride the spinal column. Here the anatomy is most variable, and the number and location of ganglia vary between patients and even from side to side in the same patient. All of the preganglionic fibers enter the chain from the L-1 level or above. As in the head, all sympathetic innervation of the lower body must pass through this one "gateway" ganglion.

The anatomy of the sympathetic system thus allows three specific centers where fibers congregate for easy blockade of their terminal branches—the stellate ganglion in the head, the celiac plexus in the abdomen, and the second lumbar plexus for the lower extremities.

Indications

The celiac plexus block is useful as a supplement to intercostal nerve blockade for abdominal anesthesia (see Chapter 9). It blocks the afferent and efferent sympathetic fibers of the abdominal viscera, which are unaffected by intercostal nerve blocks. It thus reduces the requirement for intraoperative supplementation with other anesthetic agents. The price of this technique is the hypotension that results from sympathetic blockade. More frequently, celiac plexus block (like other sympathetic blocks) is most useful in diagnosing and treating chronic pain due to malignancy (1,2), particularly abdominal pain from the pancreas (see Chapter 23).

Stellate ganglion block can be used as supplemental surgical analgesia to reduce the pain of intrathoracic procedures such as thoracoscopy. Systemic hypotension is not a problem with this more limited block. Stellate ganglion block and lumbar sympathetic block find their primary use in the management of pain problems, especially in the presence of a vascular component. Their application is more fully discussed in Chapter 23.

Drugs

Dilute concentrations of local anesthetics are sufficient to block the small unmyelinated sympathetic fibers. Lidocaine 0.5%, bupivacaine 0.25%, and equivalent doses of any of the other agents are effective. In general, larger volumes are required for ganglion blocks compared to somatic nerve blocks because of the diffuse anatomic location of the ganglia. The shorter-acting agents may be used for diagnostic blocks or in conjunction with surgical anesthesia, where prolonged sympathectomy and hypotension may be undesirable. The longer-acting agents are more appropriate when performing a series of blocks for a sympathetic dystrophy or a diagnostic block for cancer pain.

Alcohol and phenol have been used successfully as neurolytic agents on the sympathetic fibers, with the latter usually reserved for the lumbar ganglia because of concern about tissue damage to nearby blood vessels in the neck and abdomen with phenol. With stellate and lumbar ganglia blocks there is risk of neurolytic damage with either agent because of the close proximity to other nerves.

Techniques

Stellate Ganglion Block

Stellate ganglion block provides blockade of the sympathetic innervation to the head and arm. The prevertebral injection as described classically in the following list may not actually anesthetize the ganglion directly, but it may block the fibers as they emerge from this ganglion. Actual computerized tomography (CT) guidance may be needed for direct injection of the ganglion, as would be desired with neurolytic drugs.

1. The patient is placed in the supine position with the arms at the sides. A small towel or pillow is placed under the neck to provide comfortable extension of the head and neck.
2. The medial border of the sternocleidomastoid muscle on the affected side and the cricoid cartilage are marked. Approximately 2 cm lateral to the lateral edge of the cricoid cartilage, the anterior tubercle of the transverse process of the sixth cervical vertebra (Chassaignac tubercle) is gently palpated and marked. This is the most prominent tubercle in the neck. At the same distance from the midline and 1.5 to 2 cm caudad, an "X" is placed that should overlie the tubercle of the seventh cervical vertebra. This mark should fall at the medial border of the muscle body and approximately two fingerbreadths above the clavicle.
3. After aseptic skin preparation, a skin wheal is made at the "X."
4. A 22- or 25-gauge 1.5-in. needle with a 10-mL syringe attached is introduced at the mark and advanced directly posterior until bone is contacted. The muscle body and carotid sheath are retracted laterally by the index finger of the opposite hand during this maneuver (Fig. 11.1). If the tubercle is not encountered within 5 cm, the needle is redirected slightly medially. If this fails, slight caudad or cephalad angulation may be necessary. A paresthesia of the brachial plexus indicates a posterior and lateral

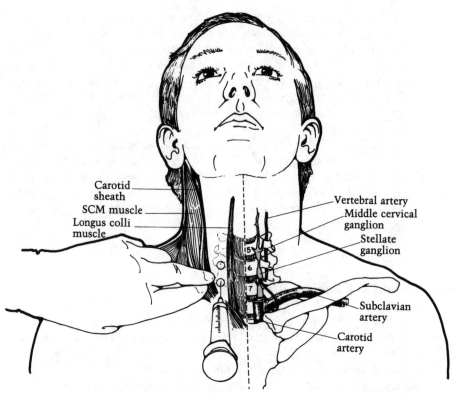

Carotid sheath

SCM muscle

Longus colli muscle

Vertebral artery

Middle cervical ganglion

Stellate ganglion

Subclavian artery

Carotid artery

Figure 11.1   **Stellate Ganglion Block**
The sternocleidomastoid (SCM) muscle and the carotid sheath are retracted laterally with one hand while the needle is introduced directly onto the lateral border of the seventh vertebral body, just medial to the transverse process. After contacting bone, the needle is withdrawn slightly and careful aspiration is performed before incremental injection.

    deviation of the needle. If the tubercle is not easily identified, the landmarks are reassessed.

5. After contacting the bone, the needle is withdrawn 2 mm and gentle aspiration is performed (Fig. 11.2). A 2-mL test dose is injected, and careful observation of mental function is performed. If no change occurs, a total of 5 to 10 mL is injected in increments with frequent aspiration and continued observation of mental status.

6. A Horner syndrome (ptosis, miosis, anhidrosis, and enophthalmos) should result within 10 minutes. Nasal congestion is also a common symptom. Although vasodilatation of the arm is not a part of the classic syndrome, it is usually associated with this block if a Horner syndrome appears.

7. As an alternative, the block can be performed at the level of the sixth cervical vertebral body, because the volume of solution injected is sufficient to spread to the fibers of the ganglion from

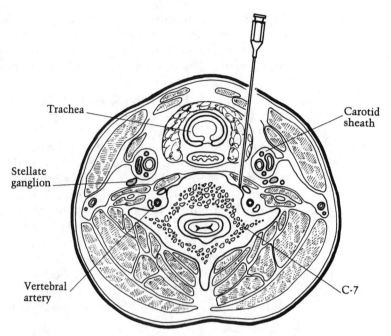

Figure 11.2

Stellate Ganglion Block, Cross Section
The needle is shown resting on the anterior border of the seventh cervical vertebra. The vascular structures of the carotid sheath as well as the vertebral artery are in close proximity. The vertebral artery is passing posteriorly at this level to enter its canal in the transverse processes, but here lies near the level of intended injection. The brachial plexus roots are also just posterior and lateral to the intended site of injection.

this level. Although this site is further from the presumed location of the ganglion, it is also further from the vertebral artery (which has moved behind the transverse process at this level), and may represent less risk of arterial injection. The technique is the same, except for the final target level.

Celiac Plexus Block

Celiac plexus block is usually performed for pancreatic pain. In addition to this classic description, there have been several alternatives proposed, but the success rate appears to be equivalent with various approaches (3).

1. The patient is placed in the prone position with a pillow under the pelvis to flatten the lumbar curve.
2. The 12th thoracic and 1st lumbar spinous processes are identified and numbered, usually by counting up from the 4th lumbar spine, which lies at or just above the line between the iliac crests. The 12th ribs are also identified and marked with an "X"

7 cm from the midline, as for intercostal block (see Fig. 9.1). A line is then drawn between these marks across the spinal column. Finally, a shallow triangle is created by connecting these points to the spinous process of the 12th vertebra (which overlies the 1st lumbar vertebral body).

3. After aseptic skin preparation, skin wheals are raised at each "X" with a small-gauge needle. Local anesthetic infiltration is carried deeper with a 22-gauge needle.

4. On each side, a 5-in. needle (6-in. needle for large patients) is introduced through the "X" and directed medially and cephalad toward the first lumbar vertebral body along the lines of the triangle previously drawn. The needles should advance at an anterior angle of approximately 45 degrees from the skin.

5. When the vertebral body is contacted, the needle is withdrawn 5 cm and the angle is steepened so that further advancement serves to "walk" the needle anteriorly off the body (Fig. 11.3). Once past the anterior border of the body, the tip is advanced a further 2 to 3 cm. The periosteum is tender, and placement may require intravenous analgesia or sedation for the patient.

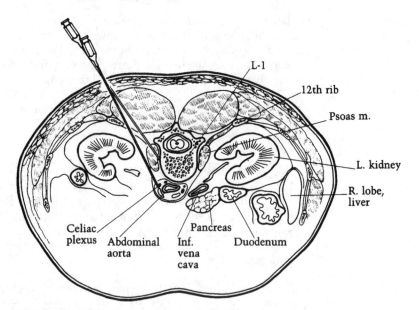

Figure 11.3   **Celiac Plexus Block**
The surface landmarks are described in Fig. 9.1. The needles are introduced into the skin at the lateral borders of the triangle, specifically 7 cm from the midline at the inferior border of the 12th rib. They are each advanced medially and superiorly (following under the angling lines of the triangle on the skin) to contact the lateral aspect of the vertebral body. They are then advanced more anteriorly to pass beyond the vertebra to the prevertebral space where the greater and lesser splanchnic nerves and their subsequent celiac plexus lie. No attempt is made to advance the needles to the anterior aspect of the vessels.

On the left side, advancement is halted as soon as aortic pulsation is perceived. If the vessel is entered, the needle is withdrawn from the vessel wall and the needle shaft is immediately cleared of blood. On the right side, the needle usually can be advanced a centimeter further than on the left. Ideally, each needle will be seen on fluoroscopy or lateral x-ray to lie at the anterior margin of the vertebral body.

6. The bony landmarks are usually sufficient localization for surgical or diagnostic blocks. For pain diagnosis, and especially if a neurolytic agent is to be injected, x-ray confirmation of needle placement should be obtained with fluoroscopy, plain films, or CT. The injection of a small volume of radiologic contrast medium at this point can confirm needle location.

7. Careful aspiration is performed, and a test dose is injected in each side to exclude subarachnoid or intravascular injection.

8. Then 20 to 25 mL local anesthetic solution is injected on each side. This volume is required because of the diffuse extent of the ganglia and the fact that this injection is still behind the aorta and vena cava, and relies on circumferential diffusion of the local anesthetic to reach the plexus and the fibers of the splanchnic nerves. If the procedure is done in conjunction with intercostal blocks, the volume or concentration may have to be reduced to avoid toxic doses of local anesthetic.

9. Blood pressure is monitored closely until the hypotensive effect disappears. If the procedure is done for diagnostic rather than surgical purposes, the patient should remain supine for at least an hour while receiving intravenous fluids, because orthostatic hypotension can be anticipated. Patients should ambulate gradually and with assistance.

Alternate Celiac Approach

Singler has described a paramedian approach in which the needles are inserted below the T-12 spinous process and 3 cm from the midline, and are advanced perpendicular to the skin (4). This technique is less likely to allow the needle to pass through the kidney, but it also makes attaining the correct depth more difficult unless x-ray confirmation is used. The plexus can also be approached anteriorly under fluoroscopic guidance with a thin needle, with apparently little risk (5). For all of the approaches, the degree of distortion of the anatomy by tumor may limit effectiveness of the block (6).

Lumbar Sympathetic Block

As in the head and arm, the sympathetic innervation of the leg can be blocked by a single injection on the "gateway" ganglion that receives the lowermost of the sympathetic fibers from the spinal cord. This is usually the second lumbar ganglion, and cadaver studies suggest that the ideal site for blockade is at the lower third of the second lumbar body or the upper third of the third lumbar body (7). Blockade at several levels also has been advocated because of the variable anatomy. If neurolytic agents are used, smaller injections at multiple levels are probably wiser.

1. The patient is placed in the prone position with a pillow under the pelvis. A skin-temperature probe may be attached to the toe to assess effectiveness of the block by following changes in skin temperature. A 3°C increase after the block confirms correct needle placement.
2. The spinous processes are identified and numbered as for celiac plexus block, as described earlier. A horizontal line is drawn through the midpoint of the second lumbar spinous process, and

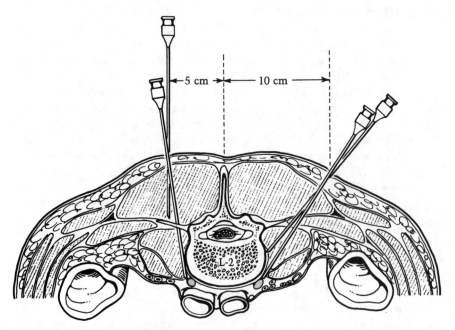

Figure 11.4   **Lumbar Sympathetic Block**

For the classic paravertebral approach, the spinous process of the second lumbar vertebra is marked along its entire extent, and a perpendicular line is drawn across its midpoint. An "X" is placed along this line 5 cm from the midline. This indicates an entry point that is slightly caudad and lateral to the point used for somatic nerve block (see Fig. 10.2), and may reduce the chance of contacting the somatic nerve. The needle is introduced as for somatic nerve block, angling first cephalad to establish the depth of the transverse process, and then being angled more perpendicular and slightly medially to approach the anterior border of the vertebral body itself. The lateral approach (*left*) is similar to celiac plexus blockade in that it starts 10 cm lateral to the midpoint of the second spinous process, and introduces the needle at a 45-degree angle to contact the vertebral body and then "walks off" further anteriorly (see Fig. 11.3).

an "X" is marked along this line 5 cm on each side of the midline (Fig. 11.4). These marks should overlie the spaces between the transverse processes of the second and third vertebrae.

3. After skin preparation, skin wheals are made at each "X." A 4-in. needle is introduced and angled 45 degrees cephalad and is advanced gently until the transverse process is contacted. This depth is noted, and the needle is withdrawn toward the skin.

4. The needle is now reintroduced perpendicular to the skin, this time angling slightly medially but passing directly anterior between the two transverse processes to a depth 5 cm beyond the identified depth of the superior transverse processes (see Fig. 10.2). Contact with the vertebral body is desirable to confirm proximity to the chain. If the vertebral body is contacted, the needle is angled slightly more laterally and "walked off" the body to the desired depth.

5. When the correct position is reached, careful aspiration and a test dose are performed on both sides. If negative, 5 to 10 mL of solution is injected on each side.

6. No solution is injected as the needle is withdrawn, because this may result in anesthesia of the second lumbar somatic nerve, which lies posterior to the sympathetic trunk just below the transverse process.

7. The block should result in vasodilation and increased skin temperature in the leg within 5 to 10 minutes, but it may take as long as 20 minutes to produce results. The presence of sensory anesthesia in the L-2 distribution on the lateral thigh indicates that solution has spread posteriorly to involve the somatic roots. This may confuse the interpretation of diagnostic pain procedures.

Alternative Lumbar Approach

The lumbar ganglia can be reached from the lateral approach, similar to the classic celiac plexus approach. This approach is less likely to directly contact the second lumbar somatic root.

1. A mark is made 10 cm lateral to and directly opposite the second lumbar spinous process. This is usually just over the last rib (Fig. 11.4).

2. A 22-gauge 6-in. needle is inserted and directed toward the body of the vertebra. On contacting bone, the needle is "walked" anteriorly until it passes the anterior edge of the vertebral body.

3. Injection here of 5 to 10 mL of local anesthetic will reach the sympathetic nerves.

Superior Hypogastric Block

The original description of Superior Hypogastric Block was given by Plancarte et al. in 1990 (8) (see Fig. 11.5) and the technique was proven useful for cancer in 1997 (9).Then in 1999, Kanazi et al. de-

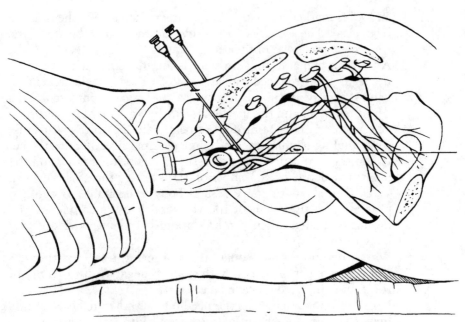

Figure 11.5   **Needle Location with Superior Hypogastric Block**
In the prone position, two 6 or 7 inch needles are inserted on each side, 5–7 cm lateral to the L4-5 interspace, and advanced 30 degrees caudad and anteriorly under fluoroscopic guidance to contact the anterolateral surface of the L5 vertebral body. The needles are advanced a further cm to pierce the anterior fascial boundary of the psoas muscle and lie in the retroperitoneal space anterior to the junction of the L5-S1.

veloped a technique for superior hypogastric plexus block using an anterior approach (10).

Complications

Intravascular Injection

Intravascular injection is the most likely complication of these procedures because of the large volumes of local anesthetic injected in close proximity to vascular structures. The greatest risk is associated with the stellate ganglion block because of the presence of the vertebral artery (Fig. 11.2); only a few milligrams of anesthetic injected here will reach the cerebral cortex immediately and produce symptoms instantly.

Hypotension

Hypotension can occur with celiac plexus block, particularly in the elderly or volume-depleted patient, such as the hypertensive. Sympathetic blocks in these patients should be approached with caution. All patients should receive generous volume loading with 10 to 15 mL per kg crystalloid through a large-bore intravenous catheter. Careful monitoring of blood pressure after the block and gradual assisted ambulation are appropriate, especially with celiac plexus blockade.

Bradycardia

Bradycardia can occur if stellate ganglion block is performed bilaterally because of loss of the cardiac accelerator fibers.

Subarachnoid Injection

Subarachnoid injection also can occur with any of these blocks and is disastrous if neurolytic agents are involved. Careful aspiration and test doses should be used, and x-ray confirmation should be obtained before celiac plexus or lumbar neurolytic injections. Local anesthetic injection in the neck or lumbar region can result in a high spinal that is usually short-lived because of the dilute concentrations used. Respiratory and cardiovascular support may be needed.

Pneumothorax

Pneumothorax can occur with a stellate ganglion block, because the dome of the pleura rises just lateral to the site of injection. Cough or chest pain on insertion of the needle should evoke suspicion and be followed by a chest x-ray. Pneumothorax also has occurred after celiac plexus block. With neurolytic celiac block, pleural effusion and shoulder pain also have been reported because of alcohol irritation of the diaphragm.

Somatic Nerve Block

Somatic nerve block can occur with either stellate or lumbar block if the needle is just slightly posterior to the sympathetic trunk. Although not serious, this is annoying and complicates the interpretation of blocks performed for diagnostic purposes. It also may delay the discharge of outpatients. If neurolytic drugs are used, this can be a more serious problem, and careful localization is essential.

Recurrent Laryngeal Nerve Block

Recurrent laryngeal nerve block can occur with stellate block. This is again more of a nuisance than a complication, but it can be uncomfortable for the patient. It is another reason to avoid bilateral blocks. If the patient does complain of difficulty swallowing or fullness in the throat, he or she should be advised not to eat or drink until the block dissipates.

Phrenic Nerve Paralysis

Phrenic nerve paralysis can occur with stellate block, but it is probably rare with the dilute concentrations of local anesthetic employed.

References

1. Practice guidelines for chronic pain management. A report by the American Society of Anesthesiologists Task Force on Pain Management, Chronic Pain Section. *Anesthesiology* 86: 995, 1997.
2. Boas, R. A. Sympathetic nerve blocks: In search of a role. *Reg. Anesth. Pain Med.* 23: 292, 1998.
3. Mercadante, S., Nicosia, F. Celiac plexus block: A reappraisal. *Reg. Anesth. Pain Med.* 23: 37, 1998.
4. Singler, R. C. An improved technique for alcohol neurolysis of the celiac plexus. *Anesthesiology* 56: 137, 1982.
5. Romanelli, D. F., Beckmann, C. F., Heiss, F. W. Celiac plexus block: Efficacy and safety of the anterior approach. *A.J.R. Am. J. Roentgenol.* 160: 497, 1993.
6. De Cicco, M., Matovic, M., Bortolussi, R., Coran, F., Fantin, D., Fabiani, F., Caserta, M., Santantonio, C., Fracasso, A. Celiac plexus block: Injectate spread and pain relief in patients with regional anatomic distortions. *Anesthesiology* 94: 561, 2001.
7. Umeda, S., Arai, T., Hatano, Y., Mori, K., Hoshino, K. Cadaver anatomic analysis of the best site for chemical lumbar sympathectomy. *Anesth. Analg.* 66: 643, 1987.
8. Plancarte, R., Amescua, C., Patt, R. B., Aldrete, J. A. Superior hypogastric plexus block for pelvic cancer pain. *Anesthesiology* 73: 236, 1990.
9. Plancarte, R., de Leon-Casasola, O. A., El-Helaly, M., Allende, S., Lema, M. J. Neurolytic superior hypogastric plexus block for chronic pelvic pain associated with cancer. *Reg. Anesth.* 22: 562, 1997.
10. Kanazi, G. E., Perkins, F. M., Thakur, R., Dotson, E. New technique for superior hypogastric plexus block. *Reg. Anesth. Pain Med.* 24: 473, 1999.

12 Brachial Plexus Blocks

The brachial plexus is conveniently arranged to allow a regional nerve block. There are several locations to achieve excellent anesthesia of the arm, shoulder, or hand with minimal patient cooperation, and many approaches have been described.

Anatomy

The ventral nerve roots of C-5 through T-1 intertwine to form a closely approximated bundle as they pass readily identifiable bony, muscular, and vascular landmarks in the neck and shoulder. At their origin in the neck, all the roots exit the spinal column in the trough between the anterior and posterior tubercle of the transverse process of the vertebral body, and pass laterally between the bodies of the anterior and middle scalene muscles. They are enclosed in a long, narrow compartment between the posterior fascia of the anterior scalene and the anterior fascia of the middle scalene muscles, facilitating blockade of the multiple nerves of the plexus with a single injection.

As the nerve roots course further distally, the upper and lower two pairs merge, forming, along with the middle C-7 root, the three trunks of the plexus. The trunks pass over the first rib behind the insertion of the anterior scalene. The subclavian artery rises from the thorax and also crosses the first rib immediately behind the anterior scalene insertion, lying just anterior to the trunks. As the trunks divide and recombine to form the divisions, cords, and terminal nerves of the arm, they closely surround the artery before departing on their unique courses.

There are three cords at the level of the coracoid process—the lateral, medial, and posterior—that arise from the two divisions. The posterior cord continues on as the *radial nerve* after giving off the axillary nerve branch. The lateral and medial cords send major branches to form the *median nerve*, and then each continues as the smaller *musculocutaneous* and *ulnar nerves*, respectively. These four major nerves of the forearm are supplemented by sensory branches of the medial brachial cutaneous nerve and the medial antebrachial cutaneous nerves, also branches of the inferior cord.

Although knowledge of these derivations is helpful, the approach to brachial plexus anesthesia is based on the reproducible landmarks of the neck: the vertebral tubercles, the first rib, or the axillary artery (Fig. 12.1). Anesthesia is thus performed at the level of the roots (interscalene), trunks (supraclavicular), or terminal nerves (axillary). Anesthesia of the roots produces a pattern that follows the dermatomal distribution, whereas blockade of the terminal nerves follows the sensory nerve distributions (see Axillary Technique, this chapter). Each injection site produces a unique pattern of

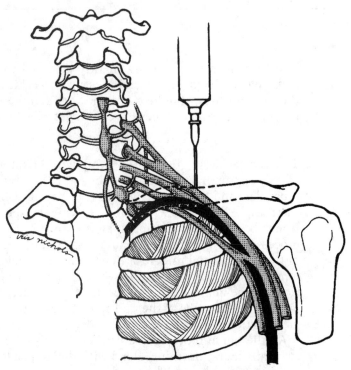

Figure 12.1   **Brachial Plexus Overview**
The ventral roots of the fifth cervical through the first thoracic spinal
nerves form the brachial plexus. The upper and lower pairs of roots
merge, creating three trunks, which join the subclavian artery as it
crosses the first rib (shown with the needle in position for a
supraclavicular block). The trunks then divide and recombine to form the
four terminal nerves of the forearm, which surround the axillary artery—
the radial, median, ulnar, and musculocutaneous.

distribution of anesthesia (1). Interscalene anesthesia is most reliable and dense on the upper roots (C5-7) and includes sensory anesthesia of the cervical plexus (C2-4). Occasionally, anesthesia is ineffective in the C8-T1 dermatome (ulnar side of arm) distribution.
This technique is thus best suited for shoulder and upper arm
surgery. The axillary block is reliable in anesthetizing the three
nerves of the hand (radial, median, and ulnar), although the musculocutaneous and medial antebrachial cutaneous nerves and their
sensory distribution in the forearm can be missed because these
nerves depart from the perivascular bundle high in the axilla. The
supraclavicular and infraclavicular blocks are performed where the
trunks and cords are most closely approximated in the fascial bundle and before branching occurs, and thus are most reliable in producing sensory anesthesia of the entire forearm and hand. They do
not reliably provide cervical plexus (shoulder) anesthesia.

A proximal fascial envelope arises from the lateral extension of the posterior fascia of the anterior scalene and anterior fascia of the middle scalene muscles, and extends from the transverse processes for a variable distance in the upper arm (Fig. 12.2). Winnie has popularized the use of this "sheath" to allow single-injection techniques for the brachial plexus and has demonstrated extensive spread of solution from single injections at all levels in the sheath (2,3). Unfortunately, fascial septa are also occasionally present distally within this sheath (4). Although they do not universally limit the spread of anesthetic solutions (5), they may defeat attempts to produce anesthesia by injection of a single bolus of solution, and may account for the less than 100% success rate of axillary anesthesia.

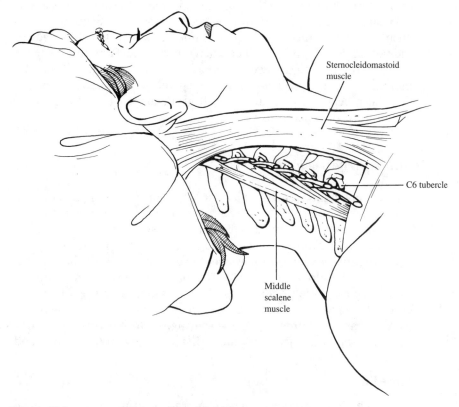

Figure 12.2   **Origins of Brachial Plexus**
The nerves of the plexus emerge from the vertebral canal through the intervertebral foramina, and pass laterally and inferior through the "trough" formed by the lateral extensions of the transverse processes of their respective vertebrae. The anterior scalene muscle attaches to the anterior tubercle of each process, whereas the middle scalene muscle completes the posterior side of the enveloping compartment by attaching to the posterior tubercle.

Drugs   Lidocaine 1% or 1.5% will provide 3 to 4 hours of anesthesia with these techniques. Mepivacaine 1.5% may provide slightly longer anesthesia, and an additional 4 hours if clonidine is added (6). If longer duration is desired, 0.5% bupivacaine, levobupivacaine, or ropivacaine will provide 12 to 14 hours of analgesia. There is no need for higher concentrations in brachial plexus anesthesia, and there is a risk of exceeding maximum recommended doses if they are employed. Epinephrine 1:200,000 will prolong the anesthesia and reduce peak systemic blood levels.

The volume to be injected has been subject to debate. Although 25 mL of solution injected directly in the neighborhood of a nerve stimulation or paresthesia will provide anesthesia for most patients, 30 to 40 mL is commonly used. The upper limit is generally recognized as 50 mL, because this quantity represents the maximum milligram dose of most of the local anesthetics employed. Although this volume may give slightly earlier onset and further spread and is advocated by some (1), Winnie et al. have shown adequate spread with 40-mL volumes in all areas of injection. Selective blockade of individual nerves may reduce the volume requirement. Because many of the techniques require an additional 5 or 10 mL of supplemental anesthetic solution for intercostobrachial branches or peripheral block of the ulnar nerve, it seems appropriate to limit injection into the sheath to 40 mL.

Techniques   *Interscalene Technique*

Indications. Interscalene injection is performed at the level of the emergence of the roots from the tubercles of their respective transverse processes. The anesthesia is most dense in the C4-7 roots, but local anesthetic spreads easily and reliably to the higher roots because the interscalene compartment is continuous with the cervical plexus. This block is thus ideal for upper arm and shoulder (acromioplasty, etc.) operations. The advantages of the incidental cervical plexus (C2-4) anesthesia are balanced by diaphragmatic paralysis and by "ulnar" (C8-T1) sparing, such that this block may require supplementation in the axilla or elbow if used for hand surgery.

Procedure

1. The patient is placed in the supine position, with the head turned slightly to the side opposite the surgical site. A small folded towel is placed under the head, and the ipsilateral hand is held at the side and extended toward the feet. The surface anatomy is identified and marked: the cricoid cartilage, the lateral border of the sternocleidomastoid (SCM) muscle, and the interscalene groove (Fig. 12.3). The latter can be located by asking

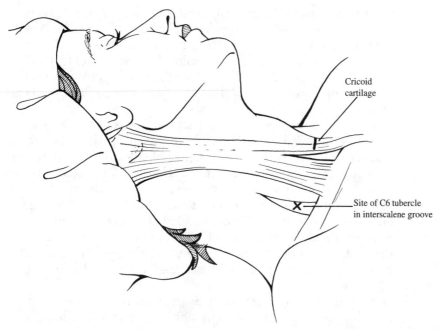

Cricoid
cartilage

Site of C6 tubercle
in interscalene groove

Figure 12.3   **Superficial Landmarks for Interscalene Brachial Plexus Block**
The sternocleidomastoid muscle is identified, and the anterior scalene
muscle found by moving the fingertips over the lateral border of the larger
muscle while it is slightly tensed. The groove between the anterior and
middle scalene muscle can usually be felt. The tubercle of the sixth
cervical vertebra, which lies at the level of the cricoid cartilage, is gently
palpated and an *"X"* marked over it.

the patient to raise the head slightly into a "sniffing" position.
Two fingers placed along the tense lateral border of the SCM and
rolled posterior will drop onto the anterior scalene muscle. The
scalene muscles lie more posterior than lateral to the SCM and
may be harder to appreciate in the heavier patient. The groove
between the scalenes can be palpated by gently rolling these fingers further posterior. The tubercle of the transverse process of
the sixth vertebral body (Chassaignac tubercle) lies in the base of
this groove at the level of the cricoid cartilage, which is commonly also the level at which the external jugular vein crosses
the posterior border of the SCM. In virtually all patients, the tubercle can be identified directly, and is a more reliable landmark
to identify the location of the nerves. This is not uncomfortable
for the patient if done gently. The location of the tubercle should
also be marked with an "X."
2. After aseptic skin preparation and draping, a skin wheal is raised
   in the interscalene groove at the level of the "X." A 1.5-in. 22-
   gauge needle is inserted in a caudad and posterior direction, an-

gling toward the tubercle. This requires that the needle be perpendicular to the skin in all planes. The hub of the needle is held between the thumb and forefinger of the dominant hand, the heel of which rests solidly on the clavicle or neck (Fig. 12.4). This fixation of the needle reduces the chance of accidental movement of the needle when a stimulator response or paresthesia is encountered.

3. The needle is advanced until a stimulator response or paresthesia is obtained or the bone is contacted. If the tubercle is reached before identifying the nerve, the needle is withdrawn almost to the skin and redirected. The path of search for the nerve is in 1-mm steps along a line perpendicular to the presumed course of the nerve (i.e., anterior to posterior); the needle tip should never be directed cephalad or medially (Fig. 12.5). This would allow entry into the intervertebral foramen, with the possibility of puncture of the vertebral artery or dura itself. A more caudad direction will increase the potential for pneumothorax.

4. On obtaining a stimulation or paresthesia in the arm (usually thumb or forearm), gentle aspiration is performed, followed by

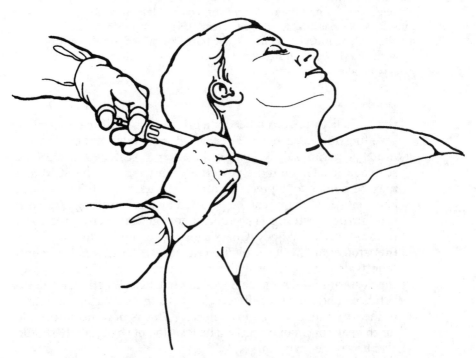

Figure 12.4   **Hand Position for Interscalene Block**
The needle is introduced into the skin at the "X" and directed inferiorly and medially seeking the tubercle while one hand resting on the clavicle exerts constant control of the depth of insertion.

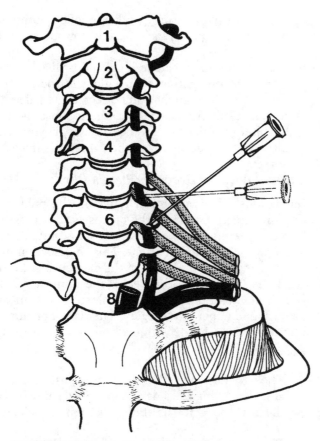

Figure 12.5   **Needle Direction for Interscalene Block**
The needle is always kept in a 45-degree angle to the spinal column.
Medial insertion will allow the point to pass into the intervertebral
foramen and produce epidural, spinal, or intraarterial injection of
anesthetic. A caudad direction will contact the pleura. Note the relation
of the vertebral artery and the nerve roots to the transverse processes.

injection of a 1 mL "test dose." If no cramping or discomfort is
produced with this test, 30 to 40 mL of anesthetic solution is injected incrementally. The needle is held in position with the
dominant hand while the 10-mL syringe is detached and refilled.
Alternatively, a 50-mL syringe of anesthetic solution is connected to the needle by a short length of intravenous extension
tubing. Aspiration is performed after each 3- to 5-mL injection,
and the patient is observed carefully for signs of intravascular injection.

5. Anesthesia is evaluated in 5 minutes, and if weakness of the biceps or sensory anesthesia of the forearm is present, surgical
preparation is begun. A Horner syndrome occasionally may develop, but more concern should be focused on possible shortness

of breath, which may indicate pneumothorax or ipsilateral phrenic nerve paralysis if the solution spreads anterior to the scalene muscles.

6. Continuous interscalene blockade is also practical (7). For this technique, an appropriate needle is introduced more cephalad in the interscalene groove, and directed caudad and medially. Upon nerve stimulation, the anesthetic dose is injected and the catheter introduced a few centimeters beyond the tip of the needle. After needle removal, the catheter is fixed to the skin.

Supraclavicular Brachial Plexus Block

Indications. This approach relies on the predictable anatomy of the three major trunks of the plexus as they cross over the first rib between the insertion of the anterior and middle scalenes just posterior to the subclavian artery. This intersection of nerves with rib occurs behind the midpoint of the clavicle and lies relatively superficial. As mentioned, this technique is most reliable in providing anesthesia of all branches of the plexus and is most appropriate for forearm and upper arm surgery. The risk of pneumothorax is higher than with the other techniques and may limit its application.

Procedure

1. The patient is placed in the supine position, with the ipsilateral arm held along the side and extended caudally (as if reaching for the knee) so as to facilitate palpation of the clavicle and scalene muscles.

2. The clavicle and scalene muscles are identified and marked, and an "X" is placed on the skin just posterior to the midpoint of the clavicle or in the interscalene groove at this level if it is palpable. The scalene muscles are identified by having the patient lift his or her head to the "sniffing" position. Fingers placed on the taut SCM muscle will then easily roll posterior onto the anterior scalene. On a thin patient, the subclavian artery or even the first rib may be identified at the base of the groove between anterior and middle scalenes.

3. After aseptic skin preparation, a skin wheal is placed in the "X," and a 1.5-in. 22-gauge needle on a three-ring syringe is introduced in a caudad direction. The syringe is held such that the axis is constantly parallel to the head, ensuring that the needle direction remains caudad and not directed medially toward the cupola of the pleura. The nondominant hand rests on the clavicle, grasping the hub of the needle between index finger and thumb to prevent unintentional misdirection with patient movement (Fig. 12.6).

4. The 1.5-in. needle is advanced to the depth of the security bead. If the first rib is not contacted, the needle is redirected in 4-mm steps laterally to locate the rib (a "safe" search pattern). If the rib

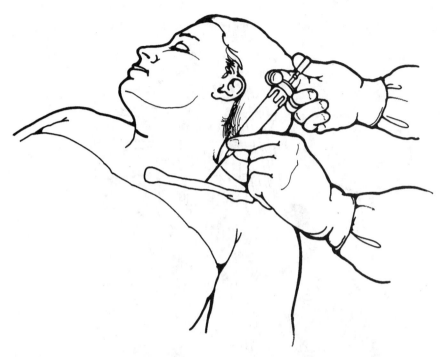

Figure 12.6   **Hand Position for Supraclavicular Block**
The needle is directed caudad behind the midpoint of the clavicle in the
interscalene groove. Again, control of depth is maintained by the hand
resting on the clavicle. The syringe is kept in the sagittal plane parallel to
the patient's head to prevent medial angulation, which increases the
chance of pneumothorax.

does not lie lateral to the "X," then careful 2-mm step exploration is performed medial to the mark. In the occasional heavy
or "bullnecked" patient, a 2-in. needle may be required in order
to reach the rib. If a sharp chest pain associated with a cough is
produced, the technique is abandoned and a chest x-ray obtained.

5. Once the rib is contacted, the needle is withdrawn almost to the
   skin and is redirected 1 to 2 mm posteriorly and reinserted to
   gently contact the rib. Vigorous repeated periosteal contact in-
   flicts pain on the patient and dulls and barbs the needle point.
   The needle direction change needs to be achieved with almost
   complete withdrawal to skin; partial withdrawal may only succeed in pushing the superficial nerve bundle ahead of the advancing needle (Fig. 12.7).

6. The rib follows an anteroposterior course in this area. The path
   of exploration is directly posterior and thus in the sagittal plane
   parallel to the longitudinal axis of the body. This is also perpendicular to the course of the nerve bundle at this point (Fig. 12.1).

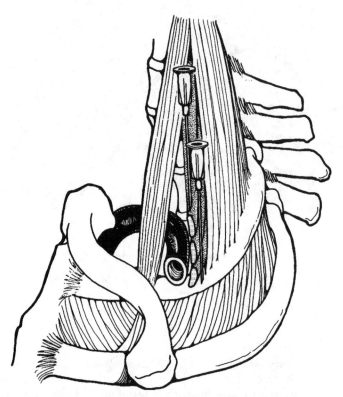

Figure 12.7   **Needle Direction for Supraclavicular Block, Lateral View**
The needle is directed downward onto the first rib, where it can be
expected to contact the three trunks of the brachial plexus as they cross
over the rib. The rib at this point lies along the anterior–posterior plane of
the body. The syringe is kept in the sagittal plane of the body. If the
needle contacts the rib without identifying the nerve, it should be
withdrawn almost completely to the skin before redirection, because
short steps along the bone may simply "push" the nerves ahead of the
needle.

Medial direction of the needle can only serve to identify the
lung. The needle is "walked" posteriorly until it falls off the
posterior angle of the rib; at this point, direction is reversed and
it is "walked" anteriorly until it passes the anterior angle of the
rib or the subclavian artery.

7. A stimulation or paresthesia may be elicited at any time. Sensa-
tions in the back or chest wall should not be accepted; successful anesthesia is greater when eliciting a motor response or
paresthesia in the hand or forearm. The patient must be instructed beforehand to report the paresthesia verbally but not to
move. The needle is immobilized immediately on the patient's
report, and local anesthetic is injected slowly. If a paresthesia is
exacerbated or the patient complains of a cramping pain, the

needle is withdrawn 1 mm and the injection is repeated. Aspiration is performed after each 3 to 5 mL of incremental injection to avoid intravascular injection.

8. A total of 30 to 40 mL is injected in the neighborhood of the first response. The septa that limit diffusion in the axillary sheath are rarely present at this level, and solution reliably spreads to the major branches of the plexus.

9. If no response is obtained in the first 10 minutes, the landmarks are reexamined and the attempt is repeated. The nerves usually lie posterior to the initial contact of the rib if difficulty is encountered. If no paresthesias are obtained, a "wall" of local anesthetic may be created by a series of four to five injections of 6 to 7 mL each as the needle is withdrawn from the rib in 3-mm steps "marching" posteriorly from the artery. This is less likely to succeed, and the alternative of an interscalene, axillary, or intravenous block should be considered.

10. If a tourniquet is to be used, a subcutaneous wheal across the axilla may be necessary to anesthetize the skin of the inner aspect of the upper arm innervated by the intercostobrachial branches. This can be achieved with 5 to 10 mL of anesthetic solution injected subcutaneously along the axillary skin crease.

Alternative Technique: Plumb-bob Approach. In an attempt to reduce the risk of contacting the lung, alternative approaches to the trunks have been devised. One such technique relies on the anatomical information that the nerves always lie superior to the lung. Positioning and preparation are the same as for the traditional approach. With the patient lying supine, the needle is introduced through the skin just above the clavicle at the point of the lateral insertion of the SCM muscle, but it is directed downward toward the floor (posteriorly), following the gravitational line that a plumb bob would follow (Fig. 12.8). If the needle is then redirected in small steps in a 15-degree arc caudad, it will contact the nerves and produce a paresthesia or motor response. Radiological studies suggest that the nerves will always be contacted before the rib or the lung (8).

Alternative Technique: Subclavian Approach. Another technique designed to reduce the risk of pneumothorax is to approach the neurovascular bundle from below the clavicle, but still at the point where the major cords are in close proximity. Multiple variations of this approach have been described, reflecting that the nerves lie considerably deeper from the skin in this area, and are not as reliably associated with clear landmarks. The original description by Raj used the C-6 tubercle and the brachial pulse to create a line that would identify the midpoint of the clavicle, where a needle was inserted and directed 45 degrees laterally (Fig. 12.9). This landmark may be too medial, and a more lateral approach with a 65-degree angulation of insertion may be superior (9). The approach described uses a more lateral point with a vertical needle insertion (10).

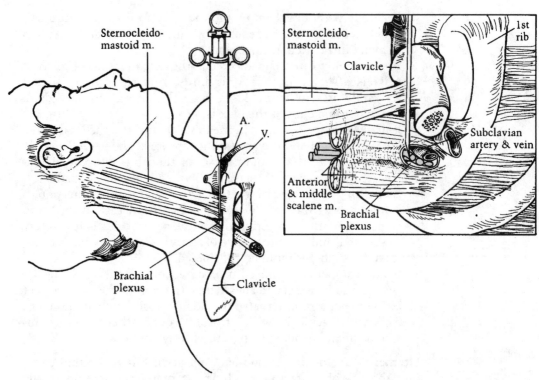

Figure 12.8   **The "Plumb-bob" Approach to the Supraclavicular Block**
The needle is introduced at the midpoint of the clavicle at a position
directly posterior. If the nerves are not encountered at the first insertion,
the needle is rotated in a caudad direction in very small steps, and will
encounter the neurovascular bundle before encountering the lung.

Procedure

1. The patient is positioned supine, with the arm in any comfortable position, including resting at the side.
2. The coracoid process is identified and marked on the skin. An
   "X" is placed 2 cm caudad and 2 cm medial to the coracoid surface mark.
3. A skin wheal is raised at this point, and a 2-in. needle introduced
   perpendicular to the skin and directed posteriorly. The average
   depth of the bundle is 1.5 in., but in heavier patients a 3- or 4-in.
   needle may be required.
4. When the nerves are identified by either a nerve stimulation or
   paresthesia in the hand, 25 to 35 mL of local anesthetic is injected. A musculocutaneous nerve response is not reliable.
5. This technique is also suitable for continuous catheter insertion.
   An appropriate needle is inserted in the same manner, and after
   identification of the neurovascular bundle, a catheter is threaded
   in a lateral direction and secured to the skin.

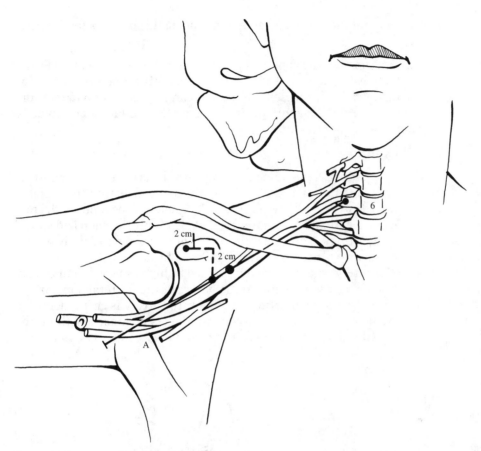

Figure 12.9   **Infraclavicular Approach**
The original description of this technique used the midpoint of the line
between the C-6 tubercle and the axillary artery (A) to mark the insertion
point of a needle directed 45 degrees laterally. A lateral approach 2 cm
medial and inferior to the coracoid process allows a more perpendicular
approach, which may reduce the chance of pneumothorax. For continuous
catheter insertion, the more medial entry and greater angulation may
allow the catheter to thread more easily and be secured to the skin more
solidly.

Axillary Technique

The axillary approach to the brachial plexus has a lower incidence
of serious complications. It usually requires multiple injections because of greater separation of the nerves. Three major nerves remain
in the neurovascular bundle (median on the superior side of the
artery, radial behind, and the ulnar inferior and posterior), but septae are now frequently present separating these nerves and frustrating single-injection techniques. Three other nerves have left the
bundle above this level. The musculocutaneous now lies in the
body of the coracobrachialis muscle, and the medial brachial cuta-

neous and medial antebrachial cutaneous lie in the subcutaneous tissue posterior to the artery.

Indications.   This approach provides anesthesia to the three terminal nerves of the hand and is thus suited for most procedures on the hand itself. With supplementation, it can be used to provide sensory anesthesia for the forearm. It is frequently the block of choice in ambulatory surgery units.

Procedure

1. The patient is positioned supine with the arm abducted at 90 degrees and flexed at the elbow, with the hand resting comfortably on a towel or pillow (Fig. 12.10). Abduction beyond 90 degrees can obscure the axillary pulse and also limit the cephalad spread of anesthetic solution because of pressure on the perivascular compartment by the rotated humeral head.
2. The artery is identified and marked as high as possible in the axilla, usually just lateral to the border of the pectoralis major.
3. After aseptic preparation and drape, the artery is again identified and gently "pinned" between two fingers of equal length on the anesthesiologist's nondominant hand (Fig. 12.11). The index and

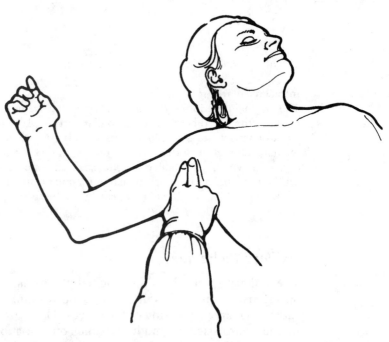

Figure 12.10   **Position for Axillary Block**
The arm is elevated (abducted) at 90 degrees at the shoulder, with the elbow flexed at a 90-degree angle and the forearm slightly elevated on a pillow. More extreme abduction may obscure the pulse, which is the critical landmark, usually easily identified by gentle palpation.

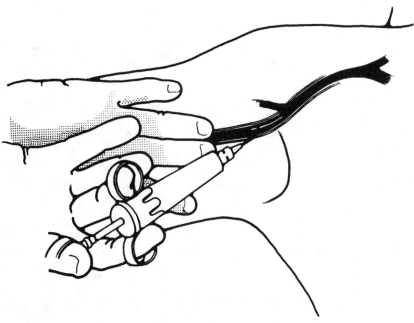

Figure 12.11   **Hand Position for Axillary Block**
Two fingers of equal length straddle the artery while the needle is
introduced along its long axis with a central angulation. The palpating
fingers serve not only to identify the vessel, but also to compress the
perivascular sheath and encourage the spread of anesthetic solution
centrally.

middle fingers are commonly used, but the middle and ring fingers are also used.
4. A skin wheal is made over the artery, and a 5/8-in. needle attached to a 10-mL three-ring syringe is introduced.
5. At this point, there are several options:
   (a) The simplest technique is *perivascular infiltration* on opposite sides of the artery (11). The needle is advanced as close as
practical to one side of the artery while aspirating (Fig. 12.12).
If no blood is obtained at a depth felt to be just beyond the
vessel, the needle is withdrawn slowly while 3 to 4 mL of
anesthetic is injected. The needle is then redirected slightly
further away from the vessel, and the process is repeated
twice, producing three injections of local anesthetic (total of
10 mL) along three parallel lines alongside the vessel, cover-
ing a depth from just behind to just in front of the artery. The
syringe is refilled, and the process repeated on the opposite
side of the vessel. After these initial injections, supplemental
anesthesia of the other nerves is produced by other injections
(see number 6, this section). After 5 minutes, evaluation of
the distal nerves is performed, and reinjection is made in the

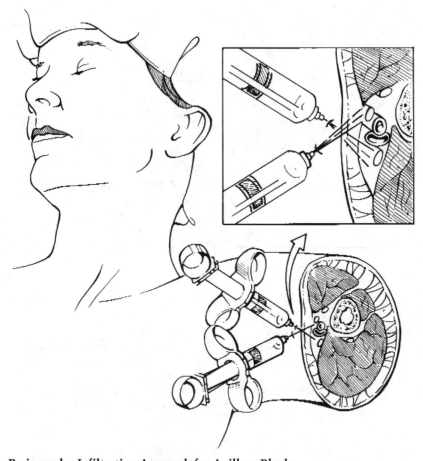

Figure 12.12   **Perivascular Infiltration Approach for Axillary Block**
The needle is introduced next to the artery with constant aspiration, and
then injection of multiple small increments is made on withdrawal in a
fanwise pattern moving away from the vessel.

areas of nerves that are not yet anesthetized. If at any time
the artery itself or a paresthesia is identified, the alternative
approaches below are then used.

(b) The *transarterial approach* is also simple and reliable. The
needle is advanced intentionally into the vessel with constant aspiration, and the advance halted as soon as blood no
longer returns. At this point, the needle is fixed, and 10 mL
is injected behind the artery, with intermittent aspiration to
ensure that the needle has not migrated back into the vessel.
The syringe is then reloaded and withdrawn back through the
vessel with constant aspiration to indicate when the needle
has just exited the anterior side of the artery. At this point, an
additional 10 mL of anesthetic is injected, followed by the

supplemental nerve injections described in number 6, this section.

(c) The *nerve stimulator* can be used in the axilla to identify the three nerves around the artery. It is more effective with the stimulator to move a distance distally, to the junction of the upper and middle third of the humerus (the *"midhumeral" approach*) (12), where all four major nerves can be blocked with separate injections (Fig. 12.13) (12). For this approach, the arm is abducted 80 degrees, and the brachial artery is identified at the junction of the upper and middle third of the arm. First, the median nerve is identified by introducing the stimulator needle next to the brachial artery on the superior side

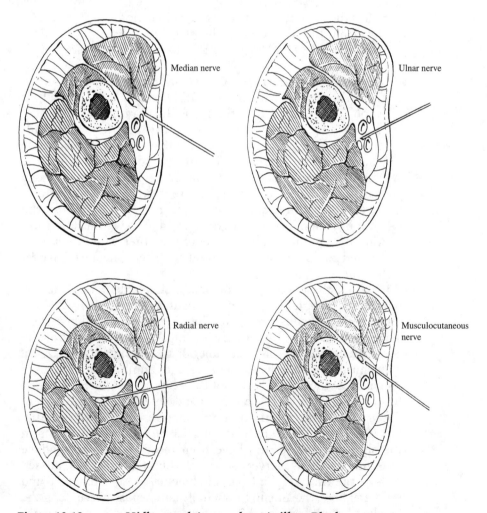

Figure 12.13   **Midhumeral Approach to Axillary Block**
At this point, the nerves are separated more than in the axilla itself, but still allow easy identification with the nerve stimulator.

in the direction of the axilla. Stimulation of the median nerve in this area produces flexion of the wrist or fingers, or pronation of the forearm. Next, the ulnar nerve can be identified by redirecting the needle from the same insertion point in a posterior and inferior direction from the artery. Stimulation of the nerve produces ulnar flexion of the wrist or the last two fingers, or adduction of the thumb. The needle is then redirected perpendicular to the skin and deep to the artery to the level of the inferior side of the humerus itself to stimulate the radial nerve. Isolated contraction of the triceps muscle due to direct stimulation can be confusing, so the nerve is better identified by extension of the wrist or fingers. Finally, the needle is redirected superior to the artery to the body of the coracobrachialis muscle, where flexion of the wrist identifies the musculocutaneous nerve. Injection of 5 to 10 mL of local anesthetic on each of the first three nerves is sufficient, whereas 5 to 6 mL may be adequate for the musculocutaneous.

(d) A fourth approach is the traditional *paresthesia technique*. Paresthesias are sought on either side of the vessel; it should be recalled that the musculocutaneous and median nerves lie superior to the artery in this position and the ulnar and radial nerves lie inferior (Fig. 12.14). Paresthesias should be sought first in the area most likely to affect the surgical field. Success is enhanced by finding at least one paresthesia on each side of the artery, although it is difficult to elicit a second paresthesia more than 5 minutes after the first injection, because partial spread of the anesthetic solution may produce hypesthesia of the other nerves. Between 10 and 20 mL of solution should be injected near each paresthesia.

6. With all of these axillary approaches, supplementation may be required to anesthetize the musculocutaneous nerve, medial antebrachial cutaneous nerve, and the intercostobrachial branches. The first is achieved by a fanwise injection in the body of the coracobrachialis muscle just superior to the artery (Fig. 12.15). This muscle can be grasped between the thumb and forefinger of one hand at the lateral border of the pectoralis while 5 mL of solution is injected with the other hand. Injection frequently produces a dull aching sensation that may resemble a paresthesia, but true nerve localization is rare. Larger-volume injections in the sheath itself (40 mL) have been recommended to produce musculocutaneous nerve anesthesia, but this nerve is missed 25% of the time. The medial antebrachial cutaneous nerve and its neighbor, the medial brachial cutaneous nerve, can be blocked by infiltration of the subcutaneous tissues just inferior to the level of the neurovascular bundle parallel to the axillary skin crease with 5 mL of solution (Fig. 12.14). Blockade of these

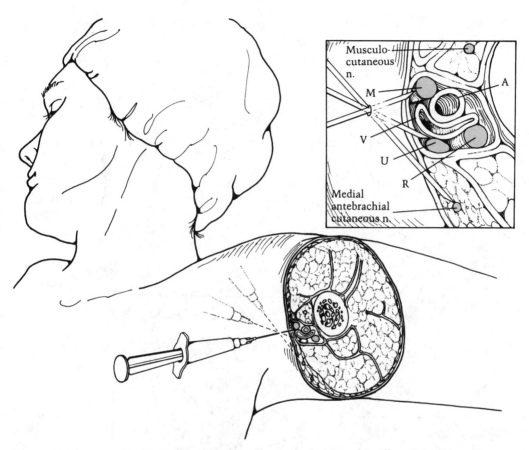

Figure 12.14   **Needle Position for Paresthesia Technique of Axillary Injection**
The median (M) and musculocutaneous nerves lie on the superior side of
the artery (A). The latter usually lies within the body of the
coracobrachialis muscle at this point. The ulnar (U) nerve lies inferior and
the radial (R) nerve is inferior and posterior to the artery. These positions
may vary with individual patients, and the medial antebrachial cutaneous
nerve usually lies in the subcutaneous tissues just inferior to the
neurovascular bundle and is anesthetized by a subcutaneous wheal along
that area, along with the intercostobrachial fibers.

nerves is usually not necessary if surgery is confined to the hand.
The use of an upper arm tourniquet may dictate block of these
nerves and the intercostobrachial fibers, which is obtained by the
same injection.

Continuous Axillary Technique

A continuous axillary technique has been described for use in patients with anticipated long-duration surgery (such as finger reim-
plantation with microsurgical techniques), or requirements for prolonged postoperative analgesia or sympathectomy. Prolonged

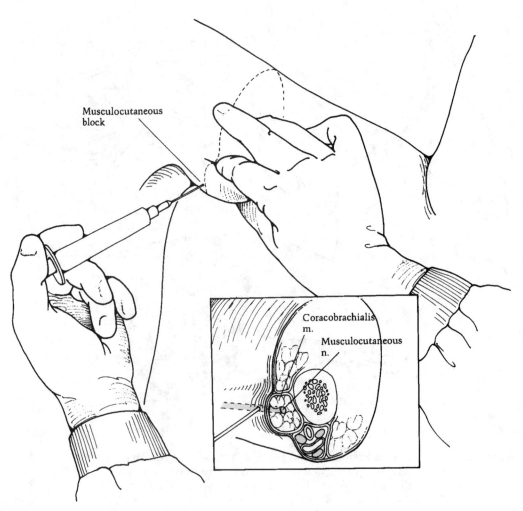

Musculocutaneous
block

Coracobrachialis
m.

Musculocutaneous
n.

Figure 12.15   **Musculocutaneous Nerve**
The musculocutaneous nerve lies in the body of the coracobrachialis
muscle. This muscle can be grabbed between the thumb and forefinger of
one hand and the nerve blocked by the injection of 5 cm³ of local
anesthetic into the body of the muscle.

anesthesia can be attained by placing a plastic intravenous catheter
in or alongside the axillary sheath and using intermittent bolus or
continuous infusions of local anesthetic drugs. The long-acting
amino-amide anesthetics will produce up to 8 hours of anesthesia
and thus can be reinjected two or three times daily. A continuous
infusion of 10 mL per hour of 0.2% to 0.25% concentration of any
of these drugs is another alternative that will provide continuous
anesthesia.

The original placement of the catheter can be performed by rely-
ing on the sensation of "popping" the catheter through the fascial

plane of the sheath, although this may be difficult in the heavier patient. Simple placement of the catheter in the groove between the biceps and triceps muscles alongside the sheath appears to be as effective. Elicitation of a paresthesia or use of a nerve stimulator may help confirm the catheter location in the difficult patient. Attempts to localize the sheath exactly also may lead to arterial puncture, potentially producing a hematoma that would interfere with spread of the local anesthetic solution.

The use of short (1.5 or 2 in.) catheters may reduce the chance of central spread of anesthetic and increase the frequency of musculocutaneous nerve sparing. A 3-in. catheter can be inserted with a flexible guidewire higher in the axilla, with a greater chance of anesthesia of all four nerves of the forearm. With appropriate sterile dressing of the catheter entry site, the catheter can be left in place for several days.

Complications

Missed Nerve Blocks

Missed nerve blocks occur from 3% to 30% of the time with these techniques (13,14) and usually involve only one or two of the terminal nerves. This can be rectified by repetition of the block (if paresthesias are not relied on), peripheral injection of the nerve (see Chapter 14), or local infiltration by the surgeon. Early identification is essential to allow appropriate correction (Figs. 12.16 and 12.17). The most common findings are absent C8-T1 anesthesia with the interscalene approach, or residual musculocutaneous or medial antebrachial cutaneous sensation with the axillary block. Anesthesia should be assessed as early as 5 minutes after completion of the injection. Onset of anesthesia with all the drugs, including bupivacaine, is within 5 minutes (1), and the absence of anesthesia in a critical nerve distribution at this time interval should lead to the formulation of alternative plans. Sometimes merely waiting another 5 minutes will allow sufficient diffusion of anesthetic solution to provide analgesia, but alternative plans should be reviewed with the patient and surgeon before an incision. If inadequate anesthesia is discovered at the time of incision (particularly on the forearm), infiltration of the wound with local anesthetic by the surgeon or intravenous narcotics by the anesthesiologist may provide the needed supplemental analgesia. General anesthesia should always be considered as a potential necessity in all regional-block patients.

Testing of the block can be performed quickly and effectively with the "push–pull–pinch–pinch" technique. The patient is asked to extend (push) the forearm against resistance (triceps, radial nerve) and then flex the arm (pull), drawing the thumb to the nose (biceps, musculocutaneous nerve). Sensory anesthesia of the hand to pinch

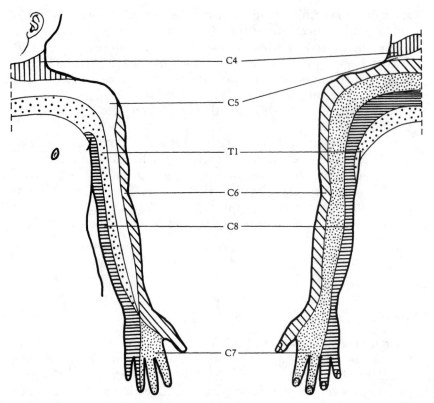

Figure 12.16   **Dermatomal Distribution of Nerve Roots in the Upper Extremity**

on the thenar (median nerve) and hypothenar (ulnar nerve) areas
will confirm block of the other two nerves. This entire sequence
can be performed in less than a minute, and the profound loss of radial muscle tone will often give the patient reassurance that the
block is working. A full 20 minutes is required for dense anesthesia
of the arm, but, fortunately, surgical preparation and draping often
provide the needed time interval. Alkalinization of the local anesthetic or performance of the block in a waiting area can further reduce onset time and improve the depth of anesthesia at the time of
incision; the most frequent cause of "failed" anesthesia is premature surgical incision.

Intravascular Injection

Intravascular injection is the most serious potential complication.
This is true for the supraclavicular and axillary techniques because
of their proximity to blood vessels, but it is a particular concern
with the interscalene technique because of the nearness of the vertebral artery to the cervical nerve roots, and the incidence is high-

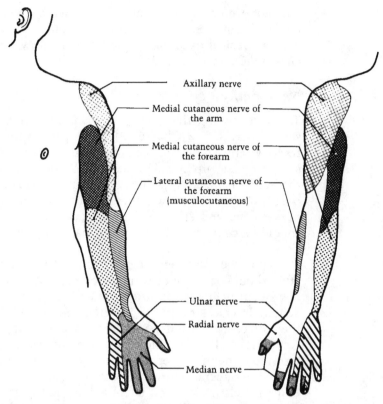

Figure 12.17   **Sensory Dermatomes of the Terminal Nerves of the Upper Extremity**
Sensation is provided by the terminal nerves as identified. This pattern is
different from the classic dermatomal distribution of the nerve roots (Fig.
12.16). Different patterns of anesthesia will develop if the block is
performed at the root level (interscalene block) or terminal nerve level
(axillary block).

est with this technique. Frequent aspiration, incremental injection,
and close observation of the patient are essential. Resuscitation gear
and intravenous access are mandatory.

Pneumothorax

Pneumothorax occurs rarely in experienced hands, being reported as
less than 1% in one series of supraclavicular blocks, but it is a risk
with this technique. It is also possible to puncture the pleura with
the interscalene approach if the needle is directed too far inferiorly.
Although the complication is not life threatening, it is painful to
the patient and a serious inconvenience, particularly if it necessitates unplanned admission of an outpatient to the hospital. The
pneumothorax is often small and may resolve spontaneously, and it

may not even be symptomatic immediately. Any patient who complains of pain in the chest or shortness of breath should be evaluated with a physical examination and a chest x-ray, and treated with a chest tube if symptomatic.

Neuropathy

Transient neuropathy is also rare, being reported as 2% or less in several series (see Chapter 3), with permanent dysfunction extremely rare. The incidence appears to be higher if paresthesias are sought with sharp (long beveled) needles or if repeated contact with the nerves is made (15). Particular attention is needed to avoid pinning the nerve roots and trunks against the bony structures during interscalene and supraclavicular blocks. As always, no injection should be continued if a cramping pain suggests intraneural injection.

If a postoperative neurologic deficit is detected, neurologic evaluation should be obtained early. Precise localization of the injury can help identify if the anesthetic injection itself was related to the deficit. Interscalene injections affect roots and dermatomes, and their effects can be differentiated from axillary injections, which affect peripheral nerves. Electromyographic testing also can help determine if the injury represents preexisting nerve damage.

Most peripheral injuries resolve spontaneously in 1 to 6 months. Empathy, close attention to follow-up, and early arrangements for physical therapy will help alleviate patient disability and dissatisfaction, although the long course of recovery is frustrating to physician and patient alike.

Hematoma Formation

Hematoma formation can occur following supraclavicular or axillary block if the artery is punctured. This is usually of little consequence, but it may discourage performance of these blocks on patients with bleeding disorders. Temporary vasospasm of the artery and occlusion of the pulse have been described after puncture, as well as occlusion of the axillary vein. These events are rare, but, again, they suggest that the minimal degree of tissue disruption is the best.

Unintentional Anesthetic Spread

Unintentional anesthetic spread is most common with the interscalene approach. The most serious problem involves injection of the anesthetic solution into the epidural or subarachnoid space, producing a high epidural or total spinal anesthetic. Although bilateral cervical and brachial plexus blocks are the most common events, total spinal anesthesia is a possibility that requires prompt recognition and treatment with ventilatory and cardiovascular support. More frequently, the anesthetic solution spreads to involve the phrenic nerve, either at its origin in the cervical roots or along its course on the anterior surface of the anterior scalene muscle. Paralysis of the ipsilateral diaphragm occurs reliably with interscalene block (16). Paralysis of one diaphragm does not represent a problem in the healthy patient, but it may not be well tolerated in the patient with respiratory disease. The sympathetic chain also lies close to the site of injection, and a unilateral Horner syndrome is not unusual. Bronchospasm caused by sympathetic blockade also has been attributed to spread of interscalene anesthesia.

Spread of anesthesia to these structures after supraclavicular anesthesia is less common, and axillary injection is associated with the least likelihood.

References

1. Lanz, E., Theiss, D., Jankovic, D. The extent of blockade following various techniques of brachial plexus block. *Anesth. Analg.* 62: 55, 1983.
2. Winnie, A. P. Interscalene brachial plexus block. *Anesth. Analg.* 49: 455, 1970.
3. Winnie, A. P., Collins, V. J. The subclavian perivascular technique of brachial plexus anesthesia. *Anesthesiology* 25: 353, 1964.
4. Thompson, G. E., Rorie, D. K. Functional anatomy of the brachial plexus sheaths. *Anesthesiology* 59: 117, 1983.
5. Partridge, B. L., Katz, J., Benirschke, K. Functional anatomy of the brachial plexus sheath: Implications for anesthesia. *Anesthesiology* 66: 743, 1987.
6. Singelyn, F., Gouverneur, J., Robert, A. A minimum dose of clonidine added to mepivacaine prolongs the duration of anesthesia and analgesia after axillary brachial plexus block. *Anesth. Analg.* 83: 1046, 1996.
7. Chelly, J., Casati, A., Fanelli, G., *Continuous Peripheral Nerve Block Techniques.* London: Mosby, 2001.
8. Brown, D. L., Cahill, D. R., Bridenbaugh, L. D. Supraclavicular nerve block: Anatomic analysis of a method to prevent pneumothorax. *Anesth. Analg.* 76: 530, 1993.
9. Klaastad, O., Lilleas, F. G., Rotnes, J. S., Breivik, H., Fosse, E. A magnetic resonance imaging study of modifications to the infraclavicular brachial plexus block. *Anesth. Analg.* 91: 929, 2000.
10. Wilson, J. L., Brown, D. L., Wong, G. Y., Ehman, R. L., Cahill, D. R. Infraclavicular brachial plexus block: Parasagittal anatomy important to the coracoid technique. *Anesth. Analg.* 87: 870, 1998.
11. Thompson, G. E. Blocking the brachial plexus. *Anaesth. Intensive Care* 15: 119, 1987.
12. Bouaziz, H., Narchi, P., Mercier, F. J., Labaille, T., Zerrouk, N., Girod, J., Benhamou, D. Comparison between conventional axillary block and a new approach at the midhumeral level. *Anesth. Analg.* 84: 1058, 1997.
13. Goldberg, M. E., Gregg, C., Larijani, G. E., Norris, M. C., Marr, A. T., Seltzer, J. L. A comparison of three methods of axillary approach to brachial plexus blockade for upper extremity surgery. *Anesthesiology* 66: 814, 1987.

14. Selander, D., Edshage, S., Wolff, T. Paresthesiae or no paresthesiae? Nerve lesions after axillary blocks. *Acta Anaesthesiol. Scand.* 23: 27, 1979.
15. Selander, D. Axillary plexus block: Paresthetic or perivascular. *Anesthesiology* 66: 726, 1987.
16. Urmey, W. F., Gloeggler, P. J. Pulmonary function changes during interscalene brachial plexus block: Effects of decreasing local anesthetic injection volume. *Reg. Anesth.* 18: 244, 1993.

13 Intravenous Regional Anesthesia

Intravenous regional anesthesia of the extremities is one of the simplest and oldest techniques available, but it still requires understanding of the involved anatomy, pharmacology, and physiology to ensure safe and effective anesthesia.

Anatomy

The peripheral nerves of the arm and leg are nourished by small blood vessels that accompany them. Distension of the venous vessels in these nerves with a local anesthetic solution will cause diffusion of the solution into the nerves and produce anesthesia as long as the concentration in the venous system remains high. This is usually attained by blocking venous flow with a proximal tourniquet, followed by distension of the venous system with a dilute solution of local anesthetic injected through a previously placed venous catheter. The anesthetic acts on the small nerves and nerve endings and to a lesser extent on the main nerve trunks.

A form of this technique of venous injection of local anesthetic was first described by August Bier. His original technique required surgical exposure of the veins. The practical application awaited the development of intravenous needles and pneumatic tourniquets, but the technique is still commonly referred to as a *Bier block.*

Indications

Intravenous regional anesthesia is suitable for many operations on the distal extremities when a proximal occlusive tourniquet can be safely applied. It provides satisfactory anesthesia for foreign-body explorations, nerve explorations, surgical repairs of lacerations, and tendon or joint repairs. Although periosteal anesthesia is not as dense as with other techniques, it can be used for bunionectomies or reduction of simple fractures.

It is not suitable if a condition such as severe ischemic vascular disease contraindicates vascular occlusion with a tourniquet. Some surgeons also may be dissatisfied with the amount of fluid exuded into the surgical field (especially if performing microscopic procedures), but a bloodless field is maintained.

The primary advantages of intravenous regional anesthesia are its simplicity and reliability. It is the easiest and most effective block of the arm for simple, short procedures, and it is thus well suited for novices and for ambulatory surgery. A drawback is the lack of postoperative anesthesia, but the rapid recovery of function in the hand is an advantage.

The block is used primarily in the arm. Although a forearm tourniquet has been employed to reduce the total dose of local anesthetic, the upper arm tourniquet remains the standard. In the leg, larger volumes of drug are required and adequate occlusion of vessels is harder to attain because of thicker muscles and the more irregular shape of the thigh. There are also concerns about intraosseous channels allowing more leakage of local anesthetic solution into the systemic circulation, and about the potential of a higher frequency of systemic reactions to anesthetics when the lower limb is blocked with this technique. Although a calf tourniquet has been advocated in reducing the total dose of local anesthetic and has been used successfully, this technique is not as popular as application to the upper extremity.

Drugs

Lidocaine is the most commonly used drug. A dilute solution is sufficient and is required if the maximum dose is to be avoided with the high volumes necessary for venous distension. A total of 50 mL of 0.5% lidocaine is the usual volume for the arm, whereas 100 mL (500 mg) is needed to distend the venous channels of the leg if a thigh cuff is used. In smaller patients, a dose of 3 mg per kg 0.5% lidocaine can be used as a guide for total dose. Mepivacaine is also effective.

Bupivacaine (0.25% in similar volumes) has been used for this block, but systemic release of this drug has been a significant problem. Ropivacaine 0.2% is an effective alternative with a greater cardiac safety margin, and may provide some residual analgesia after tourniquet release (1). The amino-ester 2-chloroprocaine is cleared even more rapidly. Its use has been associated with phlebitis in one report, but the use of an alkalinized solution produces minimal side effects and analgesia equivalent to lidocaine (2).

Additives to the local anesthetic have been investigated. Meperidine, tramadol, and ketorolac appear to provide little advantage and some side effects (3–5). Clonidine in doses of 1 μg per kg will prolong analgesia after lidocaine block (6), whereas higher doses will also reduce tourniquet pain at the expense of some systemic side effects (7).

Technique

1. The patient is placed in the supine position, and appropriate monitors are placed. These include a blood pressure cuff to obtain systolic readings to guide tourniquet settings, and intravenous access in another extremity.
2. A tourniquet is placed securely on the proximal part of the extremity to be operated on. The "double cuff" has been popularized for this block to reduce the pressure pain in the unanesthetized skin under the cuff in longer operations (see number 8, this section). The presence of two cuffs, however, requires that

they both be narrower (5 to 7 cm) than the standard blood pressure cuff (12 to 14 cm) used on the arm. Narrower cuffs do not effectively transmit the indicated gauge pressure to deep tissues, and thus venous occlusion pressures are less than presumed (8). The use of a standard wide cuff may be more desirable and more acceptable if the procedure is to last less than an hour (about the time for pressure discomfort to develop).

3. An intravenous catheter is inserted in the hand or foot to be operated on. This should be a flexible, small, 20- or 22-gauge plastic catheter placed distally from the surgical site and in a position where it will not be dislodged by the Esmarch bandage used for exsanguination. Distal placement, rather than in the antecubital fossa, is also associated with less probability of leakage under the cuff. The catheter is taped loosely in place and a small syringe or injection cap is fitted over it after a dilute heparin flush is used to clear the lumen.

4. The arm or leg is elevated to promote venous drainage and then is exsanguinated with an Esmarch bandage wrapped from the distal end up to the tourniquet itself (Fig. 13.1).

5. The tourniquet is inflated to a pressure 100 mm Hg above the systolic blood pressure, or at least 300 mm Hg. Tourniquet inflation is checked by balloting the cuff and watching the oscillation of the pressure gauge. After inflation and removal of the Esmarch wrap, adequate occlusion is confirmed by the absence of the radial or posterior tibial pulse.

   A constant-pressure gas source must be used to maintain inflation of the cuff. All cuffs have some small-volume leak, and a simple inflation of the standard blood pressure cuff with a bulb will produce a gradual decrease in cuff pressure that will allow leakage of local anesthetic with potentially catastrophic results. The cuffs must be checked before injection and frequently during the procedure.

6. The limb is returned to the neutral position, and the local anesthetic drug is injected through the previously placed catheter. The patient is warned that this will produce an uncomfortable "pins and needles" sensation for a few seconds. The injection is made slowly (90 seconds or more) to reduce this discomfort, but, more importantly, to produce a peak venous pressure that is not greater than the occluding pressure of the cuff (8). The catheter is removed if surgery will be less than an hour, and pressure is placed over the entry site until it seals. Adequate sensory anesthesia will ensue in 5 minutes.

7. Under no circumstances is the cuff deflated in the first 20 minutes after injection.

8. If the procedure exceeds 45 minutes, the double cuff may be employed. In this situation, the *proximal* cuff is inflated for the first 45 minutes of anesthesia. The distal cuff is then inflated over the tissue area that has been numbed by the local anes-

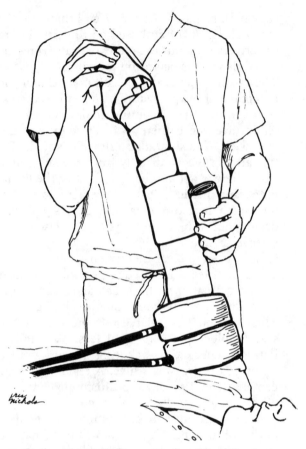

Figure 13.1   **Technique for Intravenous Regional Anesthesia**
A small intravenous catheter is placed in the hand and the tourniquet is
applied to the upper arm. A single tourniquet may be used for shorter
operations and may provide more reliable compression of the venous
system than the double-tourniquet system shown. Exsanguination of the
arm is attained by elevation and wrapping with the Esmarch elastic
bandage. The tourniquet is then inflated and the local anesthetic injected.

thetic injection, and the proximal cuff (overlying unanesthetized skin) is deflated. The adequacy of the distal cuff is
checked *before* the proximal cuff is deflated.

Although this technique allegedly reduces patient discomfort
at the area of the tourniquet, the complex procedure of shifting
the inflation adds the risk of unintentional deflation. In addition, use of the narrower cuff may not provide adequate compression to prevent the leak of fluid into the central venous system.

9. If more than 45 minutes has elapsed from the time of injection,
   anesthesia may begin to diminish. If the surgeon requires more

time, the intravenous catheter may be reinjected with local anesthetic solution after 60 to 90 minutes. This is disruptive to the surgery and potentially to the sterile field, and, because of this, for longer procedures, other regional techniques, such as brachial plexus block, are usually a more appropriate plan.

10. Deflation of the tourniquet can be performed after 45 minutes with minimal risk of systemic symptoms of local anesthetic toxicity because the drug binds to the tissues (9) (Fig. 13.2). If less than 45 minutes has elapsed, a two-stage release is recommended, where the cuff is deflated for 10 seconds and reinflated for a minute before final release. This allows a gradual washout

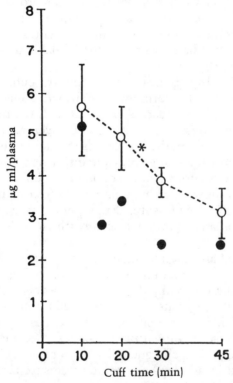

Figure 13.2   **Effect of Inflation Time on Systemic Blood Levels of Local Anesthetic after Intravenous Regional Blockade**
After release of the tourniquet, blood levels of local anesthetic increase rapidly, but are also rapidly cleared. Following 20 minutes of total inflation time, blood levels may reach toxic (symptomatic) levels; after 45 minutes, this is unlikely. The *open circles* indicate blood levels after 50 mL of 1% lidocaine; the *solid circles* indicate the lower levels achieved with 0.5% lidocaine. The tourniquet should probably not be released in less than 20 minutes with any drug, and should be released intermittently following 20 to 45 minutes of total tourniquet time. (From Tucker, G. T., Boas, R. A. Pharmacokinetic aspects of intravenous regional anesthesia. *Anesthesiology* 34: 538, 1971, with permission.)

of anesthetic. Cycling the cuff three times in this manner will delay the onset of peak blood levels, but it does not significantly reduce the level attained with a single deflation (10). As mentioned, if less than 20 minutes has elapsed, pleasant conversation should be used to fill the time until that interval has passed and a two-stage release can be performed. These steps do not guarantee the absence of systemic toxicity, however.

Complications

Systemic Toxicity

Systemic toxicity is the major risk of this procedure. The greatest danger is from an inadequate tourniquet early in the procedure when the intravenous volume and concentration are large. Every precaution must be taken to ensure a reliable tourniquet and inflation pressure source.

Even with adequate inflation, the narrow cuffs (5 to 7 cm width) used for the double-tourniquet system will sometimes allow leakage. The use of a standard width adult cuff (12 to 14 cm) provides more reliable compression of the entire venous system of the extremity, especially in the leg. Leakage is more likely if the injection is made rapidly under high pressure into a vein near the cuff (8). The least leakage occurs when injection is made into a distal vein over 90 seconds following exsanguination of the arm and inflation of the cuff to 300 mm Hg pressure. Careful monitoring of mental status is indicated for several minutes, even with an apparently functioning cuff.

Some local anesthetic remains in the veins at the end of the procedure, and tourniquet release inevitably washes drug into the systemic circulation. With lidocaine, these levels are subtoxic after 45 minutes, but dangerously high within 20 minutes after injection (9) (Fig. 13.2). This is the basis for the guidelines for tourniquet release stated. Because of variability, no safety is guaranteed, and all patients having this technique must be monitored closely at all times for possible local anesthetic toxicity. Resuscitation equipment is necessary, and an intravenous access in another extremity is indicated.

References

1. Hartmannsgruber, M. W., Silverman, D. G., Halaszynski, T. M., Bobart, V., Brull, S. J., Wilkerson, C., Loepke, A. W., Atanassoff, P. G. Comparison of ropivacaine 0.2% and lidocaine 0.5% for intravenous regional anesthesia in volunteers. *Anesth. Analg.* 89: 727, 1999.
2. Lavin, P. A., Henderson, C. L., Vaghadia, H. Non-alkalinized and alkalinized 2-chloroprocaine vs lidocaine for intravenous regional anesthesia during outpatient hand surgery. *Can. J. Anaesth.* 46: 939, 1999.

3. Acalovschi, I., Cristea, T., Margarit, S., Gavrus, R. Tramadol added to lidocaine for intravenous regional anesthesia. *Anesth. Analg.* 92: 209, 2001.
4. Reuben, S. S., Duprat, K. M. Comparison of wound infiltration with ketorolac versus intravenous regional anesthesia with ketorolac for postoperative analgesia following ambulatory hand surgery. *Reg. Anesth.* 21: 565, 1996.
5. Reuben, S. S., Steinberg, R. B., Lurie, S. D., Gibson, C. S. A dose-response study of intravenous regional anesthesia with meperidine. *Anesth. Analg.* 88: 831, 1999.
6. Reuben, S. S., Steinberg, R. B., Klatt, J. L., Klatt, M. L. Intravenous regional anesthesia using lidocaine and clonidine. *Anesthesiology* 91: 654, 1999.
7. Gentili, M., Bernard, J. M., Bonnet, F. Adding clonidine to lidocaine for intravenous regional anesthesia prevents tourniquet pain. *Anesth. Analg.* 88: 1327, 1999.
8. Grice, S. C., Morell, R. C., Balestrieri, F. J., Stump, D. A., Howard, G. Intravenous regional anesthesia: Evaluation and prevention of leakage under the tourniquet. *Anesthesiology* 65: 316, 1986.
9. Tucker, G. T., Boas, R. A. Pharmacokinetic aspects of intravenous regional anesthesia. *Anesthesiology* 34: 538, 1971.
10. Sukhani, R., Garcia, C. J., Munhall, R. J., Winnie, A. P., Rodvold, K. A. Lidocaine disposition following intravenous regional anesthesia with different tourniquet deflation technics. *Anesth. Analg.* 68: 633, 1989.

14 Peripheral Nerve Blocks of the Upper Extremity

Occasionally, anesthesia of a single nerve of the shoulder, forearm, hand, or digit is required. More commonly, supplementation of a single terminal branch is required after a partially successful brachial plexus block. Central block is more effective, but peripheral approaches are possible and sometimes easier for a single nerve distribution.

Anatomy

Two of the proximal branches of the brachial plexus are occasionally blocked to provide supplemental anesthesia—the suprascapular nerve and the musculocutaneous (as described in Chapter 12). The suprascapular nerve arises from the superior cord formed by the fifth and sixth cervical roots, and passes obliquely laterally under the trapezius to cross through the supraspinous notch to the back of the scapula. It provides sensory fibers to the shoulder joint and motor fibers to the supraspinatus muscle, which assists the deltoid in elevating the arm. It also provides motor innervation to the infraspinatus muscle, which externally rotates the humerus (a useful marker for nerve stimulator localization), but it has only a small area of surface sensory innervation on the shoulder.

Distally, the three terminal nerves to the hand travel mostly in muscle compartments, but they have reliable bony landmarks at the elbow and wrist, where the muscles are less prominent as they cross the joints. The terminal digital nerves are easily found.

At the elbow, the ulnar nerve is superficial in the groove of the medial condyle of the humerus and the olecranon process. Paresthesias are so easily elicited with pressure that this area is well known as the "funny bone." The median nerve is deeper, but it reliably passes just medial to the brachial artery above the skin crease of the antecubital fossa. The radial and lateral cutaneous nerves of the forearm cross the elbow joint laterally between the biceps tendon and the insertion of the brachioradialis. The former lies close to the humerus itself in this groove, whereas the latter is superficial and has already begun to branch into terminal distribution fibers.

On the palmar surface of the wrist, the three nerves of the hand are again easily found. The ulnar nerve crosses the wrist joint by passing above the ulnar styloid in company with the ulnar artery. The median nerve lies in the middle of the wrist, deep between the tendons of the palmaris longus and flexor carpi radialis (the prominent tendons when the wrist is flexed). The radial nerve begins branching proximal to the wrist, but it can be found in company with the radial artery and with several of its branches passing superficially dorsally over the joint and through the anatomic "snuffbox" on the back of the hand.

The digital nerves are the terminal sensory branches that course alongside the phalanges as a dorsal and a ventral branch on the side of each finger. They are easily blocked as long as care is taken not to compromise their accompanying arteries.

Indications

Suprascapular nerve block is primarily used to provide analgesia of the shoulder joint following shoulder surgery. It can accelerate discharge after shoulder surgery performed under general anesthesia (1), but is generally already blocked when an interscalene block is performed for this surgery.

Distal block techniques are best suited to supplementing brachial plexus anesthesia, which generally produces denser and longer anesthesia of the forearm. Occasionally, a single nerve is missed with one of the blocks. For forearm surgery, the nerves involved (musculocutaneous and medial antebrachial cutaneous) have already branched extensively at the level of the elbow, and local infiltration of the surgical site is often the best alternative. For hand surgery, a supplemental injection of the involved major terminal nerve at the elbow or wrist can "save" the block.

The more peripheral nerve blocks may be desirable in the patient with coagulation problems when central injections around the subclavian or axillary artery are undesirable. These peripheral techniques also may be useful for minor localized procedures in one nerve distribution, such as wound exploration or repair, simple cyst removal, or scar revision.

Digital nerve block is the simplest form of anesthesia for finger lacerations or drainage of subungual hematomas, but the anesthesia is not as dense as with more proximal blocks. Vasoconstrictors are avoided in this peripheral area.

Drugs

Any of the lower concentrations of short-, intermediate-, or long-duration local anesthetics are appropriate, such as 1% lidocaine or its equivalent, depending on the desired duration of anesthesia. Epinephrine is specifically contraindicated in the digital nerve block and is generally not needed for the other blocks.

Techniques

Suprascapular Block

This block is most easily performed with the patient in the sitting position, and thus is best introduced before shoulder surgery if it is to be used for postoperative analgesia after general anesthesia.

1. The patient is asked to sit and lean forward, resting on a Mayo stand or high table if sedation has been given.
2. The spine of the scapula is identified and marked along its length, forming an oblique line heading up and out toward the shoulder. The midpoint of the spine is identified by drawing a second line vertically from the inferior tip of the scapula (Fig. 14.1). The upper outer quadrant formed by the intersection of these two lines is then bisected by a third line extending an inch from the intersection, where an "X" is drawn.
3. A 4-in. needle is introduced at the "X" and inserted perpendicular to the skin to gently contact the scapula. The needle is then "walked" superior and medially to enter the suprascapular notch. Once the notch is located, the needle is advanced 1 cm.
4. At this point, 10 mL of local anesthetic can be injected with a high probability of success. Paresthesias of the shoulder joint can

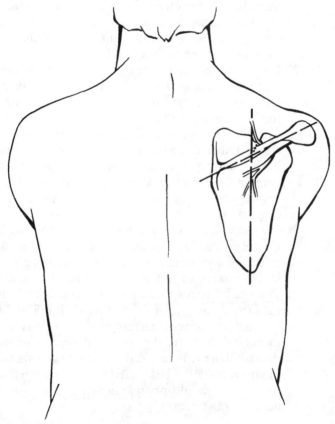

Figure 14.1   **Suprascapular Nerve Block**
The spine of the scapula is marked, and the midpoint identified by the intersection of the line from the tip of the scapula. The notch lies approximately 1 in. above and lateral to the intersection of these lines.

be sought, or the nerve can be stimulated to produce rotation of the humerus.

Elbow Block

Three separate injections are required. Because the branches of the sensory nerves of the forearm have already ramified extensively and cross this joint superficially in a diffuse subcutaneous network, good sensory anesthesia of the forearm itself is difficult to obtain. Blockade of the major nerves here really produces only anesthesia of the hand and is not significantly different from block at the wrist itself. Thus, these techniques are not often employed.

1. For the ulnar nerve, the patient's elbow is flexed approximately 30 degrees and the sulcus of the median condyle of the humerus is identified. Excessive flexion may allow the nerve to roll laterally out of the groove. With a 25-gauge needle, 3 to 5 mL of local anesthetic is injected below the fascia into the groove. Paresthesias may be sought, but are not needed. Intraneural injection or excessive pressure in this tight space should be avoided to reduce the chance of nerve injury.

2. For the median nerve, the elbow is extended and a line is drawn across the arm between the two condyles of the humerus, usually two fingerbreadths above the flexion crease. The pulsation of the brachial artery is identified at the medial aspect of this line. A 1.5-in. 25-gauge needle is inserted on the ulnar side of the artery and directed inward toward the humerus. For the most reliable anesthesia, paresthesias are sought, but they may be unobtainable if partial anesthesia already exists. If they are not found, a "wall" of 5 to 7 mL of solution is placed alongside and deep to the artery.

3. For the radial nerve, the tendon of the biceps is identified along the intracondylar line by asking the patient to flex the muscle. With the arm then extended, a needle is inserted lateral to the biceps tendon in the groove between it and the brachioradialis. The needle is advanced slightly cephalad and medial to contact the lateral condyle of the humerus, and 5 to 7 mL of solution is injected in a fanwise pattern as the needle is withdrawn. A paresthesia will improve the chance of successful anesthesia, because the radial nerve is less easily located than are the median and the ulnar nerves. An additional 3 to 5 mL injected subcutaneously in the groove should provide anesthesia for the lateral cutaneous nerve of the forearm.

Wrist Block

Three separate areas on the palmar surface of the joint must be injected (Fig. 14.2).

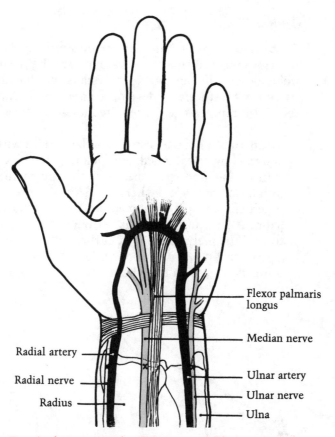

Figure 14.2   **Terminal Nerves at the Wrist**
The median nerve lies just to the radial side of the flexor palmaris longus.
The ulnar and radial nerves lie just "outside" their respective arteries.
The radial nerve has already begun branching at this level and must be
blocked by a wide subcutaneous ridge of anesthetic.

1. The ulnar nerve is blocked with a 25-gauge needle inserted just
   on the ulnar side of the ulnar artery and advanced between it and
   the flexor carpi ulnaris to the ulnar styloid. As the needle is
   withdrawn, 3 to 5 mL of solution is injected.
2. For the median nerve, the tendons of the flexor palmaris longus
   and the flexor carpi radialis are identified by flexing the wrist. A
   needle is inserted between them to the deep fascia, and 3 to 5 mL
   is injected again as the needle is withdrawn.
3. The radial nerve has already branched as it reaches the wrist. In
   addition to injecting 3 mL of solution along the lateral border of
   the radial artery two fingerbreadths above the wrist, a superficial
   ring of solution must be laid from this point extending dorsally
   over the border of the wrist and into the "snuffbox" area created
   by the extensor tendons of the thumb.

Digital Block

The terminal nerves of the fingers are similar and can be blocked by injections on each side of the base of each digit. The most common problem with this form of anesthesia is that insufficient time is allowed for anesthesia to develop before a procedure is undertaken. Ten to 15 minutes may be required for adequate analgesia.

1. The patient's hand is rested on a flat surface with the palm down and the fingers extended. For each finger, an "X" is placed on the skin of the web space between the metacarpal heads. This is usually at the point where the skin texture changes from the rough character of the dorsal hand to the smooth texture of the palm. A 25-gauge needle is introduced here and directed down toward the metacarpal head of the digit to be blocked (Fig. 14.3). Then 1 to 2 mL of solution is injected along the ventral head and 1 mL is injected along the dorsal head to anesthetize both the

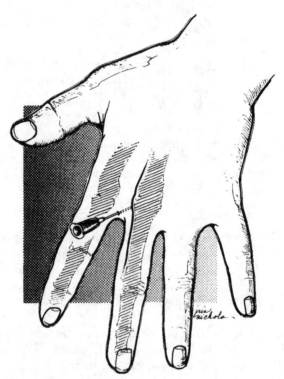

Figure 14.3   **Digital Nerve Block**
A 25-gauge needle is inserted into the dorsal aspect of the web space at a 45-degree angle at the level of the change in skin texture and advanced until the bone is gently contacted. The needle is withdrawn 3 to 4 mm and 2 mL of solution *without epinephrine* is injected in a volar direction and 1 mL is injected along the dorsal aspect of the phalanx.

dorsal and ventral branches. Both sides of each digit must be blocked. For the "outside" aspects of the index and little fingers, the injection is made along the appropriate borders of the hand at the level of the metacarpal heads.

2. For the thumb, similar injections are made on each side of the metacarpal head.

3. No epinephrine is used in these terminal digit blocks.

Complications

Ischemia

Ischemia of the digits is the most serious complication, and it can be prevented by avoiding vasoconstrictors and excessive volumes of injection in digital blocks.

Neuropathy

Neuropathy with any of these techniques is more likely if paresthesias are sought. Higher concentrations of anesthetic solutions may be implicated in their occurrence (see Chapter 3). Intraneural injection (pain on injection) increases this possibility.

Reference

1. Ritchie, E. D., Tong, D., Chung, F., Norris, A. M., Miniaci, A., Vairavanathan, S. D. Suprascapular nerve block for postoperative pain relief in arthroscopic shoulder surgery: A new modality? *Anesth. Analg.* 84: 1306, 1997.

15 Lumbo–Sacral Plexus Blocks

The lumbosacral plexus shares features with the brachial plexus that make single-injection anesthesia possible, but the lumbosacral anatomy is not as conducive to plexus anesthesia as that in the neck. The differences make single-injection techniques more difficult and less reliable, especially when spinal, epidural, and caudal techniques offer effective alternatives. Nevertheless, unilateral anesthesia is occasionally indicated or axial block is contraindicated. On the positive side, postoperative analgesia in the lower extremity is superior to the upper extremity because peripheral nerve blocks last longer in this area, and there are several nerve blocks amenable to continuous catheter insertion that have demonstrated superior analgesia, even when compared to epidural infusions.

Anatomy

The motor and sensory innervation of the lower extremities arises from the nerve roots of the second lumbar through the third sacral spinal segments. The upper branches (L2-4) form the lumbar plexus, which divides into the lateral femoral cutaneous, femoral, and obturator nerves (Fig. 15.1). These supply the upper leg, with a branch of the femoral (the saphenous nerve) extending medially below the knee. The lower roots (L4-S3) form the two major trunks of the sciatic nerve, the tibial and the common peroneal nerves (Fig. 15.2). These provide the bulk of innervation below the knee (Fig. 15.3).

As in the brachial plexus, the nerve roots leave the foramina in a fascial plane between two muscles, composed here of the anterior fascia of the quadratus lumborum muscle and the posterior fascia of the psoas muscle. For the sciatic roots, the posterior border of the compartment becomes the ilium itself. Unfortunately, the "sheath" anatomy is not as convenient here as in the neck. The branches of the lumbar plexus (except the femoral) leave the compartment early in their course, and the sciatic components are protected by the sacral bones in their initial course. Single-injection anesthesia is possible, but the thick muscles of the back make identification of this nerve compartment more difficult. The practical approach to lower-extremity anesthesia thus consists of separate injections for the posterior (sciatic) and anterior (lumbar plexus) branches.

The lumbar plexus branches course anteriorly as they traverse the pelvis (Fig. 15.1). The femoral nerve alone continues in a fascial compartment as it courses behind the psoas and then into the groove between the psoas and the iliacus muscle until it passes under the inguinal ligament. Here it lies just posterior and slightly lateral to the femoral artery, a useful and reliable landmark. Closely

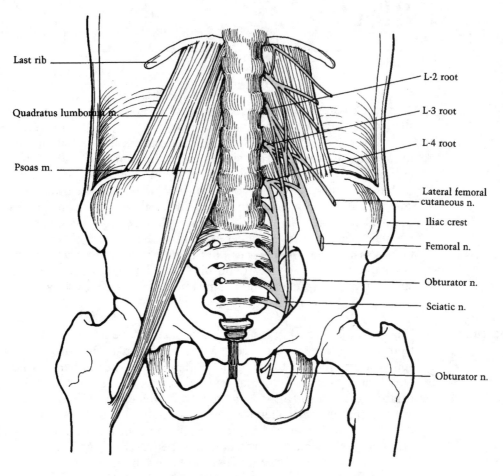

Last rib

Quadratus lumborum m.

Psoas m.

L-2 root

L-3 root

L-4 root

Lateral femoral
cutaneous n.

Iliac crest

Femoral n.

Obturator n.

Sciatic n.

Obturator n.

Figure 15.1   **Psoas Compartment Anatomy**

The roots of the lumbar plexus emerge from their foramina into a fascial plane between the quadratus lumborum muscle posteriorly and the psoas muscle anteriorly. The origin of the lumbosacral plexus is broader than the corresponding brachial plexus in the neck. The lumbar roots form the lateral femoral cutaneous, femoral, and obturator nerves, as shown, and are more likely to be blocked by an injection into this fascial compartment. The lower sacral roots form the sciatic nerve, but they lie in a compartment with a bony posterior and cannot be easily reached by a single injection.

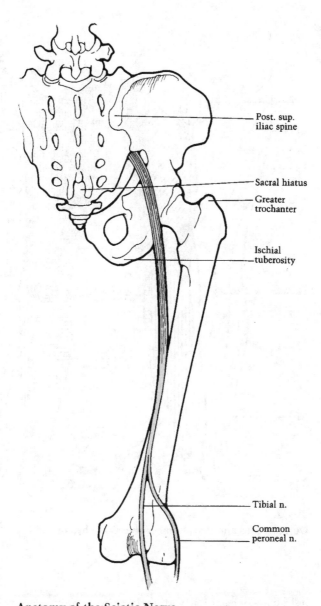

Post. sup.
iliac spine

Sacral hiatus

Greater
trochanter

Ischial
tuberosity

Tibial n.

Common
peroneal n.

Figure 15.2   **Anatomy of the Sciatic Nerve**
The nerve exits the pelvis through the sciatic notch and travels behind
the femur to bifurcate just above the knee into the tibial and common
peroneal nerves.

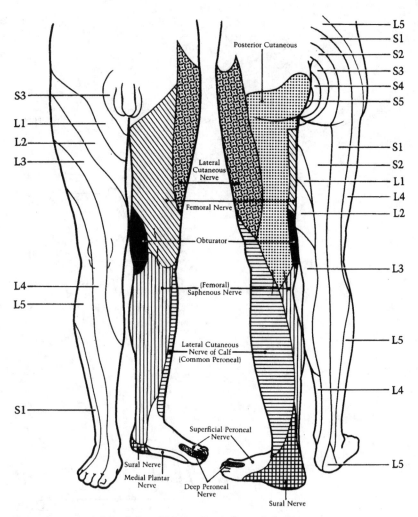

Figure 15.3   **Dermatomes and Peripheral Nerve Branches of the Leg**

below (or occasionally slightly above) the ligament, it branches into several portions, with the main trunk continuing medially across the knee as the saphenous nerve to provide sensory innervation to the medial calf all the way to the ankle and medial aspect of the foot. In contrast, the lateral femoral cutaneous nerve leaves the fascial sheath early and migrates laterally to emerge under the inguinal ligament medial to the anterosuperior iliac spine. From here, its terminal branches provide sensory supply to the lateral thigh. The third branch, the obturator, remains medial and posterior in the pelvis and emerges under the superior ramus of the pubis to pass through the obturator foramen to supply motor and sensory fibers to the medial thigh and the medial border of the knee.

The sciatic nerve is the largest nerve in the body. It is really the union of two major trunks. The roots of L-4 through S-2 form the lateral trunk, the common peroneal nerve, whereas other branches of L-4 through S-3 form the medial trunk, the tibial nerve. The conjoined bundle travels on the anterior surface of the ilium and then exits the pelvis posteriorly through the greater sciatic notch, passing anterior to the piriformis muscle and between the ischial tuberosity and the greater trochanter of the femur (Fig. 15.2). It descends behind the femur to divide into its two constituents at the upper end of the popliteal fossa. The peroneal nerve provides innervation to the anterior calf and dorsum of the foot, whereas the tibial branches remain posterior and serve the sole of the foot (see Chapter 16).

Indications

Sciatic nerve block alone often can provide anesthesia for the sole of the foot and most of the dorsum except for the medial area innervated by the saphenous branch of the femoral nerve. This is a good technique for surgery of the toes, although supplementation is often required if a thigh tourniquet is applied. In this case, femoral and lateral femoral cutaneous anesthesia is usually sufficient supplementation (1).

For knee surgery, combined sciatic–femoral block is sufficient for outpatient knee arthroscopy (2). For knee replacement surgery, single-injection (3) or continuous femoral nerve analgesia (4,5) provide superior postoperative pain relief and rehabilitation. For outpatient knee surgery, single-injection femoral nerve block provides 18 to 24 hours of analgesia following anterior cruciate ligament repair (6). Femoral nerve block is also effective for analgesia after hip surgery (7) or acute hip fracture (8).

If injections of the separate branches are awkward or painful because of fractures or other injuries, the upper plexus can be reached with a large-volume injection in the psoas compartment. This is not as reliable as an axial block, but there are times when the latter is contraindicated because of infection or coagulopathy.

Continuous catheter techniques are possible with psoas block, femoral nerve block, and sciatic anesthesia, and can offer prolonged analgesia without the side effects usually associated with central neuraxial analgesic techniques.

Intravenous regional anesthesia is also possible in the lower extremity (see Chapter 13), although the larger volumes required make it more hazardous.

Drugs

All of the local anesthetic agents used in the leg may have a longer duration than equivalent doses in the brachial plexus. Lidocaine or mepivacaine in 1.5% or 2% concentration may provide 3 hours of surgical anesthesia, but as much as 4 to 6 hours of analgesia. Ropivacaine 0.75% will have a similar onset, but longer analgesia (11 to 14 hours) (1,9). Bupivacaine or levobupivacaine 0.5% with epinephrine has a slower onset, but produces sciatic anesthesia for 18 to 24 hours or longer. Lower concentrations are suitable if less motor blockade is needed. Clonidine added to these peripheral nerve blocks in small doses (1 μg per kg) will prolong analgesia by 25% (10).

Techniques

The common techniques for anesthetizing the nerves of the lumbar and sacral roots near their origin or near the hip joint are described here; more peripheral blocks are detailed in Chapter 16.

Psoas Compartment Block

Theoretically, the simplest approach to the lumbosacral plexus is injection into the psoas compartment or sheath. The fascial planes of the posterior border of the psoas muscle and the anterior border of the quadratus lumborum form the envelope that encloses the nerve roots in a manner similar to the scalene muscles in the neck. This approach usually anesthetizes the lumbar branches of the plexus, but usually does not provide adequate anesthesia of the sciatic plexus.

1. The patient is placed prone or in the lateral position, and the spinous processes of the lumbar vertebrae are identified. An "X" is placed on the skin 5 cm lateral to the third lumbar spinous

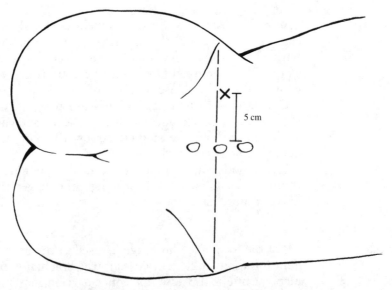

Figure 15.4   **Skin Landmarks for Psoas Compartment Block**

process, similar to the technique described for lumbar paravertebral block (Chapter 10), or along the intercristal line between the
iliac crests (Fig. 15.4).

2. A skin wheal is raised at the "X," and a 4-in. needle is advanced
perpendicular to the skin (Fig. 15.5). The compartment can be
identified by a loss of resistance to injection of fluid or air, as
with entry to the epidural space. The compartment and nerve
roots should be encountered at 7 to 10 cm of depth, depending on
the girth of the patient. A stepwise search is performed in the
cephalad–caudad plane (perpendicular to the known path of the

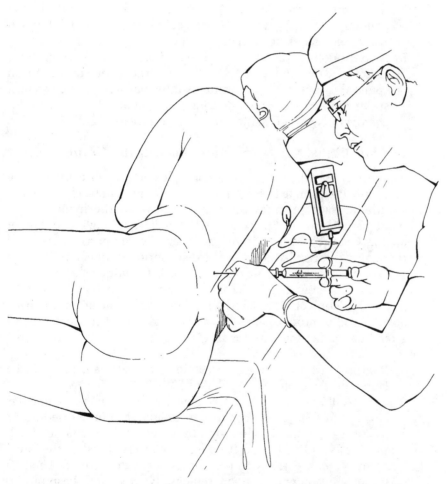

Figure 15.5 **Psoas Compartment Block**
A 4-in. needle is advanced perpendicular to the skin at the "X" until a
loss of resistance (similar to an epidural injection) is obtained. At this
point, compartment entry can be confirmed by eliciting a response to a
nerve stimulator. A catheter can be inserted if continuous analgesia is
desired.

nerve) to obtain a nerve stimulator response or a paresthesia. If the transverse process of the vertebra is encountered, the needle is merely angled caudally to bypass this landmark. Medial angulation will allow the possibility of dural puncture and is avoided.

3. In some patients, the distinct "pop" or release may suffice for localization. This is rare and not as reliable as obtaining a motor response or paresthesia to document the presence of the needle in the nerve compartment.

4. When entry into the compartment is confirmed, aspiration and a test dose are used to confirm the absence of intravascular placement. Then 40 mL of the desired local anesthetic solution is injected, and 15 to 20 minutes is allowed for spread to the roots of the lumbosacral plexus. Anesthesia of the femoral, lateral femoral cutaneous, and obturator nerves is predictable, but sciatic anesthesia is not usually produced.

5. A continuous catheter can be inserted using a large-gauge stimulator needle, and taped in place on the skin similar to an epidural catheter (11). Continuous infusions will provide analgesia in the lumbar plexus distribution, and are thus suitable for postoperative analgesia for hip or knee surgery (12).

Lumbar Plexus Single-Injection Block at the Groin

The three branches of the lumbar plexus theoretically can be blocked with a single injection if a large volume can be placed in the sheath that accompanies the femoral nerve to the inguinal ligament, producing a "three-in-one" block. Although the fascial anatomy suggests a continuity between the compartments of the three nerves, actual studies of the distribution of injectate (13) and measurements of nerve blockade with this technique show that the obturator and branches of the sacral plexus are usually not included in the single-injection block (14,15). Still, single injections are used at this level to produce anesthesia and analgesia of the femoral and lateral femoral cutaneous nerve (11).

1. Preparation for a femoral nerve block is made as described (see Femoral Nerve Block, this chapter).

2. The needle is inserted in a cephalad rather than perpendicular angulation (Fig. 15.6). For this technique, a motor response or paresthesia is sought alongside the artery. When it is obtained, the needle is fixed in position and the artery distal to the entry point is compressed with the fingers of the other hand. Then 40 mL of solution is injected incrementally after careful aspiration, thus theoretically forcing the large volume of solution centrally.

3. If continuous anesthesia is desired, a 14- or 16-gauge intravenous catheter can be inserted in the sheath with a similar technique, or a 20-gauge catheter can be directed cephalad with a Seldinger technique or threaded through a large-bore stimulator needle (Figure 15.6).

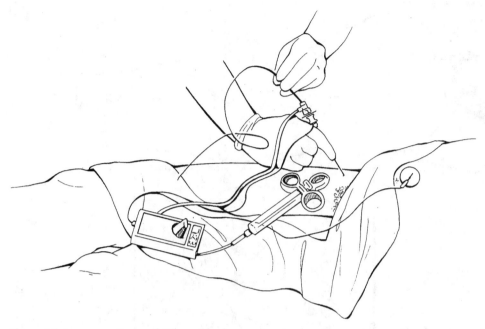

Figure 15.6   **Femoral Nerve Block**
The needle is introduced lateral to the artery and a motor response or a paresthesia is sought. If a large needle is used, a continuous catheter can be inserted.

Sciatic Nerve Block, Posterior Approach

For block of the sciatic nerve, needle localization of the nerve by means of paresthesias or nerve stimulator as it emerges from the sciatic notch is the classic technique.

1. The patient is placed in the lateral position with the leg to be blocked on the upper side (Fig. 15.7). The upper knee and hip are flexed approximately 45 degrees, and the patient is rolled slightly anteriorly. The superior aspect of the greater trochanter of the hip is marked along with the posterosuperior iliac spine. The trochanter must be identified precisely, which is sometimes difficult in the obese patient. A line is drawn between these two marks.

2. A perpendicular line is drawn from the midpoint of this line extending 5 cm caudally. A large "X" is marked here. This spot should overlie the superolateral border of the U-shaped sciatic notch. A second line drawn from the trochanter to the sacral hiatus of the caudal canal should intersect this "X." In the taller patient, an extension of the perpendicular line may be necessary to create an intersection, and the nerve may lie closer to the point where the lines meet.

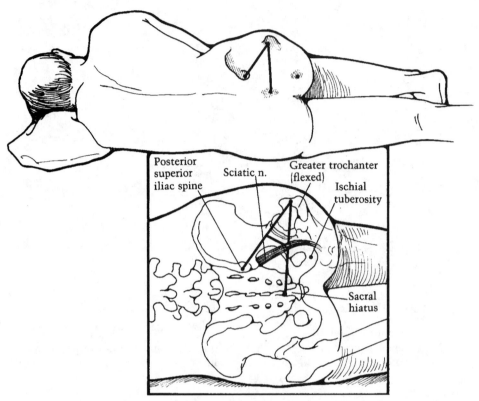

Figure 15.7   **Sciatic Nerve Block, Classic Posterior Approach**
With the patient in the lateral position and the hip and knee flexed, the
muscles overlying the sciatic nerve are stretched to allow easier
identification. The nerve lies beneath a point 5 cm caudad along the
perpendicular line that bisects the line joining the posterior superior iliac
spine and the greater trochanter of the femur. This is also usually the
intersection of that perpendicular with another line joining the greater
trochanter and the sacral hiatus.

3. After aseptic preparation, a skin wheal is raised at the "X" and a
   4-in. needle is introduced perpendicular to all planes of the skin.
   The needle is advanced gently until a motor response or paresthesia is obtained, or bone is encountered. If bone is encountered, the depth and location are noted. The nerve will lie only
   slightly deeper. The bone is usually the lateral border of the
   notch, and it indicates that more medial angulation is needed.
   The needle is withdrawn almost to the skin and redirected along
   a line perpendicular to the presumed course of the nerve until it
   is located. If bone is again encountered, the location is noted and
   a mental map of the rim of the sciatic notch is constructed. The
   nerve emerges from the medial side to the center of the notch
   and curves downward to course midway between the trochanter

and the ischial tuberosity. Drawing this imagined path can aid the search pattern in the difficult patient.

4. If the bone is at the full depth of the needle, a longer (6 in.) needle may be necessary. Blind infiltration is rarely successful. Reassessment of the landmarks is advised if more than 10 minutes is required for success.

5. When a motor response or paresthesia is obtained in one of the main trunks, 25 mL of local anesthetic is injected while the needle is held immobile. Redirecting the needle slightly to produce a second stimulation in the distribution of the other nerve and dividing the dose appears to improve the quality of the block (16). If the patient experiences pain or a cramping sensation in the leg on injection, the needle is withdrawn until the sensation disappears.

6. Continuous infusion is also possible if a Tuohy needle is used to introduce a catheter with the same technique (11).

Sciatic Nerve, Lithotomy Approach

If the patient cannot turn to the lateral position, the nerve can be approached in the supine position if an assistant is available to hold the leg in flexion.

1. With the patient in the supine position, an assistant flexes the hip and holds the leg up at 90 degrees. A line is drawn from the greater trochanter to the ischial tuberosity, and an "X" is marked at the midpoint.

2. After aseptic preparation, a skin wheal is raised and a 4-in. needle is introduced at the "X." A motor response or paresthesia is sought along the direction of the line (perpendicular to the course of the nerve), and 25 mL of anesthetic is injected when the nerve is located.

Sciatic Nerve, Anterior Approach

If the hip cannot be flexed, the nerve can be sought anteriorly in the supine position. A greater distance must be traversed by the needle, with a corresponding decrease in accuracy and reliability. This is the least reliable approach.

1. With the patient in the supine position, the line joining the anterosuperior iliac spine and the pubic tubercle is drawn. A second line is drawn parallel to this one starting at the level of the greater trochanter of the femur and extending medially. The upper line is divided into thirds, and a perpendicular line is drawn from the junction of the medial and middle thirds to the bottom line; an "X" is placed at the intersection.

2. A 6-in. needle is introduced at the "X" and advanced directly posterior until the lesser trochanter of the femur is contacted.

The needle is then redirected, "walked" medially off the bone, and advanced 2.5 cm further, searching for a motor response or paresthesia of the sciatic nerve.

3. A 25-mL volume of local anesthetic is injected in the vicinity of the nerve. If the nerve is elusive, the local anesthetic may be injected 2.5 cm beyond the lesser trochanter, with the hope that the fascial compartment contains the nerve, but the reliability of anesthesia is obviously decreased.

Femoral Nerve Block

The femoral nerve is approached in its reliable position just lateral and posterior to the femoral artery below the inguinal ligament.

1. With the patient in the supine position, an "X" is placed immediately lateral to the femoral artery pulse 2.5 cm below the inguinal ligament (Fig. 15.8). At this level, usually near the inguinal crease, the nerve lies closer to the artery than at the level of the ligament itself (17).
2. After aseptic preparation, a skin wheal is made at the "X" and a 22-gauge 1.5- or 2-in. needle is introduced perpendicularly. As the needle is passed, the index finger of the opposite hand identifies the femoral pulsation so that the needle lies immediately lateral to the vessel. In a thin patient, 2.5 cm of needle depth is sufficient to reach the area of the nerve. When the hands are removed, the needle should be close enough to the vessel to display visible movement with each pulsation.
3. A 10-mL syringe of local anesthetic is attached, and careful aspiration is performed. Then 3 to 5 mL of anesthetic is injected as the needle is withdrawn 1.5 cm, and again as it is reinserted 1.5 cm slightly laterally (away from the artery). This procedure is repeated with a second syringe of anesthetic, so that a total of 20 mL is injected in a fanlike pattern lateral to the artery. For this technique, paresthesias are not necessary and are rarely encountered. The pattern of injection produces a generous wall lateral and superficial to the main nerve to ensure anesthesia of superficial sensory branches that leave the main trunk at or above the inguinal ligament.
4. If the artery is entered, the needle is merely withdrawn and redirected laterally.
5. Alternatively, a nerve stimulator can be used, which searches for quadriceps contraction. Injection of 25 mL of anesthetic will produce anesthesia within 20 minutes. If the nerve stimulator is used to produce multiple responses of the various branches of the femoral nerve trunk (vastus medialis, vastus intermedius, and vastus lateralis), smaller quantities of anesthetic can be placed on each of the major branches and faster onset of blockade ensues (18).

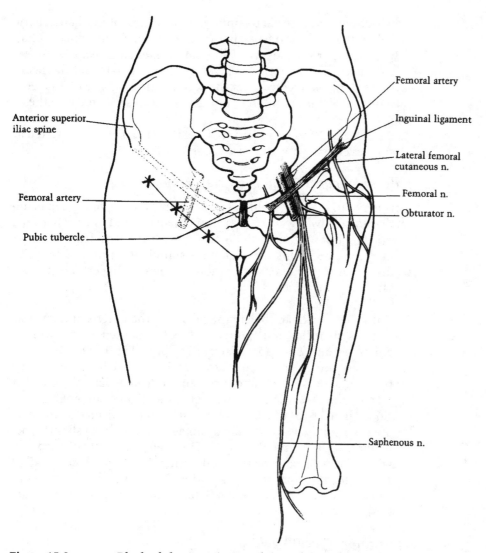

Figure 15.8   **Block of the Anterior Lumbosacral Branches in the Groin**
The lateral femoral cutaneous nerve emerges approximately 2.5 cm medial to the anterior superior iliac spine and is best blocked along that line 2.5 cm caudad to the anterior superior iliac spine. The femoral nerve emerges alongside and slightly posterior to the femoral artery, and is again easily approached approximately 2.5 cm below the inguinal ligament. On that same line, the obturator nerve emerges from the obturator canal, but it is deeper and less reliably located.

6. Another alternative is to simply inject 25 mL of local anesthetic below the level of the fascia iliaca. A needle is introduced a half inch lateral to the artery at this same level and advanced to feel two distinct penetrations of fascia, the fascia lata and the fascia iliaca. Drug is injected after the second release (14,15). This technique is useful in children, but also produces reliable anesthesia in adults.

7. As described above, a continuous catheter can also be inserted at this level using any of these techniques.

Lateral Femoral Cutaneous Nerve Block

This nerve to the lateral thigh has a variable course, but it can be reliably blocked by a wall of anesthesia medially and inferiorly to the anterior iliac spine, and usually occurs with standard femoral nerve block. Blockade of this nerve alone is sufficient for muscle biopsies of the thigh in patients with whom malignant hyperthermia susceptibility is suspected.

1. With the patient in the supine position, the anterosuperior iliac spine is identified and marked. An "X" is marked on the skin 2.5 cm below and 2.5 cm medial to this spine (Fig. 15.8).

2. After aseptic preparation, a 22-gauge 1.5-in. needle is introduced through a skin wheal and directed 45 degrees laterally until it pierces the fascia lata. This is felt as a slight "popping" sensation. Then 3 to 5 mL of anesthetic solution is injected as the needle is withdrawn slowly, and again as it is reinserted slightly medially to again pierce the fascia. The needle is "walked" medially while injecting on insertion and withdrawal to produce a wall of 15 to 20 mL of anesthetic solution 5 cm wide extending both above and below the fascia lata. Again, no paresthesias are sought.

Obturator Nerve Block

Anesthesia of this nerve is more challenging because of the deeper location and the early branching of the nerve. Again, a wide wall of anesthetic solution is employed to block the path of the nerve with the traditional approach; a smaller volume of anesthetic solution is required if a nerve stimulator is used to locate the nerve precisely. Isolated blockade of this nerve is sometimes useful in treating spasticity of muscles of the lower leg.

1. With the patient in the supine position, the pubic tubercle is identified and the lateral border is marked. An "X" is marked 1.5 cm below and 1.5 cm lateral to the tubercle. Note that if a line is drawn from the tubercle to the anterosuperior iliac spine, the marks for all three branches of the lumbar plexus lie approximately 2.5 cm lower and also in a line (Fig. 15.8).

2. After aseptic preparation, a skin wheal is raised and a 22-gauge 3-in. needle is introduced slowly until it contacts bone. This should be the inferior ramus of the pubis, and redirection of the needle slightly lateral and caudad will move it off the bone and into the obturator foramen (Fig. 15.9). The needle is advanced a further 2 to 3 cm. After aspiration, 5 mL of anesthetic is injected as the needle is withdrawn, and again as it is reinserted with a slight lateral direction. This process is repeated to produce a wall of 20 mL of solution across the path of the nerve in the foramen.
3. Alternatively, a nerve stimulator can be used to search for the nerve in this area, and 10 mL of solution is injected when an adductor response is elicited in the thigh.

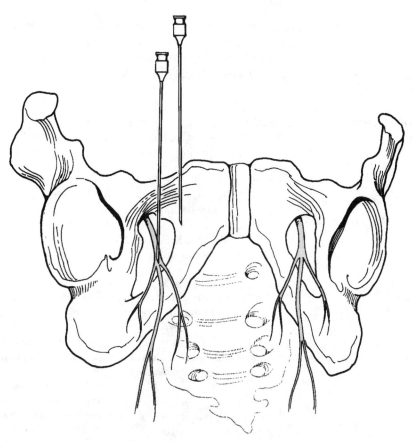

Figure 15.9   **Obturator Nerve Anatomy**
A 3-in. needle is introduced perpendicular to the skin at the "X" indicated in Fig. 15.5, 1.5 cm below and lateral to the pubic tubercle. When it contacts the inferior ramus of the pubis, it is redirected slightly lateral and caudad to enter the obturator foramen. A "wall" of anesthesia is then created by injection of 20 mL of anesthetic as the needle is withdrawn and reinserted more laterally. Localization is more difficult because the nerve does not lie in close proximity to a bony or vascular landmark.

Complications

Systemic Toxicity

Systemic toxicity is best avoided by frequent aspiration and incremental injection combined with heart rate monitoring with epinephrine-containing solutions. Large total volumes are required if multiple nerves (as in the four-nerve combination) are blocked, and systemic toxicity is possible from slow absorption in these patients. Careful attention must be paid to the total milligram dose when large volumes are injected, and lower concentrations are mandatory if safe limits are not to be exceeded.

Neuropathy

Neuropathy can be produced by intraneural injection or may rarely be associated with needle trauma. It should not be confused with the extremely long duration of anesthesia that is possible with bupivacaine in the sciatic distribution.

References

1. Fanelli, G., Casati, A., Beccaria, P., Aldegheri, G., Berti, M., Tarantino, F., Torri, G. A double-blind comparison of ropivacaine, bupivacaine, and mepivacaine during sciatic and femoral nerve blockade. *Anesth. Analg.* 87: 597, 1998.
2. Casati, A., Cappelleri, G., Fanelli, G., Borghi, B., Anelati, D., Berti, M., Torri, G. Regional anaesthesia for outpatient knee arthroscopy: A randomized clinical comparison of two different anaesthetic techniques. *Acta Anaesthesiol. Scand.* 44: 543, 2000.
3. Allen, H. W., Liu, S. S., Ware, P. D., Nairn, C. S., Owens, B. D. Peripheral nerve blocks improve analgesia after total knee replacement surgery. *Anesth. Analg.* 87: 93, 1998.
4. Capdevila, X., Barthelet, Y., Biboulet, P., Ryckwaert, Y., Rubenovitch, J., d'Athis, F. Effects of perioperative analgesic technique on the surgical outcome and duration of rehabilitation after major knee surgery. *Anesthesiology* 91: 8, 1999.
5. Singelyn, F. J., Gouverneur, J. M. Extended "three-in-one" block after total knee arthroplasty: Continuous versus patient-controlled techniques. *Anesth. Analg.* 91: 176, 2000.
6. Mulroy, M. F., Larkin, K. L., Batra, M. S., Hodgson, P. S., Owens, B. D. Femoral nerve block with 0.25% or 0.5% bupivacaine improves postoperative analgesia following outpatient arthroscopic anterior cruciate ligament repair. *Reg. Anesth. Pain Med.* 26: 24, 2001.
7. Singelyn, F. J., Vanderelst, P. E., Gouverneur, J. M. Extended femoral nerve sheath block after total hip arthroplasty: Continuous versus patient-controlled techniques. *Anesth. Analg.* 92: 455, 2001.
8. McGlone, R., Sadhra, K., Hamer, D. W., Pritty, P. E. Femoral nerve block in the initial management of femoral shaft fractures. *Arch. Emerg. Med.* 4: 163, 1987.
9. Casati, A., Fanelli, G., Borghi, B., Torri, G. Ropivacaine or 2% mepivacaine for lower limb peripheral nerve blocks. Study Group on Orthope-

dic Anesthesia of the Italian Society of Anesthesia, Analgesia, and Intensive Care. *Anesthesiology* 90: 1047, 1999.
10. Casati, A., Magistris, L., Fanelli, G., Beccaria, P., Cappelleri, G., Aldegheri, G., Torri, G. Small-dose clonidine prolongs postoperative analgesia after sciatic-femoral nerve block with 0.75% ropivacaine for foot surgery. *Anesth. Analg.* 91: 388, 2000.
11. Chelly, J., Casati, A., Fanelli, G., *Continuous Peripheral Nerve Block Techniques*. London: Mosby, 2001.
12. Chudinov, A., Berkenstadt, H., Salai, M., Cahana, A., Perel, A. Continuous psoas compartment block for anesthesia and perioperative analgesia in patients with hip fractures. *Reg. Anesth. Pain Med.* 24: 563, 1999.
13. Marhofer, P., Nasel, C., Sitzwohl, C., Kapral, S. Magnetic resonance imaging of the distribution of local anesthetic during the three-in-one block. *Anesth. Analg.* 90: 119, 2000.
14. Capdevila, X., Biboulet, P., Bouregba, M., Barthelet, Y., Rubenovitch, J., d'Athis, F. Comparison of the three-in-one and fascia iliaca compartment blocks in adults: Clinical and radiographic analysis. *Anesth. Analg.* 86: 1039, 1998.
15. Ganapathy, S., Wasserman, R. A., Watson, J. T., Bennett, J., Armstrong, K. P., Stockall, C. A., Chess, D. G., MacDonald, C. Modified continuous femoral three-in-one block for postoperative pain after total knee arthroplasty. *Anesth. Analg.* 89: 1197, 1999.
16. Bailey, S. L., Parkinson, S. K., Little, W. L., Simmerman, S. R. Sciatic nerve block. A comparison of single versus double injection technique. *Reg. Anesth.* 19: 9, 1994.
17. Vloka, J. D., Hadzic, A., Drobnik, L., Ernest, A., Reiss, W., Thys, D. M. Anatomical landmarks for femoral nerve block: A comparison of four needle insertion sites. *Anesth. Analg.* 89: 1467, 1999.
18. Casati, A., Fanelli, G., Beccaria, P., Cappelleri, G., Berti, M., Aldegheri, G., Torri, G. The effects of the single or multiple injection technique on the onset time of femoral nerve blocks with 0.75% ropivacaine. *Anesth. Analg.* 91: 181, 2000.

16 Peripheral Nerve Blocks of the Lower Extremity

For surgery of the foot itself, the branches of the sciatic and femoral nerves can be blocked below the hip, either at the knee or at the ankle.

Anatomy

The two main branches of the sciatic nerve pass behind the femur as separate trunks enclosed in a single epineural sheath. They separate in the popliteal fossa to form the tibial and common peroneal nerves. The upper border of this fossa lies at the peak of the triangle formed by the biceps femoris and semitendinosus muscles behind the knee. The actual separation of the trunks occurs somewhere between the popliteal crease and 10 cm above this level (1). Here the nerves lie midway between the skin and the femur and superficial to the popliteal vessels. The branches of the tibial and common peroneal nerves then ramify into the muscles of the anterior and posterior tibial compartments. The terminal branches to the foot itself can be identified as they cross the ankle joint, where the mass of bone displaces the nerves superficially again. The major trunk to the sole of the foot is the posterior tibial nerve, which lies just anterior and medial to the Achilles tendon, coursing with the posterior tibial artery just behind the tibial bone at the level of the medial malleolus. The major branch to the dorsum of the foot, the deep peroneal nerve, also accompanies its artery (the anterior tibial) as it crosses the very front of the ankle joint behind the tendon of the extensor hallicus longus and also just above the tibial bone. The other two branches of the sciatic nerve are quite superficial. The superficial peroneal branches splay across the front of the ankle joint, while the sural nerve to the lateral border of the foot lies subcutaneously behind the lateral malleolus.

The femoral nerve sends one terminal sensory branch to the foot. The saphenous nerve crosses the knee joint medially and passes superficially over the head of the tibia. It is superficial again as it passes anterior to the medial malleolus to provide sensation to a variable area of the medial border of the foot.

Indications

Ankle block is sufficient for most operations of the foot itself, including bunionectomy and neuroma excision. Some local infiltration of the periosteum may be necessary. If a calf tourniquet is to be used (or if fewer injections are preferred), the knee approach is appropriate and effective (2,3). The latter is also simpler for the patient and the anesthetist, although it will include loss of some motor

217

ability in the foot. This limitation is not as severe as with the blocks at the hip region, because the thigh muscles are spared by these techniques.

Drugs

Lower concentrations of the intermediate- or long-duration amino-amides are ideal for these blocks. As in sciatic block, 0.5% bupivacaine or ropivacaine may produce anesthesia for 12 to 24 hours at the ankle (4), and 15 to 18 hours at the knee (5). A high concentration is not necessary for the usual foot procedures. Clonidine in doses of 10 μg per mL will significantly prolong the duration of lidocaine analgesia (6).

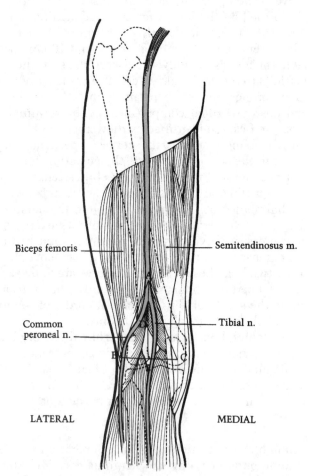

Biceps femoris

Semitendinosus m.

Common peroneal n.

Tibial n.

LATERAL

MEDIAL

Figure 16.1

Popliteal Fossa Block
The two major trunks of the sciatic bifurcate in the popliteal fossa 7 to 10 cm above the knee. A triangle is drawn using the heads of the biceps femoris and the semitendinosus muscles and the skin crease of the knee; a long needle is inserted 1 cm lateral to a point 6 cm cephalad on the line from the skin crease that bisects this triangle.

Techniques Blockade at the knee is a simple and effective procedure that is very useful for ambulatory surgery; it can be performed with either nerve stimulator or paresthesia technique, from either the posterior or lateral approach. The lateral approach may take a little longer, but both approaches produce good anesthesia (7).

Popliteal Fossa Block: Posterior Approach

1. The patient is placed in the prone position, and the popliteal fossa is outlined by drawing a line over the interior borders of the biceps femoris muscle and the tendon of the semitendinosus. The base of the triangle is formed by the skin crease behind the knee. If the muscles are poorly defined, the patient can assist by flexing the knee 20 or 30 degrees.
2. The triangle is then bisected by a perpendicular line from the base to the apex. Six centimeters up this line an "X" is drawn 1 cm lateral to the bisecting line (Fig. 16.1).
3. After skin is prepared and a local anesthesia skin wheal is raised, a 3-in. needle is inserted through the "X" and directed 45 degrees cephalad (Fig. 16.2). If a motor response or paresthesia is not obtained, the needle is withdrawn back to the skin and redirected in a search pattern perpendicular to the course of the nerve. The nerve should lie midway between the skin and the bone.
4. When a motor response or paresthesia is obtained, the needle is withdrawn slightly and 30 to 40 mL of local anesthetic is in-

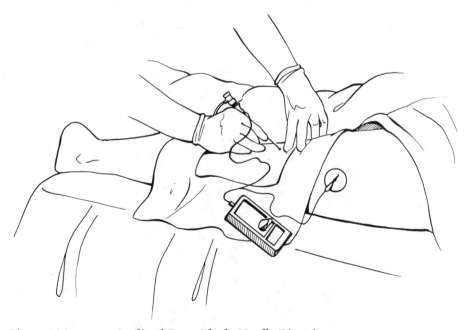

Figure 16.2 **Popliteal Fossa Block, Needle Direction**
The needle is inserted at the point described in Fig. 16.1 and angled 45 degrees cephalad. The nerves will usually be contacted halfway between the skin and the femur.

jected. If pain or cramping is felt on injection, the needle is withdrawn further.

5. For prolonged analgesia, a continuous catheter can be inserted
   through a large-bore stimulator needle or with a Seldinger technique (8), as with femoral nerve catheters.

6. The femoral branches can be blocked by subcutaneous injection
   of 5 to 10 mL of solution over the medial tibial head just below
   the knee. This is advisable if surgery will involve the medial aspect of the foot or if a tourniquet will be used on the calf. Adequate anesthesia should ensue 20 minutes after injection.

Popliteal Fossa Block: Lateral Approach

1. With the patient in the supine position, the groove between the
   biceps femoris and vastus lateralis muscles is located on the lateral side of the leg, and an "X" is drawn at the level of the upper
   border of the patella.

2. After skin anesthesia, a 4-in. needle is introduced at this point
   (Fig. 16.3) and directed 30 degrees posterior (Fig. 16.4), and a motor response or paresthesia is sought in the foot (5,9). Foot move-

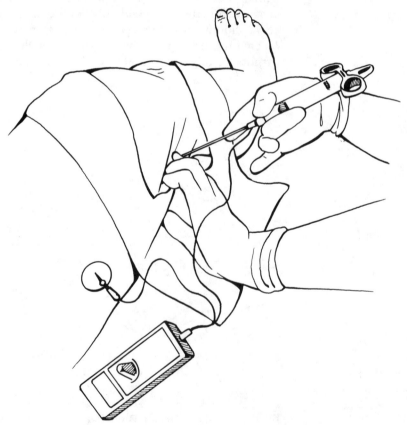

Figure 16.3   Lateral Approach

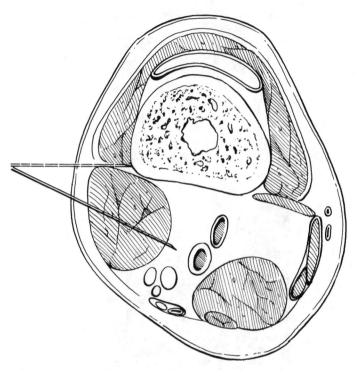

Figure 16.4   **Cross-sectional View of Lateral Approach**

ment in response to the nerve stimulator will lead to successful block, but a higher frequency of success can be obtained by searching for two separate responses (dorsal flexion or eversion for the common peroneal, and plantar flexion or eversion for the tibial) and making two injections (10). Injection of 30 to 40 mL of local anesthetic on a single response, or 10 mL on each separate response, is sufficient.
3. As with the posterior approach, separate injection of the femoral nerve is required.

Ankle Block

The ankle-block technique involves more injections and thus may be more time consuming, but it can be performed without seeking paresthesias. A ring of anesthesia is produced that blocks all five branches of the foot (Fig. 16.5). Alternatively, for distal operations, local blockade of terminal branches can be performed.

1. *Posterior tibial nerve.* This can be performed with the patient in the prone or supine position. If the patient is supine, the knee is flexed to bring the sole of the foot flat on the bed surface. A 1.5-in. 23- to 25-gauge needle is introduced at the level of the medial

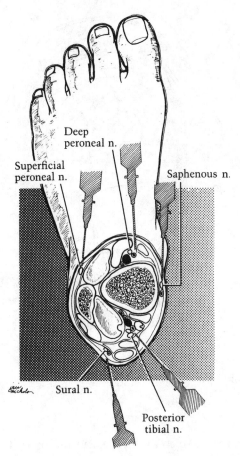

Figure 16.5   **Ankle Block**
Injections are made at five separate nerve locations. The superficial peroneal nerve, the sural nerve, and the saphenous nerve are usually blocked simply by subcutaneous infiltration, because they may have already generated many superficial branches as they cross the ankle joint. Paresthesias can be sought in the posterior tibial nerve or the deep peroneal, but the bony landmarks will usually suffice to provide adequate localization for the deeper injections.

malleolus just behind the posterior tibial artery pulsation and is directed 45 degrees anteriorly to seek a paresthesia in the sole of the foot. Then 5 mL of anesthetic will be sufficient if the nerve is located. If the nerve is not located, 10 mL can be injected in a fan-shaped area in the triangle formed by the tibia, the artery, and the Achilles tendon.

2. *Sural nerve.* With the patient still either prone or supine with the knee flexed, 5 mL more is injected superficially behind the lateral malleolus to fill the groove between the malleolus and the calcaneous.

3. *Saphenous nerve.* Next, 5 mL is injected around the saphenous vein at the level of the medial malleolus between the skin and the bone itself.
4. *Deep peroneal nerve.* Moving to the front of the ankle, a needle is inserted into the deep planes below the fascia just lateral to the anterior tibial artery at the level of the skin creases and 5 mL more is injected. If the artery is not palpable, the tendon of the extensor hallicus longus can be used as a landmark.
5. *Superficial peroneal branches.* A subcutaneous ridge of anesthetic solution is laid down from the anterior tibia around to the lateral malleolus (overlying the previous injection of the deep peroneal nerve and continuing laterally to meet the previous injection for the sural nerve). A total of 5 to 10 mL may be required to cover the 2 to 3 in. necessary to catch all of these superficial fibers.

Complications

Neuropathy

Neuropathy is the most likely problem with peripheral nerve blocks. Sharp-beveled needles, multiple paresthesias, and excessive concentrations of anesthetic should be avoided, as well as direct intraneural injection. With ankle block, care must be exercised not to pin the nerve against the bones with the needle at the time of injection. The use of epinephrine with a distal injection near the terminal sensory nerves of the toes should be avoided.

References

1. Vloka, J. D., Hadzic, A., April, E., Thys, D. M. The division of the sciatic nerve in the popliteal fossa: Anatomical implications for popliteal nerve blockade. *Anesth. Analg.* 92: 215, 2001.
2. Hansen, E., Eshelman, M. R., Cracchiolo, A., 3rd. Popliteal fossa neural blockade as the sole anesthetic technique for outpatient foot and ankle surgery. *Foot Ankle Int.* 21: 38, 2000.
3. Singelyn, F. J., Gouverneur, J. M., Gribomont, B. F. Popliteal sciatic nerve block aided by a nerve stimulator: A reliable technique for foot and ankle surgery. *Reg. Anesth.* 16: 278, 1991.
4. McLeod, D. H., Wong, D. H., Vaghadia, H., Claridge, R. J., Merrick, P. M. Lateral popliteal sciatic nerve block compared with ankle block for analgesia following foot surgery. *Can. J. Anaesth.* 42: 765, 1995.
5. Zetlaoui, P. J., Bouaziz, H. Lateral approach to the sciatic nerve in the popliteal fossa. *Anesth. Analg.* 87: 79, 1998.
6. Reinhart, D. J., Wang, W., Stagg, K. S., Walker, K. G., Bailey, P. L., Walker, E. B., Zaugg, S. E. Postoperative analgesia after peripheral nerve block for podiatric surgery: Clinical efficacy and chemical stability of lidocaine alone versus lidocaine plus clonidine. *Anesth. Analg.* 83: 760, 1996.

7. Hadzic, A., Vloka, J. D. A comparison of the posterior versus lateral approaches to the block of the sciatic nerve in the popliteal fossa. *Anesthesiology* 88: 1480, 1998.

8. Singelyn, F. J., Aye, F., Gouverneur, J. M. Continuous popliteal sciatic nerve block: An original technique to provide postoperative analgesia after foot surgery. *Anesth. Analg.* 84: 383, 1997.

9. Vloka, J. D., Hadzic, A., Kitain, E., Lesser, J. B., Kuroda, M., April, E. W., Thys, D. M. Anatomic considerations for sciatic nerve block in the popliteal fossa through the lateral approach. *Reg. Anesth.* 21: 414, 1996.

10. Paqueron, X., Bouaziz, H., Macalou, D., Labaille, T., Merle, M., Laxenaire, M. C., Benhamou, D. The lateral approach to the sciatic nerve at the popliteal fossa: One or two injections? *Anesth. Analg.* 89: 1221, 1999.

17 Airway

Anesthesiologists frequently intubate patients for whom the routine thiobarbiturate–succinylcholine induction technique is not appropriate. Adequate regional or topical anesthesia of the nasal and pharyngeal airway makes the painless passage of nasal or oral endotracheal tubes or fiberoptic bronchoscopes possible in these patients.

Anatomy

Sensory fibers of the nasal mucosa arise from the middle division of the fifth cranial nerve by means of the sphenopalatine ganglion. This major branch lies under the nasal mucosa posterior to the middle turbinate (Fig. 17.1). Fibers from this ganglion also provide sensory innervation for the superior portion of the pharynx, uvula, and tonsils. These fibers can be blocked proximally by direct injection of the maxillary branch of the trigeminal nerve, but they are more easily approached by transmucosal topical application of local anesthetic.

The ninth cranial nerve (glossopharyngeal) provides the sensory innervation of the oral pharynx and supraglottic regions, as well as the posterior portion of the tongue. This nerve can be blocked by direct submucosal injection behind the tonsillar pillar, but it is more easily approached by topical anesthesia of its terminal branches in the mouth and throat.

Sensation in the larynx itself above the vocal cords is provided by the superior laryngeal branch of the vagus. This nerve departs the main vagal trunk in the carotid sheath and courses anteriorly, sending an internal branch that penetrates the thyrohyoid membrane. Behind this membrane, the nerve branches to provide sensory innervation to the cords, epiglottis, and arytenoids.

Below the vocal cords, sensory innervation is provided by branches of the recurrent laryngeal nerve, which also provides motor fibers to all but one of the intrinsic laryngeal muscles. Sensation in the trachea itself is also a function of the recurrent laryngeal nerve. Although direct blockade of this nerve is possible (and is seen as a side effect of several other regional-block techniques in the neck), topical anesthesia is again the simplest approach.

Indications

In the presence of facial trauma or distortion of the upper airway by abscess or malignancy, it is safer to perform tracheal intubation with the patient awake or lightly sedated. This is also appropriate in the presence of a history of previously difficult intubation, cervical radiculopathy, and severe respiratory distress. Familiarity with these techniques is suggested by the American

225

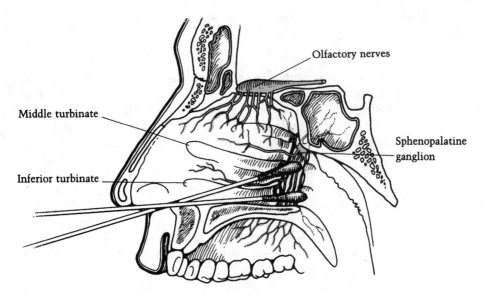

Figure 17.1   **Nasal Airway Anesthesia**
Cotton pledgets soaked with anesthetic are inserted along the inferior and
middle turbinates to produce anesthesia of the underlying sphenopalatine
ganglion by transmembrane diffusion of the solution. Wide pledgets are
needed to provide maximal topical anesthesia and vasoconstriction of the
nasal mucosa as well.

Society of Anesthesiologists (ASA) guidelines for airway management (1,2).

Nasal mucosal anesthesia is useful if a nasal tube is passed, and
is particularly helpful if a vasoconstrictor is used to reduce the
chance of mucosal bleeding. Anesthesia of the mouth and oral
pharynx will allow introduction of both the laryngoscope and the
tube down to the level of the epiglottis, and is also helpful when
transesophageal echocardiography is performed on a patient who
is awake. Anesthesia of the larynx and trachea themselves (by
blockade of the branches of the vagus nerve) allows the patient to
tolerate insertion of the tube or fiberoptic scope below the cords
without coughing or bucking (3), and will reduce the significant
cardiovascular responses usually associated with tracheal intubation. Blockade of laryngeal sensation may be contraindicated,
however, if there is concern about vomiting and aspiration. Tracheal anesthesia is also unwise if preservation of active cough reflexes is desired.

Airway anesthesia is also useful in facilitating diagnostic fiberoptic laryngoscopy, and may help agitated intubated patients in intensive care units tolerate the presence of an endotracheal tube.

Drugs   Direct blockade of the superior laryngeal nerves can be performed by infiltration with local anesthetic agents such as 1% or 1.5% lidocaine. The other innervation of the airway is just as easily approached by topical anesthesia. Higher concentrations of local anesthetics are required for topical application to overcome the usual slow penetrance of the drugs across mucosal membranes. Commercial preparations of local anesthetics (such as 10% flavored lidocaine) are available as oral sprays, but the delivered quantity cannot be measured. A better approach is to nebulize a known quantity of anesthetic (such as 10 mL of 4% lidocaine) with an atomizer such as those used in otolaryngology. Lidocaine 4% and tetracaine 0.5% to 1% are available for transtracheal injection or oral topical application in this manner. These high concentrations carry the obvious risk of rapidly exceeding the maximum recommended doses of these agents. This problem is further compounded by the common practice of using unmeasurable quantities of several different drugs for the multiple blocks performed.

Nasal anesthesia carries the additional requirement for vasoconstriction to reduce the incidence of bleeding from the nasal mucosa. Cocaine 4% has been the traditional agent of choice because it is the only local anesthetic with intrinsic vasoconstrictor properties. Because of cocaine's high toxicity and abuse potential, the use of 3% lidocaine with 0.25% phenylephrine may be a better alternative for nasal topical anesthesia.

Technique Airway anesthesia can be performed with the patient in the supine position, but it is often more comfortable for the patient if it is done with the head slightly elevated or in the sitting position.

1. For the nasal mucosa, cotton pledgets on long applicators are soaked in 4% cocaine (or a mixture of lidocaine–phenylephrine) and inserted gently into both nares. The first applicator is inserted directly posterior along the inferior turbinate to the posterior pharyngeal wall (Fig. 17.1). A second applicator is inserted with a slight cephalad angle to follow the middle turbinate and again is advanced to its full depth until it touches the mucosa over the sphenoid bone. Anesthesia is performed bilaterally, because the object is to provide anesthesia of the branches of the sphenopalatine ganglion as well as topical anesthesia of the mucosa itself. Two to 3 minutes of contact time is usually required to provide adequate penetration of the agent into the mucosa. Cotton-tipped applicator sticks are available in most operating rooms, and are tolerated by patients. The more generous sized pledgets used by otolaryngologists are less comfortable, but more effective in providing adequate surface area for delivery of the anesthetic.

2. While the nasal applicators are in place, the superior laryngeal nerves are blocked bilaterally. The patient's head is extended, and the thyroid cartilage and hyoid bone are identified. The index finger retracts the skin down over the superior ala of the thyroid cartilage, and the skin is wiped with an alcohol swab. A 23- or 25-gauge needle on a 5-mL syringe filled with 1% lidocaine is inserted onto the tip of the cartilage. The index finger then releases the skin traction, and the needle is "walked off" the cartilage superiorly and is inserted just through the firm thyrohyoid membrane. The tip now lies in the loose areolar tissue plane beneath the membrane (Fig. 17.2). After aspiration to detect unwanted intravascular placement, 2.5 mL is injected into the plane beneath the membrane. This sequence is repeated on the opposite side.

   Alternatively, the needle can be inserted onto the posterior (greater) cornu of the hyoid bone and "walked" caudad off the bone onto the membrane.

   If a transtracheal injection (step 4) is to be performed, this syringe and needle can be used to inject a final 0.3-mL local-anesthetic intradermal wheal over the cricothyroid membrane in the midline of the neck.

3. The mouth and pharynx are anesthetized topically. A total of 4 mL 4% lidocaine or 0.5% tetracaine is placed in an atomizer. The tongue is sprayed with local anesthetic, and then the patient is asked to gargle with the residue. Next, the numbed tongue is grasped with a dry gauze sponge and gently held with one hand. The patient is then in-

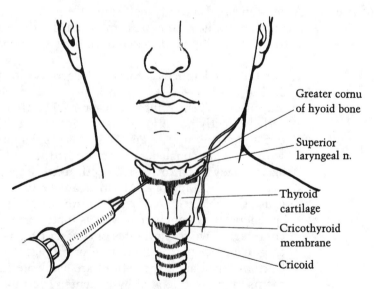

Figure 17.2 **Superior Laryngeal Nerve Block**
The 23- to 25-gauge needle is introduced onto the superior border of the lateral wing of the thyroid cartilage. It is then gently advanced off the cartilage to drop through the thyrohyoid membrane. After gentle aspiration to exclude intravascular injection, 2 to 3 mL of local anesthetic are injected into the space below the membrane.

structed to pant vigorously ("like a puppy") while the rest of the local anesthetic is sprayed into the posterior pharynx with each inspiration. The anesthesia provided by the superior laryngeal block should allow the patient to aspirate the nebulized anesthetic without gagging and will provide some tracheal anesthesia.

4. Direct submucosal injection into the base of the anterior tonsillar pillar will produce denser anesthesia and gag suppression (2). After initial topical anesthesia, the tongue is retracted medially with a tongue depressor, revealing the inferior curve of the anterior tonsillar pillar (Fig. 17.3). A 25-gauge spinal needle is used to

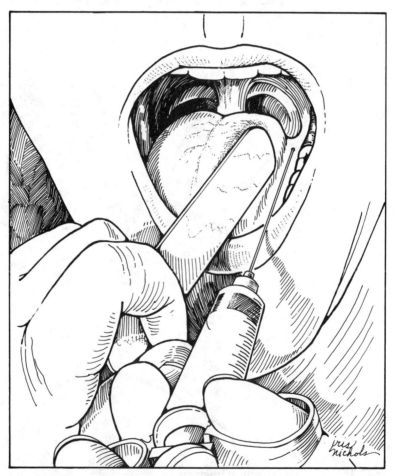

Figure 17.3   **Glossopharyngeal Nerve (Lingual Branch) Block**
The tongue is pushed medially with a tongue depressor, and a spinal needle is inserted into the base of the anterior tonsillar pillar 0.5 cm lateral to the base of the tongue and advanced 0.5 cm deep. After aspiration of the needle, 2 mL of local anesthetic is injected. Both sides need to be injected for adequate block of the gag reflex. A three-ring syringe makes aspiration easier, and the use of a 3-in. (spinal) needle allows better visualization of the injection site while the hand remains outside the mouth.

inject 2 mL of 1% lidocaine 0.5 cm below the mucosa at a point 0.5 cm lateral to the base of the tongue itself. The longer length of the spinal needle will allow easier control by permitting the syringe itself to remain outside the mouth. Aspiration is performed before injection to detect intravascular placement or advancement of the needle through the posterior border of the pillar. Bilateral injection is needed to block both lingual branches of the glossopharyngeal nerve. The risks of intravascular injection and the greater discomfort make simple topical anesthesia a better choice for most patients.

5. Finally, the trachea is topically anesthetized by transtracheal injection. A 20-gauge plastic intravenous catheter with a metal

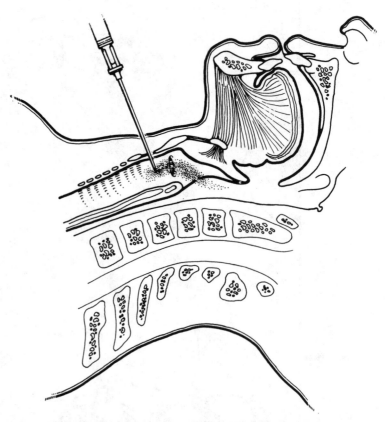

Figure 17.4 **Transtracheal Injection**
A 20-gauge intravenous catheter is introduced through the cricoid membrane. After tracheal entry is confirmed by air aspiration, the metal introducer is removed, and a syringe is attached to the plastic needle, which is left in place. Four mL of topical anesthetic is injected as the patient inspires; the inward air flow will carry the solution down the trachea, and the usual reflex cough will spread it up to the undersurface of the vocal cords.

stylet is introduced through the cricothyroid membrane through the previously injected skin wheal (Fig. 17.4). Entry into the trachea is confirmed by aspiration of air. The metal stylet is removed, and a syringe with 4 mL 4% lidocaine is attached to the plastic cannula remaining in the trachea. The lidocaine is injected as the patient inspires; the spray will produce a cough that will spread the solution up the trachea to the level of the cords.

6. As an optional addition to the topical anesthesia of the nasal passages, the applicators can be removed and a soft rubber nasal airway coated with lidocaine cream can be inserted. If a series of these nasal airways are introduced in sequentially larger sizes, they will dilate the nasal passages and will help lubricate them for eventual passage of an endotracheal tube. With a large airway in place, a final spray of nebulized lidocaine by this route will be delivered almost directly to the vocal cords.

7. If the nasal airways are not used, the nasal applicators are removed and endotracheal tube insertion is begun. The interval required for the other blocks is usually sufficient to allow development of nasal and oral anesthesia. If the trachea itself was not anesthetized, the anesthesiologist must be ready to administer rapidly acting intravenous sedation or anesthesia to blunt the cardiovascular and coughing reflexes that will occur when the tube passes below the cords.

Complications

Systemic Toxicity

Systemic toxicity is the most likely adverse outcome, owing to absorption rather than intravascular injection. Although not all the local anesthetic is absorbed, the total quantities used, as shown in Table 17.1 are significant.

Resuscitation equipment should be at hand, and the patient must be observed closely during the block and for at least 20 minutes after completion of the block.

Table 17.1   **Common Dosages Used for Airway Anesthesia**

Drug	Amount (cc)	Concentration	Total Milligrams	Percentage Maximum Recommended Dose
Cocaine	3	4%	120	60
Tetracaine	5	1%	50	25
Lidocaine	5	1%	50	
	4	4%	160	40

Epistaxis

Epistaxis may occur even with the use of a vasoconstrictor in the nose. Gentle insertion and generous lubrication of the tube will reduce this possibility, whereas the presence of a deformity or coagulopathy will increase the risk.

Aspiration

Aspiration of gastric contents may occur if anesthesia of the cords and trachea is created in the presence of reflux or active vomiting. These techniques should be used with caution (or not at all) if there is significant risk of aspiration.

References

1. Practice guidelines for management of the difficult airway. A report by the American Society of Anesthesiologists Task Force on Management of the Difficult Airway. *Anesthesiology* 78: 597, 1993.
2. Benumof, J. L. Management of the difficult adult airway. With special emphasis on awake tracheal intubation. *Anesthesiology* 75: 1087, 1991.
3. Graham, D. R., Hay, J. G., Clague, J., Nisar, M., Earis, J. E. Comparison of three different methods used to achieve local anesthesia for fiberoptic bronchoscopy. *Chest* 102: 704, 1992.

18 Facial and Head Nerve Blocks

Surgery of the head is rarely performed with regional anesthesia alone, but facility with blockade of the nerves of the head is useful in many diagnostic and therapeutic pain procedures.

Anatomy

Sensory fibers to the posterior scalp arise from the upper cervical roots and course upward over the occiput as the greater and lesser occipital nerves (Fig. 18.1). These nerves can be blocked superficially on the posterior scalp or more centrally by blockade of the deep cervical plexus (see Chapter 19). The anterior portion of the scalp and the face are innervated by the branches of the trigeminal nerve. The three main branches of this cranial nerve are the ophthalmic, maxillary, and mandibular. These produce (respectively) the three main terminal sensory nerves of the face: the supraorbital, the infraorbital, and the mental (Fig. 18.2). These nerves can be blocked at their superficial foramina or more centrally just beyond their trifurcation and exit from the skull.

The trigeminal nerve arises from the base of the pons and sends its sensory fibers to the large gasserian (or semilunar) ganglion on the superior margin of the petrous bone just above the foramen ovale. Direct alcohol neurolysis of this ganglion for total trigeminal ablation has been practiced in the past. The risks of intracranial spread of the neurolytic solution are significant. Radiofrequency ablation by a neurosurgeon using fluoroscopic guidance is more common today.

The three branches of the ganglion depart the skull through separate exits. The uppermost ophthalmic nerve enters the orbit through the sphenoidal fissure. Its main branch, the frontal nerve, bifurcates into the supraorbital and supratrochlear nerves. The former exits the superior border of the orbit at the supraorbital notch, whereas the latter departs the orbit more medially (Fig. 18.3).

The middle branch of the trigeminal, the maxillary nerve, is also purely sensory, but it is somewhat larger than the ophthalmic nerve. It exits the skull through the foramen rotundum and crosses the sphenomaxillary fossa medial to the lateral pterygoid plate to reenter the bone of the floor of the orbit in the infraorbital canal (Fig. 18.2). In the fossa, it gives off the sphenopalatine branches medially to the pharynx (see Chapter 17), and the orbital and posterior dental branches. The anterior dental branches arise from the main trunk while in the canal. The infraorbital nerve that finally emerges

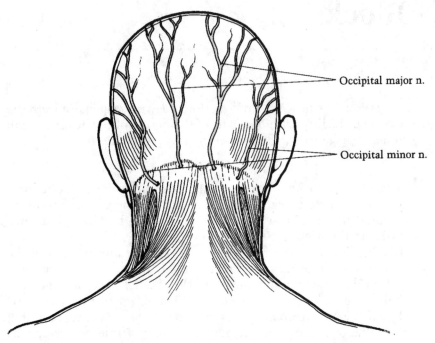

Occipital major n.

Occipital minor n.

Figure 18.1   **Occipital Nerve Block**
The greater and lesser branches of the occipital nerve emerge from under
the muscles at the level of the nuchal ridge on the posterior scalp. They
can be easily blocked by a subcutaneous ridge of anesthetic solution.

from the infraorbital foramen just below the eye branches into the
palpebral, nasal, and labial nerves.

The mandibular branch is the largest branch of the ganglion, and
it exits the skull through the foramen ovale. It lies just posterior to
the lateral pterygoid plate of the sphenoid bone. It contains the only
motor fibers of the trigeminal, the branches to the muscles of mastication. These nerves are carried by an anterior branch that separates from the nerve just after its exit from its cranial foramen. The
posterior branch gives off an early auriculotemporal nerve that provides sensory innervation to the auricular and temporal regions of
the lateral scalp. The main trunk continues as the inferior alveolar
nerve to the lower jaw. Its terminal branch is the mental nerve,
which exits the mental foramen to supply the lower lip and jaw (Fig.
18.2).

All three of the main trunks lie deep and are well protected by the
skull, the mandible, and the zygomatic arch. The terminal branches
are superficial, and their foramina are relatively easily identified.
Conveniently, the three external foramina lie in the same sagittal
plane (Fig. 18.3).

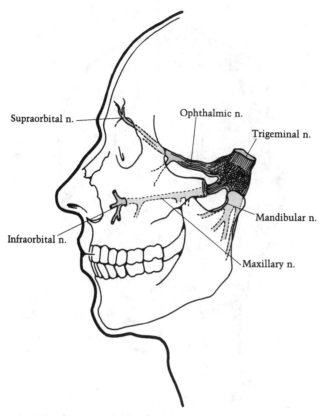

Figure 18.2
Trigeminal Nerve, Sagittal View
Each of the three main branches of the trigeminal nerve exits the skull through its own foramen and provides sensory innervation of the face and jaw.

Indications
Surgical indications for anesthesia of any of these pathways are rare. Performance of cranial burr holes on the debilitated patient can be done with occipital nerve blocks and field infiltration. Generally, anesthesia of the branches of the trigeminal nerve is used only in attempts to diagnose and treat pain complaints. Occasionally, a patient with tic douloureux involving a branch of the trigeminal nerve will respond to block of the nerve with local anesthetic or a neurolytic agent. Incapacitating pain of malignancy also can be relieved by a neurolytic block, although the advent of radiation, chemotherapy, and radiofrequency ablation techniques has made this requirement rare. Occipital nerve block is occasionally useful in relieving some headaches, but it is rarely an adequate long-term therapy.

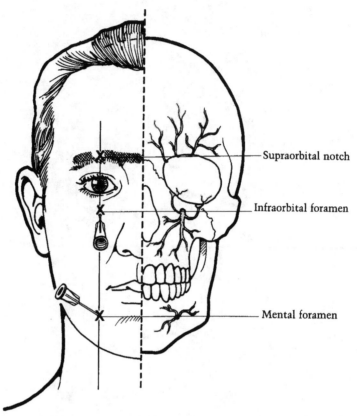

Figure 18.3

Terminal Branches of the Trigeminal Nerve
Each of the three terminal branches (the supraorbital, infraorbital, and mental) exits its respective bony canal in the same sagittal plane, approximately 2.5 cm from the midline. The infraorbital canal is angled slightly cephalad, whereas the mental canal can be entered if the needle is directed medial and slightly caudad.

Drugs

Any of the local anesthetics in lower concentrations are appropriate for facial or head blocks. Bupivacaine or ropivacaine 0.25% are probably best for diagnostic blocks, because their longer duration may help differentiate some physiologic pain complaints from those of psychological origin and may help the patient who is considering a neurolytic procedure.

Alcohol is the preferred neurolytic agent for facial blocks (see Chapter 23), but this therapy is usually reserved for patients who are not candidates for radiofrequency ablation.

Techniques

Occipital Nerve Block

The greater and lesser occipital nerves emerge from under the muscles of the neck on each side to become superficial at the level of the nuchal line, the prominent ridge of bone extending from the mastoid to the external occipital protuberance (Fig. 18.1).

1. The patient is asked to sit with the head flexed toward the chest.
2. The external occipital protuberance is palpated, and an "X" is marked on the involved side at this level just lateral to the insertion of the erector muscles of the neck (usually 2.5 cm laterally from the midline).
3. After the skin is wiped with an alcohol swab, a 23-gauge needle is inserted at the "X" and is advanced gently until it contacts the bone. It is withdrawn slightly, and a ridge of 3 mL of local anesthetic is injected under the mark and on either side of it.
4. If lesser occipital nerve block is also desired, the needle is then angled anteriorly and laterally along the skull, and the subcutaneous injection is extended from this area forward to the area of the mastoid process. A total of 6 to 8 mL will usually suffice.
5. Care is taken not to advance the needle under the angle of the occiput toward the foramen magnum.
6. If anesthesia of the entire scalp is desired, the subcutaneous wheal is carried around the entire circumference of the scalp, but it is angled so that it crosses above the ear on each side and extends at this same level anteriorly.

Facial Anesthesia

The three terminal sensory branches of the trigeminal nerve can be blocked at their respective foramina. For all three blocks, the patient lies supine with the head slightly elevated.

1. For the supraorbital nerve, the supraorbital notch is palpated along the superomedial rim of the orbit, usually 2.5 cm from the midline. Paresthesias should be elicited in the notch if a neurolytic agent is to be injected, but, for simple anesthesia, 2 mL can be injected in the area. For medial (supratrochlear) anesthesia, a line of superficial infiltration at the level of the orbital rim should be continued medially to cross the midline.
2. The infraorbital nerve exits its foramen just below the inferior orbital rim and at the same distance from the midline as the supraorbital notch (approximately 2 cm from the lateral border of the nose). The foramen can be palpated directly or discovered with a gentle, exploring 23-gauge needle. The needle should be introduced through a skin wheal 0.5 cm below the anticipated level of the opening, because the canal angles cephalad from this point (Fig. 18.3). Once the foramen is identified, 2 mL of local anesthetic is injected at the orifice. If a neurolytic agent is used, paresthesias are necessary and 1 mL alcohol is sufficient.
3. The mental nerve canal of the mandible also lies 2.5 cm from the midline, usually about midway between the upper and lower borders of the mandible. Again, the opening usually can be pal-

pated directly, but it can be marked with an approximate "X" and explored for gently with a 23-gauge needle. The canal angles medially and inferiorly such that needle insertion should not be perpendicular to its opening but should start 0.5 cm above and 0.5 cm lateral to the orifice (Fig. 18.3). Injection of 2 mL of anesthetic in the foramen will anesthetize the nerve. If a neurolytic agent is used, paresthesias are again necessary and smaller quantities are sufficient. In older patients, resorption of the mandibular bone will cause the foramen to lie relatively more superiorly along the mandible.

Maxillary Nerve Block

When tic douloureux or neuralgia of the middle division (presenting as both facial and upper dental pain) requires more proximal block, the maxillary nerve is blocked in the sphenopalatine fossa.

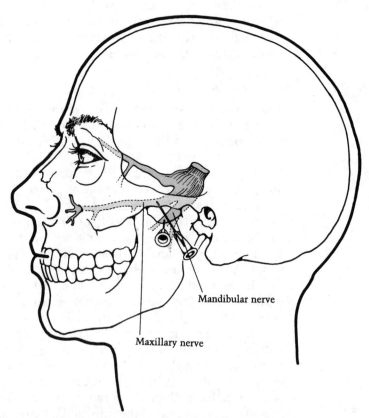

Mandibular nerve

Maxillary nerve

Figure 18.4   **Lateral View of Major Branches of the Trigeminal Nerve**
The maxillary and mandibular branches emerge from the skull medial to the lateral pterygoid plate, which serves as the landmark for their identification. A needle introduced onto the plate can be advanced anterior for the maxillary nerve and posterior for the mandibular nerve.

1. The patient lies supine with the head turned slightly away from the side to be blocked.
2. The zygomatic arch is identified and marked. The patient is then asked to open and close the mouth slowly while an index finger explores the upper border of the mandible. The mandibular notch will be felt moving up and down anterior to the temporo-mandibular joint at the midpoint of the zygoma (Fig. 18.4). An "X" is marked over the notch at its deepest point.
3. After aseptic preparation, a skin wheal is raised at the "X."
4. A 7.5-cm needle is introduced through the "X" and directed 45 degrees cephalad and slightly anterior, aiming at the imagined position of the back of the globe of the eye itself.
5. When the pterygoid plate is contacted, the needle is withdrawn and redirected slightly anteriorly. When the needle succeeds in passing anterior to the pterygoid plate, the nerve lies about 1 cm deeper (Fig. 18.5). Paresthesias to the nose or upper teeth confirm the appropriate location.

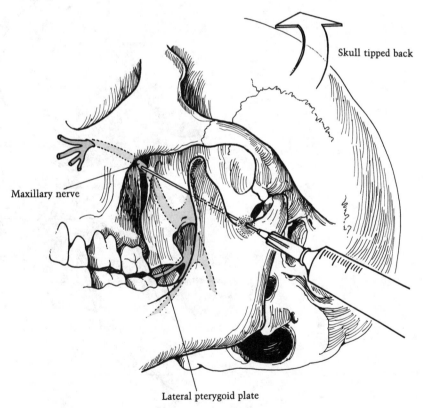

Skull tipped back

Maxillary nerve

Lateral pterygoid plate

Figure 18.5   **Lateral Approach to the Maxillary Nerve**
The needle is introduced through the skin just over the notch of the mandible and is directed anterior and cephalad to identify the pterygoid plate. As the needle is advanced anteriorly off the plate, the maxillary nerve is encountered before it reenters the skull in the infraorbital canal in the base of the orbit.

6. If paresthesias are not obtained, anesthesia can be achieved by injecting 5 mL into the fossa 1 cm deep to the plate. For a neurolytic block, a paresthesia is essential, and 1 mL alcohol will suffice. Alcohol injection is painful, and the head must be secured by an assistant during the injection to prevent movement. Sedation or analgesia is appropriate after localizing paresthesias are obtained.

Mandibular Nerve Block

The mandibular nerve also can be blocked for neuralgia, tic problems, or cancer pain, but anesthesia here may induce some weakness of the muscles of mastication.

1. The position and superficial landmarks are the same as for the maxillary nerve (steps 1 to 3; Fig. 18.4).

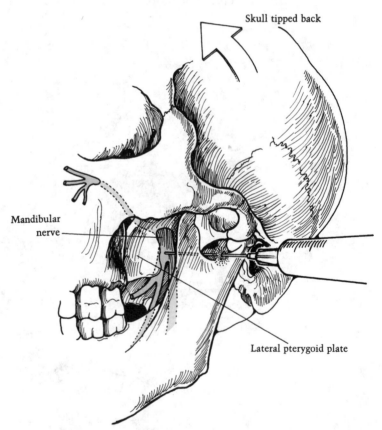

Skull tipped back

Mandibular nerve

Lateral pterygoid plate

Figure 18.6   **Lateral Approach to the Mandibular Nerve**
The needle is introduced in the same manner as for maxillary nerve block, but it is directed posteriorly. After contacting the pterygoid plate, it is directed further posteriorly until it passes behind the plate, where it should encounter the nerve.

2. A 5-cm needle is introduced through the skin wheal and directed medially and slightly posteriorly (Fig. 18.6). Less cephalad angulation is required. The needle will usually be perpendicular to the skin in all planes.
3. The needle is advanced until bone is contacted. This will be the posterior border of the lateral pterygoid plate. The needle is redirected posteriorly off the plate and should contact the nerve 0.5 to 1.0 cm deep to this point.
4. Paresthesias of the jaw or teeth confirm identification of the nerve. If not obtained, they may be sought by gently exploring cephalad and caudad. In the absence of paresthesias, 5 to 10 mL of solution may be injected 0.5 cm deep to the posterior border of the plate with reasonable confidence that it will produce anesthesia. Careful aspiration and test doses are required because of the proximity of the middle meningeal artery.
5. If alcohol is to be used, 1 mL will suffice, but paresthesias are essential. Again, injection is painful, and the same precautions should be employed as with the maxillary block.

Complications

Systemic Toxicity

Systemic toxicity is possible because of the proximity of blood vessels to many of these nerves. Unintentional injections under pressure into the arterial circulation of the head can produce rapid high intracerebral levels and convulsions. Careful aspiration and incremental injection are needed.

Spread of Anesthetic

Spread of anesthetic is occasionally seen, most commonly to the facial nerve when large volumes are injected to block the mandibular nerve. Retrobulbar block of the nerves in the orbit is also possible when maxillary nerve block is performed. These are of little consequence unless a neurolytic agent is used, but blindness can result if the optic nerve is damaged with a neurolytic agent.

Hematoma Formation

Hematoma formation is also possible in these highly vascular areas, but, again, it is rarely of long-term consequence. Easily reversible defects of coagulation mechanisms should probably be treated before employing these techniques.

19 Cervical Plexus Blocks

The nerve roots of the second, third, and fourth cervical vertebrae supply sensory and motor fibers to the neck and posterior scalp. Direct plexus anesthesia provides the usual motor and sensory anesthesia to its distribution. The anatomy of the superficial plexus allows blockade of just the sensory fibers.

Anatomy

The cervical vertebrae are unusual in that their elongated transverse processes include a medial passage for the ascent of the vertebral artery and a well-formed trough (sulcus) for the emergence of their respective nerve roots lateral to the artery (Fig. 19.1). Each sulcus has a posterior and anterior tubercle, which often can be palpated easily in the neck. The anterior divisions of the second through fourth roots form an extensive plexus that provides motor innervation for the muscles of the neck and sensation for the occipital region, the neck below the mandible, and the shoulder above the clavicle. The most significant motor fibers are the contributions of the third, fourth, and fifth roots to the phrenic nerve.

All of the fibers emerge (like the brachial plexus) between the anterior and middle scalene muscles. The anterior scalenes are attenuated at this level but still form a landmark for the cervical plexus, as they do for the brachial plexus. The cervical motor branches curl around the lateral border of the anterior scalene muscle and proceed caudad and medially toward the muscles of the neck, giving anterior branches to the sternocleidomastoid (SCM) muscle as they pass behind it. The sensory fibers also emerge from behind the scalene, but they continue laterally and emerge superficially under the posterior border of the SCM to ramify to both the anterior and posterior skin of the neck.

Indications

Superficial cervical plexus anesthesia provides sensory anesthesia to the skin of the neck and shoulder above the clavicle and is useful for providing superficial anesthesia for thyroidectomy or tracheostomy incisions. If motor relaxation is desired, deep cervical plexus blockade is required. Even with deep plexus anesthesia, the surgeon may occasionally need to supplement the block with local anesthesia, particularly around the upper pole of the thyroid, which has some sensory innervation from cranial nerves. Blockade does provide good postoperative analgesia (1). It is also possible to perform carotid surgery with this block, although some local infiltration of the glossopharyngeal branches around the carotid sinus may be required. Superficial plexus block alone appears to be sufficient for this surgery (2).

243

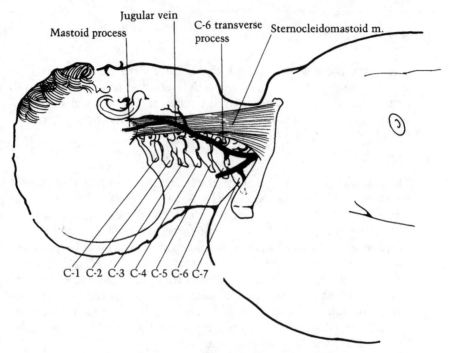

Figure 19.1   **Anatomy of Deep Cervical Plexus Block**
The transverse processes lie under the lateral border of the
sternocleidomastoid muscle, each with a distal trough or sulcus that
defines the path of nerve exit.

Shoulder anesthesia can be obtained with deep cervical plexus anesthesia, but is usually provided by the interscalene approach to the
brachial plexus, which inevitably blocks the lower cervical fibers. The
latter approach may even be preferable in shoulder surgery patients
owing to the motor relaxation of the arm. Cervical plexus block can
be combined with thoracic epidural anesthesia for breast surgery.

Drugs   For surgery, any of the intermediate- or long-acting amino-amides
are appropriate. Lower concentrations are sufficient for the superficial (sensory) block, but higher concentrations such as 1.5% lidocaine or 0.5% bupivacaine (or ropivacaine) will give better motor
anesthesia with deep plexus block. All of the drugs will demonstrate a slightly shortened duration in the neck compared to other
peripheral areas because of the generous blood supply of the region.

Techniques   For both deep and superficial blocks, the patient is placed supine
with a small towel under the occiput and the head turned to the side
opposite the one to be blocked.

Deep Cervical Plexus Anesthesia

1. The mastoid process is identified and marked, as is the transverse process of the sixth cervical vertebra. This is the most prominent tubercle in the neck, and it lies at the level of the cricoid cartilage.
2. A line is drawn between these two points, indicating the plane of the transverse processes of the cervical vertebrae (Fig. 19.2). The lateral border of the SCM muscle is also marked.
3. Starting 1.5 cm below the mastoid, gentle palpation is used to identify the tubercle of the second vertebra just posterior (about 0.5 cm) to the first line. An "X" is placed over this process.
4. The third and fourth processes are identified and marked in the same fashion by moving 1.5 cm caudad for each level. The third mark should fall approximately at the level of the junction of the external jugular vein and the SCM muscle.
5. After aseptic preparation, a skin wheal is raised at each of the three "X" marks.
6. A 3.5-cm 22-gauge needle is introduced perpendicular to the skin and is directed posterior and slightly caudad at each "X" until it rests on the transverse process. A palpating finger of the opposite hand helps in guiding the placement.
7. Placement on the transverse process is confirmed by "walking" the needle caudad and cephalad; it should slip off the bone of the process rather than continuing to contact bone, as it would if on the vertebral body (Fig. 19.1). The latter situation is undesirable because the needle is not near the nerve, but is more likely to produce intravascular or subarachnoid injection.

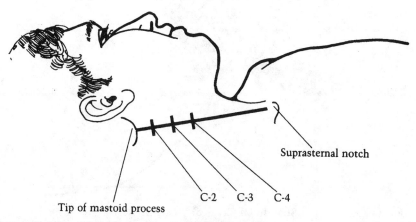

Suprasternal notch

C-2   C-3   C-4

Tip of mastoid process

Figure 19.2   **Superficial Landmarks for Cervical Plexus Block**
A line is drawn from the mastoid process to the prominent tubercle of the sixth cervical vertebra. The transverse processes of the second, third, and fourth cervical vertebrae lie 0.5 cm posterior to this line, and at 1.5-cm intervals below the mastoid.

8. A syringe is attached to each needle in turn while it is securely held in place just above the transverse process. Then 3 to 5 mL of anesthetic solution is injected in small increments with frequent aspiration and assessment of the patient's mental status.
9. Onset of anesthesia should occur within 5 minutes.

An alternative is to use a variation of the interscalene technique with a nerve stimulator. A single stimulating needle is introduced into the groove between the muscles at the C4-5 level (at the upper border of the thyroid cartilage). Stimulation of the levator scapulae muscle produces elevation and internal rotation of the scapula, and injection of a single bolus of 40 mL of anesthetic produces plexus blockade (3).

Superficial Cervical Plexus Anesthesia

Superficial cervical plexus anesthesia is performed with the patient in the same position as for deep plexus anesthesia.

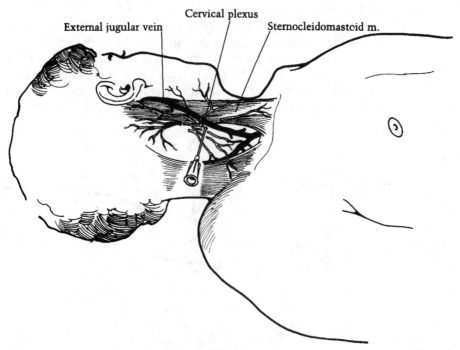

Figure 19.3   **Superficial Cervical Plexus Block**
The sensory fibers of the plexus all emerge from behind the lateral border of the sternocleidomastoid muscle. A needle inserted at its midpoint, usually where the external jugular vein crosses the muscle, can be directed superiorly and inferiorly to block all of these terminal branches.

1. An "X" is made at the level of the transverse process of the fourth cervical vertebra, as described, or simply at the junction of the external jugular vein with the posterior border of the SCM muscle.
2. After aseptic preparation, a skin wheal is made at the "X."
3. A 5-cm needle is introduced through the wheal, and local infiltration is performed along the posterior border of the SCM muscle 4 cm above and below the level of the "X" (Fig. 19.3). This may require 10 mL of anesthetic solution to block all of the superficial sensory fibers.

Complications

Central Nervous System Toxicity

Central nervous system toxicity is the most serious consequence of deep cervical plexus block, owing to the proximity of the vertebral artery to the injection site. Multiple careful aspirations are required, and injections should be in small increments (1.0 to 1.5 mL), with careful monitoring of the patient's mental status.

Spinal Anesthesia

Spinal anesthesia is also easily produced because the cervical roots carry long sleeves of dura through their intervertebral foramina. These may be entered easily if the needle is directed cephalad in the sulcus. Maintaining a caudad direction helps prevent entry of the needle too far medially. Again, careful aspiration and incremental injection are appropriate.

Phrenic Nerve Block

Phrenic nerve block is inevitable, and deep cervical plexus block should be used with caution in any patient who is dependent on the diaphragm for ventilation. Fortunately, most patients have adequate tidal ventilation from their intercostal muscles, and many phrenic nerve blocks are simply undetected. Bilateral blockade obviously increases the possibility that this complication may become symptomatic.

Recurrent Laryngeal Nerve–Vagus Nerve Block

Recurrent laryngeal nerve–vagus nerve block also can occur and, again, is a troublesome but not serious complication. The only potential problem is the inability to assess laryngeal function following thyroidectomy.

Hematoma Formation

Hematoma formation in the neck also can occur if a major vessel is entered. This is distressing only when it interferes with the anticipated surgery, as in the case of carotid endarterectomy.

References

1. Dieudonne, N., Gomola, A., Bonnichon, P., Ozier, Y. M. Prevention of postoperative pain after thyroid surgery: A double-blind randomized study of bilateral superficial cervical plexus blocks. *Anesth. Analg.* 92: 1538, 2001.
2. Pandit, J. J., Bree, S., Dillon, P., Elcock, D., McLaren, I. D., Crider, B. A comparison of superficial versus combined (superficial and deep) cervical plexus block for carotid endarterectomy: A prospective, randomized study. *Anesth. Analg.* 91: 781, 2000.
3. Merle, J. C., Mazoit, J. X., Desgranges, P., Abhay, K., Rezaiguia, S., Dhonneur, G., Duvaldestin, P. A comparison of two techniques for cervical plexus blockade: Evaluation of efficacy and systemic toxicity. *Anesth. Analg.* 89: 1366, 1999.

20 Ophthalmic Anesthesia

Surgery of the eye is usually performed with regional anesthesia, or even topical anesthesia for simple cataract extraction. Ophthalmology patients are frequently older and more likely to have systemic diseases, and they are most likely to profit from regional blockade without heavy systemic sedation or general anesthesia.

Anatomy

Sensation in the eye is transmitted through afferent fibers from the cornea and conjunctiva, which pass through the ciliary ganglion in the retrobulbar space to the first branch (ophthalmic division) of the fifth cranial nerve. Motor innervation of the extraocular muscles is through the motor fibers of the third (oculomotor) cranial nerve to all of the muscles of the eye except the lateral rectus (innervated by the sixth [abducens] nerve) and the superior oblique (innervated by the fourth [trochlear] nerve). The oculomotor and abducens motor nerve fibers pass through the muscle cone in the retrobulbar space with the ciliary ganglion. The trochlear lies outside the cone on the superior medial side of the orbit. The motor fibers of the seventh (facial) nerve control contraction of the orbicularis oculi muscles. These fibers emerge from the base of the skull near the mastoid process and travel anteriorly from the tragus of the ear to ramify into the muscles surrounding the orbit.

Indications

The anesthesiologist can provide regional anesthesia for ophthalmic surgery by a combination of local infiltration of the facial nerve and blockade of the motor and sensory branches of the posterior orbit by means of a peribulbar or retrobulbar block. Facial nerve block will produce both sensory anesthesia of the periorbital area and motor block of the lid. Bulbar block creates the akinesia needed for cataract extraction, enucleation, and other superficial ophthalmic procedures, as well as sensory anesthesia of the terminal branches of the trigeminal nerve in the ciliary ganglion.

Drugs

For seventh nerve blockade, lidocaine or mepivacaine in 1% concentrations is adequate. For the retrobulbar and peribulbar blocks, higher concentrations are used to provide good muscular block. Lidocaine 2% is adequate for short cases, but 0.75% bupivacaine or ropivacaine (either alone or mixed with 2% lidocaine) will provide good akinesis and longer analgesia. The potential advantages of dense motor block must be weighed against the risk of intravascular injection in this area. Hyaluronidase (7.5 units per mL) is added to retrobulbar injections to promote spread of the anesthetic through the muscle cone. Epinephrine 1:200,000 may be added, but does not appear to provide any advantage with bupivacaine. The adjustment of the pH with sodium bicarbonate has been shown to speed the onset of bupivacaine and reduce the need for supplemental blocks with the peribulbar technique.

Technique

For bulbar blocks, intravenous sedation is useful to provide analgesia, amnesia, and patient cooperation, which is an important factor in reducing the chance of globe injury. Many drugs have been employed, but the shortest duration of sedation (such as a small propofol bolus) is ideal in this population. With the high frequency of associated disease and age in these patients, monitoring and supplemental oxygen are advisable if sedation is used. Once the block is injected, these patients generally do not require further sedation during the procedure.

Facial Nerve Blockade

The facial nerve can be blocked at any point from the terminal fibers near the eye, to its exit from the cranium at the base of the skull.

1. A simple approach to the terminal branches is to insert a 1.5-in. needle through a skin wheal 2 cm lateral to the orbital rim. The needle is advanced first superior toward the upper orbital rim, and 3 to 4 mL of anesthetic injected as it is withdrawn to the insertion point. It is then redirected toward the inferior orbital rim, and a repeat injection is made (Fig. 20.1). Sensory blockade of the lid is achieved by a subcutaneous injection of 1% lidocaine or mepivacaine through this single skin puncture.
2. The classic van Lint approach is slightly more medial, at a point 2 cm posterior to the lateral canthus of the eye (Fig. 20.2). Three mL of local anesthetic is injected as the needle is withdrawn to the entry point. The needle is left in the skin and redirected inferiorly and anteriorly, with a similar injection of 3 mL on withdrawal. The two injections should produce a "V" bordering the eye. An additional 2 mL can be injected deeper at the apex of the "V" to provide anesthesia of deeper fibers.
3. An alternative approach, described by Atkinson, is to insert the needle over the zygomatic arch at the level of the lateral orbital rim and advance it subcutaneously upward toward the top of the ear. Three to 4 mL of local anesthetic can be injected as the needle is withdrawn.
4. More proximal block of the facial nerve (near the ear), as described by O'Brien, will also produce paresis of the orbicularis oculi, and may be less likely to produce periorbital ecchymoses, which are disturbing to the patient and family. A needle is inserted 1 cm

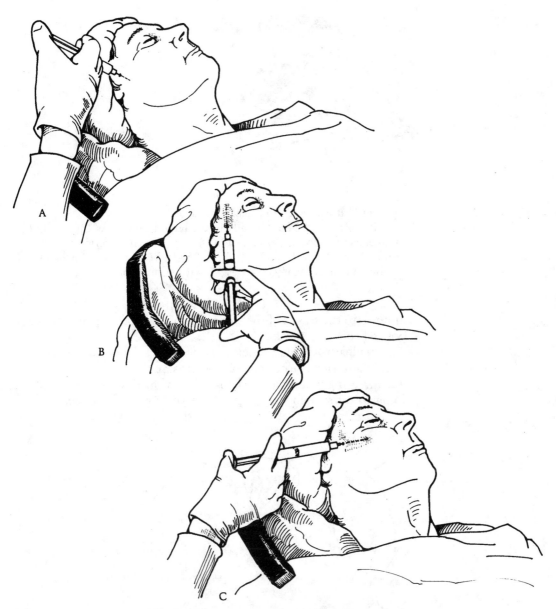

Figure 20.1   **Modified Atkinson Approach to Facial Nerve Block**
The needle is inserted 2 cm lateral to the lateral border of the orbit,
which is usually 2 to 3 cm further lateral than the van Lint approach.
Infiltration is first performed with 2 or 3 mL as the needle is withdrawn
up from its first contact with the bone (**A**). Local anesthetic is then
injected superiorly (**B**) and inferiorly (**C**) from this point to catch the
spreading fibers of the facial nerve as they surround the eye. This
approach has less chance of producing periorbital ecchymosis than the
classic van Lint approach, and it is less likely to produce a total facial
paralysis as would be obtained with a more proximal (O'Brien or
Nadbath–Rehman) approach.

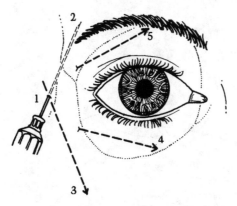

Figure 20.2   **Classic van Lint Approach to Facial Blockade**
The needle is inserted 2 cm laterally to the lateral canthus of the eye and
subcutaneous injection is performed in the superior and inferior borders of
the orbit. (From Hersh, P. S. *Ophthalmic Surgical Procedures.* Boston:
Little, Brown and Company, 1988. P. 17, with permission.)

anterior to the tragus of the ear, and 2 mL of local anesthetic is de-
posited subcutaneously.
5. The Nadbath-Rehman block is performed by inserting a 5/8-in.
needle anterior to the mastoid process at the base of the skull,
and directing it superior and posterior in the direction of the sty-
lomastoid foramen (as if aiming for the top of the opposite ear

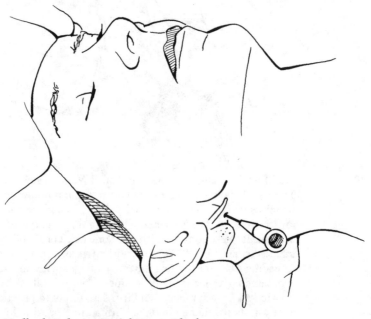

Figure 20.3   **Nadbath-Rehman Facial Nerve Block**

through the skull) (Fig. 20.3). After careful aspiration to avoid the nearby carotid artery, the needle is fixed and 3 mL of local anesthetic is injected.

Both of these latter techniques produce unneeded sensory and motor blockade of the lower face. The resulting facial drooping may be disconcerting to the patient and family, but is considered a trade–off compared to the risk of ecchymosis (black eye) associated with the more distal techniques. The choice of injection site is a compromise between these side effects. An alternative is to avoid facial nerve injection by using large volumes of anesthetic with the peribulbar technique.

Retrobulbar Block

1. Instillation of topical local anesthetic to the conjunctiva is usually performed as an associated step. Tetracaine 1% or other ophthalmologic preparations are all adequate.
2. The inferior border of the orbital rim is located at a point approximately one-third of the distance from the lateral to the medial canthus (Fig. 20.4). This point is usually directly inferior to the lateral border of the dilated pupil. The eye is held in neutral forward gaze; upward medial deviation may rotate the optic nerve and vessels into the intended path of the needle (1).
3. A 1.5-in. 23-gauge blunt-tipped needle is introduced perpendicularly into the skin and advanced directly posterior parallel to the floor of the orbit. The tip will usually lie opposite the equator of the globe, just below the skin.
4. After the needle is advanced past the equator of the globe, it is angled superonasally at approximately a 45-degree angle to pass into the muscular cone (Fig. 20.5). Entry into the muscle body will cause the globe to rotate inferiorly, rotating the eye down 15 to 30 degrees. Once the needle passes through the muscle body into the cone, there is an abrupt release of this traction, and the globe springs back to a neutral position. If this release is not obtained, the needle is withdrawn and reinserted.
5. After careful aspiration, 3 to 4 mL of anesthetic is injected slowly. There should be no resistance to injection if the needle is in the cone. Resistance might indicate undesirable intramuscular placement, and the needle should be repositioned if it is felt.

   Scleral perforation should be suspected if the patient complains of pain on injection. Many blocks are performed with sedation, which may mask this sign. Other indications are continued movement of the globe with needle movement once the muscle body is penetrated. Special blunt-tipped needles, which are designed to reduce the chance of perforation of the globe, are available for retrobulbar block, but the best protection is to avoid too shallow an angle when advancing the needle. The greatest risk exists with

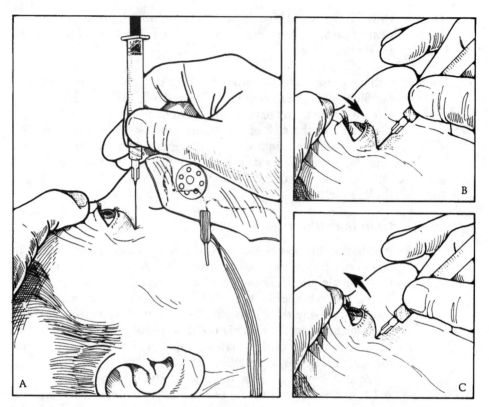

Figure 20.4   **Retrobulbar Block**
A: The needle is inserted perpendicular to the skin at the lateral border
of the dilated pupil just above the inferior orbital rim. B: Once the skin
is penetrated, the angle of the needle is changed to approximately 45
degrees cephalad and advanced until the globe rotates down as the needle
tip enters the muscle cone. C: When the tip penetrates into the central
cone, the globe will dramatically rotate back to the neutral position. At
this point, 3 mL of the local anesthetic mixture is injected into the
retrobulbar area.

the myopic patient with an elongated globe. The axial length
should be evaluated in all of these patients, and a steeper angle
maintained in any patient whose axial length exceeds 25 mm.
6. Gentle pressure is applied to the globe for 5 minutes to facilitate
spread of the solution, but it is released every 30 seconds to preserve retinal blood flow.
7. A slightly larger volume of anesthesia will produce more reliable
block of the trochlear nerve (motor innervation of the superior
oblique muscle), which lies outside the muscle cone containing
the other motor nerves and the ciliary ganglion. Sparing of this
muscle is not usually a problem because of its limited motion. If
troublesome intorsion of the eye persists after classic retrobulbar
block, the trochlear nerve can be blocked by injection of an ad-

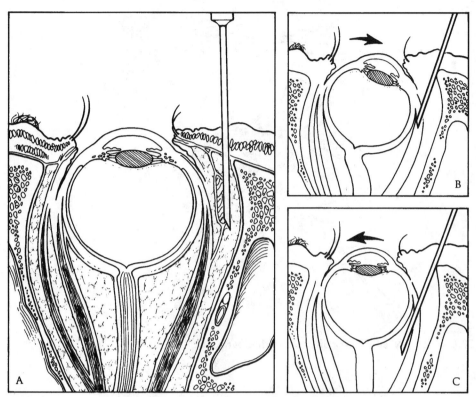

Figure 20.5 **Needle Direction Associated with Retrobulbar Injection**
The three positions (**A**, **B**, **C**) correspond to the stages in Fig. 20.4.

ditional 1 mL of anesthetic above the globe near the superior oblique muscle.

Peribulbar Block

Because of concern about the potential for retrobulbar hemorrhage and globe perforation with the classic retrobulbar approach, the technique of peribulbar injection has been described. Anatomical studies suggest that the cone of muscles is not a closed space with dense septae, but that there is easy access to the ciliary ganglion from outside the muscles (2). The peribulbar needle does not enter the muscle cone, and thus theoretically this approach reduces the chance of complications. This presumed reduction of risks is balanced by a slower onset of anesthesia and a need for reinjection of 25% to 35% of these patients (1,3,4) compared to 10% with retrobulbar injections.

1. Topical anesthesia is produced as for retrobulbar injection.
2. A 1.5-in. 25-gauge needle is inserted through the conjunctiva at the inferior temporal area above the inferior orbital rim (Fig. 20.6).

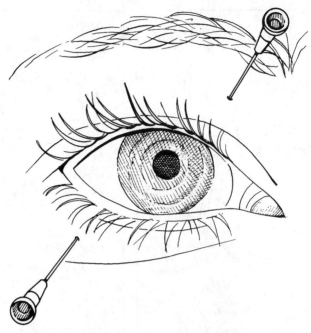

Figure 20.6   **Needle Entry Sites for Peribulbar Block**

The needle is advanced in a slight upward direction (parallel to the rising orbital floor at this level) without any attempt to enter the cone, and 4 to 5 mL of local anesthetic is injected.

3. The needle is reinserted in the superior nasal area just below and medial to the supratrochlear notch, and an additional 4 to 5 mL is injected. Again, insertion is basically tangential to the globe without any attempt to enter the cone. With both injections, the needle is advanced only 1 in. into the orbit. This is generally sufficient to reach behind the equator of the globe, but the insertions are both tangential to the globe and are unlikely to enter the cone.

4. The onset of anesthesia is slower, and the block needs to be assessed at 10 minutes for potential supplemental injection. Loss of vision does not always occur with this approach, but seventh nerve anesthesia is often obtained by diffusion of the anesthetic into the subcutaneous tissues of the upper lid without the need for separate injection.

Complications

Retrobulbar Hematoma Formation

Hemorrhage is the most frequent complication of retrobulbar blockade and occurs as often as 1% of cases in some reported series, although it appears to be less frequent in larger series (4). Easily reversible defects of coagulation mechanisms should be reversed before retrobulbar injection. Retrobulbar hemorrhage during ophthalmic anesthesia is a serious complication, which may interfere with retinal blood supply if excessive pressure develops. Signs include immediate proptosis, increased pressure in the globe, and appearance of subconjunctival blood. Monitoring of retinal pulsations and postponement of surgery are warranted, and drainage via lateral canthotomy by the surgeon may be needed to relieve pressure.

Brain-Stem Anesthesia

Spread of the anesthetic to the brainstem area is less common (less than 0.5%), but it is more life threatening because of the potential development of apnea. The mechanism is unclear, but it may be due to the spread of anesthetic along the optic nerve to the central brain stem. Shortness of breath and dysphagia may be presenting signs. Ventilation and supportive therapy will usually suffice until the symptoms resolve.

Systemic Toxicity

Systemic toxicity is possible because of the proximity of the retinal artery. Unintentional injections under pressure into the arterial circulation of the head can produce rapid high intracerebral local anesthetic blood levels and convulsions. Careful aspiration and incremental injection are needed.

Oculocardiac Reflex

Any stretch of the extraocular muscles can produce reflex bradycardia and should be treated immediately with atropine to block the vagal component.

Perforation of the Globe

Perforation of the globe can occur, even with blunt-tipped needles and even with the peribulbar technique, but is generally less than 0.1% in frequency. Risk factors also include elongated globe, multiple injections, previous scleral buckling, and the use of long-beveled needles (1). It can be recognized by movement of the globe when the needle is moved prior to injection. Perforation will also usually produce pain and restlessness. Surgery should be canceled and appropriate ophthalmologic care rendered.

Intramuscular Injection

Direct injection of the local anesthetic into the muscle body can produce muscle destruction and ultimate paresis (4). Fortunately, this is rare and can be avoided by halting any injection that meets resistance.

References   1. Wong, D. H. Regional anaesthesia for intraocular surgery. *Can. J. Anaesth* 40: 635, 1993.
2. Ripart, J., Lefrant, J. Y., de La Coussaye, J. E., Prat-Pradal, D., Vivien, B., Eledjam, J. J. Peribulbar versus retrobulbar anesthesia for ophthalmic surgery: An anatomical comparison of extraconal and intraconal injections. *Anesthesiology* 94: 56, 2001.
3. Ali-Melkkila, T. M., Virkkila, M., Jyrkkio, H. Regional anesthesia for cataract surgery: Comparison of retrobulbar and peribulbar techniques. *Reg. Anesth.* 17: 219, 1992.
4. Hamilton, R. C., Gimbel, H. V., Strunin, L. Regional anaesthesia for 12,000 cataract extraction and intraocular lens implantation procedures. *Can. J. Anaesth.* 35: 615, 1988.

21 Pediatric Regional Anesthesia

Linda Jo Rice

Although regional techniques have similar advantages in pediatric patients as in adults, the methods used for performing these techniques in adults must be modified. There are obvious differences in anatomy and drug dosages, as well as patient cooperation. Children, especially young children, require a general anesthetic or deep sedation in order to accept placement of a block. This attention to the psychological well-being of the child must extend through the intraoperative period; children do not tolerate being awake and holding still in the scary operating room, even if their block is adequate for the surgical procedure (1). Because of this need for deep sedation or general anesthesia prior to block placement, two individuals are usually required: one to place the block and the other to monitor the child. All techniques, whether regional or general, have risks, and these risks must be weighed against the potential benefits of employing these techniques in anesthetized children, just as in adults. Fortunately, the most frequent regional techniques employed for the common surgical procedures in children are relatively simple. This chapter has a primary emphasis on how regional techniques performed in children differ from the previously described adult techniques. There are many excellent reviews of pediatric regional anesthetic techniques for those who wish to pursue these techniques in more detail (2–5).

Topical Blocks

Several local anesthetic preparations will penetrate intact skin (6). Eutectic mixture of local anesthetics (EMLA) is a combination of 5% lidocaine and 5% prilocaine that, when covered with an occlusive dressing and left undisturbed for 60 to 90 minutes, provides anesthesia to a depth of 5 mm. Numby Stuff is a device that allows iontophoresis of lidocaine 2% and epinephrine providing similar anesthesia of intact skin about 20 minutes after application. This device employs a small electric current to provide the iontophoresis that some younger children find objectionable. Both EMLA and Numby Stuff allow placement of an intravenous (i.v.) catheter, painless access to an implanted i.v. catheter, or other superficial procedures. All topical local anesthetic preparations have the limitation that they must be placed over the area to be anesthetized, and they

259

take varying amounts of time to become effective. If the anesthesiologist misses the vein and has to go elsewhere, the skin at the new location will not be numb.

Topical local anesthetics have also been successfully employed to provide anesthesia for exposed mucous membranes. Oral mucous membranes can be anesthetized in order to allow earlier placement of oral airways or laryngoscopy in infants and children with potentially difficult airways. Topical intratracheal lidocaine (1 to 2 mg per kg) is often employed following induction of general anesthesia in infants who require diagnostic direct laryngoscopy in order for the otolaryngologist to view vocal cord movement.

Topical 0.5% lidocaine or 0.25% to 0.5% bupivacaine has been utilized during circumcision repair to provide effective postoperative analgesia (7). EMLA has also been employed for anesthesia for newborn circumcisions because it can penetrate the intact foreskin. Application of other local anesthetics must be done following amputation of the foreskin in order to expose the mucous membranes that will absorb these local anesthetic preparations. Because this is a topical technique, only enough local anesthetic is required to contact all of the "target" mucous membrane. If jelly or ointment is employed, parents need to be reassured regarding the appearance of the wound, because the sight of the dried local anesthetic mixed with a tinge of blood may be unsettling. Repeated administration of the local anesthetic every 6 hours for 2 days will provide effective postoperative analgesia (8).

Topical local anesthetics have also been employed to provide effective postoperative analgesia for children undergoing hernia or hydrocele repair. Here, 0.25% to 0.5% bupivacaine or ropivacaine 0.2% to 0.5% in enough volume to fill the wound is instilled at the end of surgical dissection, just prior to wound closure, and is left in contact with the exposed ilioinguinal nerve and surrounding muscle tissue for 1 minute (9). The resulting analgesia is equivalent to a more formal block of the ilioinguinal nerve.

Ilioinguinal and Iliohypogastric Nerve Block

This block provides analgesia equivalent to that of caudal blockade for children undergoing inguinal hernia, hydrocele, or orchidopexy repair (Fig. 21.1). The ilioinguinal nerve is usually exposed by the surgeon during surgical dissection.

Technique

These nerves can be blocked by topical techniques, as described above. A formal block of the nerves can be performed following induction of general anesthesia (10). An alternative technique, where the surgeon infiltrates the wound edges at the end of dissection

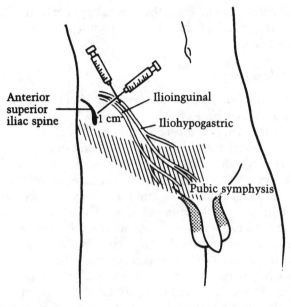

Figure 21.1

Ilioinguinal and Iliohypogastric Block
A 23- to 25-gauge needle is inserted 1 cm medial to the anterior superior iliac spine, and a wall of anesthesia is created by injecting in a fanlike fashion along the muscle wall from the ilium to the border of the rectus. A total of 5 to 10 mL of 0.25% bupivacaine will provide anesthesia for the ilioinguinal (crosshatched) and the iliohypogastric (stippled) innervation. (From Yaster, M., Maxwell, L. G. Pediatric regional anesthesia. *Anesthesiology* 70: 324, 1989, with permission.)

(which also instills local anesthetic into the wound) is more effective than when the surgeon infiltrates the skin edges prior to closing the skin. Bupivacaine 0.25% to 0.5% is most often employed, in a dose of 5 to 10 mL depending on patient size. Ropivacaine 0.5% has also been employed in children for this block.

Complications

Three to 5% of children receiving this block by techniques other than application of topical anesthesia may demonstrate transient blockade of the femoral nerve, with temporary inability to stand due to loss of quadriceps strength.

Penile Block   This block is useful for perioperative analgesia for boys undergoing circumcision or hypospadias repair. Although the American Academy of Pediatrics does not endorse circumcision, it does endorse the use of local anesthetics if the family desires a circumcision in the neonatal period. Both the topical application of EMLA cream and the ring block of the penis are simple and have minimal risk to the newborn.

Technique

The simplest way to block the dorsal penile nerves is to place a subcutaneous wheal of 0.25% to 0.5% bupivacaine *without epinephrine* that rings the base of the penis (11). This subcutaneous block places local anesthetic just superficial to the tough Buck fascia that surrounds the corpora, and the dorsal nerve, arteries, and veins of the penis. The local anesthetic diffuses across this fascia to provide anesthesia. Another technique involves blockade of the dorsal penile nerves in the subpubic area (Fig. 21.2) (3). This involves downward traction on the penis, and the injection of local anesthetic under Scarpa fascia (which is continuous with Buck fascia in the shaft of the penis). Two injections are made 0.5 to 1 cm lateral to the midline below the symphysis pubis. A 23- to 25-gauge needle is inserted slightly medially and caudally until the characteristic "pop" is felt as the needle traverses Scarpa fascia just below the pubis and 2 to 5 mL of local anesthetic is injected.

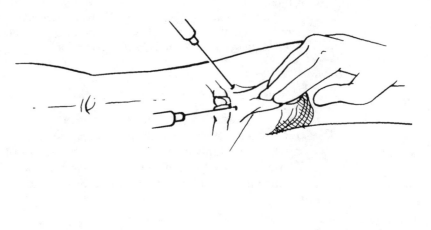

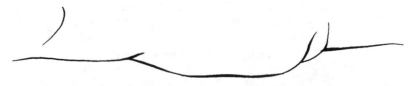

Figure 21.2   **Suprapubic Penile Block**
The penis is retracted downward and injections are made on each side of the base, 0.5 to 1 cm lateral to the midline and below the symphysis pubis. The needle is inserted slightly medially and caudally to pierce Scarpa fascia.

Complications

There have been no complications observed with the ring technique. Blockade of the dorsal penile nerve deep to Buck fascia in the shaft of the penis has been associated with decreased perfusion to the tip of the glans penis.

Caudal Block   The single-injection caudal block is one of the most popular and versatile pediatric regional anesthetic techniques. Placement of a catheter allows continuous infusion of local anesthetic or local anesthetic and opioid mixture.

A combination of caudal blockade supplemented with light regional anesthesia allows for a quicker wake-up due to a lesser need for volatile anesthetic agents.

Anatomy

Caudal blocks are technically much easier to perform in children than in adults. There is less fusion in the region of the sacral hiatus, and less distortion of the bony landmarks in infants and children, who have not developed the gluteal fat pad that is common at puberty. This poorly developed gluteal musculature and limited amount of subcutaneous fat means that landmarks defining the sacral hiatus are not obscured.

The fifth sacral cornua are very prominent, lying well above the gluteal cleft. The sacrococcygeal ligament is not calcified in the infant or child; indeed, the distinct "pop" one encounters is quite similar to the tactile sensation experienced when entering a peripheral vein with an 18-gauge i.v. catheter in an adult. The dural sac ends between the second and third sacral vertebrae, whereas the length of the sacrum is reduced in proportion to the overall size of the child. It is possible to pierce the fragile sacrum or perform a dural puncture in an infant; most catastrophic complications of caudal block have occurred in infants less than 10 kg in weight. Meticulous attention to technique is vital in these small patients (12).

Indications

A caudal block combined with a light general anesthetic provides excellent perioperative analgesia for children undergoing sacral segment surgery (circumcision, rectal dilation, clubfoot repair), as well as most other surgeries below the diaphragm. This list includes commonly performed groin surgeries, such as herniorrhaphy, orchidopexy, and hydrocele repair. Children undergoing lower-extremity orthopedic procedures or urologic procedures also enjoy profound postoperative analgesia provided by a caudal block.

Caudal blocks are usually placed following induction of general anesthesia, and placement of an i.v. catheter. Only a very light plane of general anesthesia is required once the block has taken effect. The time spent placing the block prior to the beginning of surgery is recovered at the end of surgery because the child awakens so quickly.

Drugs

Bupivacaine 0.25% provides minimal motor blockade with adequate sensory blockade. The total dose of bupivacaine should not exceed 3 mg per kg. Ropivacaine 0.2% to 0.25% in doses that do not exceed 2 mg per kg have also been employed (13). An easy calculation of volume is that employed by Armitage (14): 0.5 mL per kg for sacral blockade, 0.75 mL per kg for lower-thoracic segments, and 1.25 mL per kg for upper-thoracic levels of blockade.

Technique

The block is usually performed following the induction of general anesthesia.

1. The patient is turned into the lateral position, and the hips and knees are flexed similar to the position that would be appropriate for performance of a lumbar puncture (Fig. 21.3).

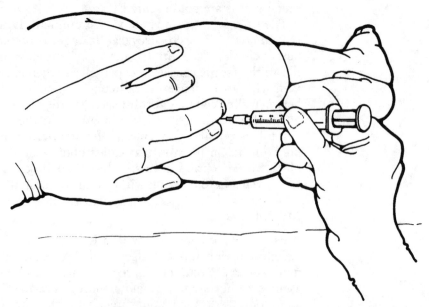

Figure 21.3

Pediatric Caudal Anesthesia, Lateral Position
This technique is performed following the induction of general anesthesia and placement of an intravenous catheter. It is easily done in children in either the lateral or the prone position. The sacrococcygeal membrane is easily identified with the characteristic "pop," and the injection is made after advancing the needle 1 to 2 mm.

2. The sacral cornua and hiatus should be palpated and marked; this should result in a "C" figure above the cleft of the buttocks, in the midline, with the open part of the "C" facing caudad.

3. A "no-touch" technique or sterile gloves may be used after aseptic preparation of the area with povidone–iodine. A 1-in. 23-gauge needle or 22-gauge i.v. needle/catheter is inserted into the sacrococcygeal ligament at a 60-degree angle. The bevel should be maintained in a ventral position to avoid puncture of the anterior wall of the sacrum. A distinct "pop" will be felt as the needle punctures the membrane; the needle hub and syringe are then dropped into a plane parallel to the spinal axis, and the needle shaft is advanced an additional 2 mm to be certain that the entire bevel of the needle is in the caudal space or the intravenous catheter is advanced easily into the caudal space.

4. After aspiration, the local anesthetic solution is injected in aliquots into the caudal space. It is important to stabilize the needle so that pressure on the plunger does not advance the needle into the caudal space. Frequent aspiration and fractionated injection of local anesthetic is the best safeguard against undetected intravascular injection, because test doses are unreliable in children (12,15,16). Fifty percent of children will have analgesia for up to 12 hours if adequate doses are employed.

Complications

Dural puncture with resultant total spinal anesthesia is possible. Careful stabilization of the needle and frequent gentle aspiration will assist in avoiding this complication. Dysrhythmias and cardiac arrest have occurred, usually in infants less than 10 kg. Extensive experience in older children prior to use of this technique in infants is recommended.

Infraorbital Nerve Block

This simple block provides profound pain relief for 12 to 18 hours in children undergoing cleft lip or palate repair or other surgery on the anterior hard palate, lower eyelid, side of nose, or upper lip (17). Even though plastic surgeons employ local anesthetic injected directly into the surgical site, the duration of the local anesthetic is not as long as with this peripheral nerve block.

Anatomy

The infraorbital notch lies on a line connecting the supraorbital and mental foramina and the pupil of the eye (Fig. 18.3).

Technique

There are two techniques for blocking this nerve. Both are field blocks and are not intended to be injected in the notch or in the nerve. The first is to locate the infraorbital foramen with the index finger of the nondominant hand—approximately 0.5 cm from midpoint of lower orbital margin. A 25-gauge needle inserted perpendicular to the notch will touch bone; the needle is then withdrawn slightly so that the injection is not intraosseous, and 0.25 to 0.5 mL of local anesthetic is injected. A small skin wheal should be visible. The second technique is transoral and will leave no mark on the face. The lip is elevated and a 1.5-in. 25-gauge needle is guided over the incisor toward the nondominant index finger to locate the infraorbital notch until the tip of the needle is felt in the area of the notch. Be careful not to stick yourself in the finger. Inject 1 to 1.5 mL of local anesthetic. If this technique is planned, it should be performed prior to the surgery so that there is no risk of disruption of the surgery by the manipulation of the upper lip.

Extremity Blocks

The basic techniques of extremity blockade in infants and children are similar to those used in adults, with one difference: infants and children will not cooperate, because of fear of needles and general suspicion of medical personnel. Therefore, sedation or light general anesthesia and a nerve stimulator are both important in neural blockade in infants and children. The principles of use of the nerve stimulator are detailed in Chapter 5.

Indications

Upper-extremity blocks can provide muscle relaxation and analgesia for the reduction of fractures as well as in the immediate perioperative period following an open procedure. A femoral nerve block, alone or in conjunction with a lateral femoral cutaneous nerve block, or an inguinal paravascular ("three-in-one") block can provide anesthesia for muscle biopsy. Femoral nerve blockade also provides excellent analgesia and muscle relaxation for children with femur fractures. With the addition of a sciatic block, all lower-extremity surgery is possible. Usually, however, caudal blockade with its single needle is preferred for lower-extremity surgery in the pediatric population.

Drugs

A combination of 0.5% lidocaine with 0.12% tetracaine and epinephrine 1:200,000 provides effective anesthesia and analgesia for up to 12 hours, although 0.25% bupivacaine can also be employed.

Table 21.1   **Drug Doses and Volumes for Pediatric Regional Techniques**

Agent	Maximum Doses (mg/kg) with Added Epinephrine 1:200,000
Lidocaine	7–10
Bupivacaine	2–3
Compound	
Lidocaine	5
Tetracaine	2

Peripheral nerve block	Volume (mL/kg)[a]
Axillary	0.33
Interscalene	0.25
Inguinal paravascular	0.50
Sciatic	0.20

[a]Volume of 0.25% bupivacaine or lidocaine—tetracaine.

This combination works well when performing blocks with a nerve stimulator because of the rapid onset of the lidocaine; bupivacaine is less reliable. It must be remembered that toxicities are additive when compounding local anesthetics (Table 21.1).

There is little experience with ropivacaine in extremity blocks for pediatric patients.

Techniques

Arm Block.   The easiest approach to the brachial plexus is the axillary approach. The technique is the same as in adults (see Chapter 12). A nerve stimulator is useful, but simple infiltration on either side of the easily palpable artery will usually produce adequate anesthesia. Appropriate volumes of local anesthetics are noted in Table 21.1; these volumes usually include blockade of the musculocutaneous nerve.

Leg Block.   The femoral nerve block is described in Chapter 15; few modifications are required for pediatric patients. Again, a nerve stimulator is useful, but simple infiltration along the artery is effective.

The sciatic nerve is more easily blocked more peripherally than in the classic Labat description. Children rarely have the gluteal fat pad developed at puberty; one can frequently see their sciatic groove. Place the child in the lateral (Sims) position; the ankle of the upper leg is placed on the knee of the lower leg. Locate and mark the greater trochanter and the ischial tuberosity of the upper leg. A 22-gauge needle (3.5-in. spinal needle, if the child is big enough) is connected to a nerve stimulator, and inserted midway between the two landmarks until dorsiflexion or plantar flexion of the foot is noted. All flexion should be abolished with 1 mL of local anesthetic solution if the needle is in the proper place. Motor activity above the knee is most likely due to direct muscle stimulation and is not a reliable indicator that the needle is in the proper position.

Conclusions

Just because we can perform a technique does not mean that it is the best choice for the patient. Although these techniques are very safe, they are not without risk (18,19). Thoughtful consideration of the risk and benefits of any technique are the responsibility of all caregivers. Optimum analgesia is achieved by "hitting the pain monster with a 1-2-3 punch." Preoperative administration of acetaminophen or nonsteroidal antiinflammatory drugs, followed by appropriate regional analgesia, will only provide optimum analgesia if postoperative instructions include timely use of oral analgesics so that effective blood levels are achieved before the block wears off—because the block wears off about midnight.

References

1. Dalens, B., Hasnaoui, A. Caudal anesthesia in pediatric surgery: Success rate and adverse effects in 750 consecutive patients. *Anesth. Analg.* 68: 83, 1989.
2. Broadman, L. M., Rice, L. J. Neural blockade for pediatric surgery. In Cousins, M. J., Bridenbaugh, P. O., Eds., *Neural Blockade in Clinical Anesthesia and Management of Pain*, 3rd ed. Philadelphia: Lippincott, 1998.
3. Dalens, B. J. Regional anesthesia in children. In Miller, R. D. M., Ed., *Anesthesia*, 5th ed. New York: Churchill Livingstone, 2000.
4. Rice, L. J. Regional anesthesia. In Motoyama, E., Davis, P., Eds., *Smith's Anesthesia for Infants and Children*, 6th ed. St. Louis: Mosby, 1995.
5. Sethna, N. F., Berde, C. B. Pediatric regional anesthesia. In Gregory, G. A., Ed., *Pediatric Anesthesia*. New York: Churchill Livingstone, 1994.
6. Squire, S. J., Kirchhoff, K. I., Hissong, K. Comparing two methods of topical anesthesia used before intravenous cannulation in pediatric patients. *J. Pediatr. Health Care* 14: 68, 2000.
7. Andersen, K. H. A new method of analgesia for relief of circumcision pain. *Anaesthesia* 44: 118, 1989.
8. Tree-Trakarn, T., Pirayavaraporn, S., Lertakyamanee, J. Topical analgesia for relief of post-circumcision pain. *Anesthesiology* 67: 395, 1987.
9. Casey, W. F., Rice, L. J., Hannallah, R. S., Broadman, L., Norden, J. M., et al. A comparison between bupivacaine instillation versus ilioinguinal/iliohypogastric nerve block for postoperative analgesia following inguinal herniorrhaphy in children. *Anesthesiology* 72: 636, 1990.
10. Langer, J. C., Shandling, B., Rosenberg, M. Intraoperative bupivacaine during outpatient hernia repair in children: A randomized double blind trial. *J. Pediatr. Surg.* 22: 267, 1987.
11. Broadman, L. M., Hannallah, R. S., Belman, B., Elder, P. T., Ruttiman, U., et al. Post-circumcision analgesia—a prospective evaluation of subcutaneous ring block of the penis. *Anesthesiology* 67: 399, 1987.
12. Veyckemans, F., Van Obbergh, L. J., Gouverneur, J. M. Lessons from 1100 pediatric caudal blocks in a teaching hospital. *Reg. Anesth.* 17: 119, 1992.

13. Koinig, H., Krenn, C. G., Glaser, C., Marhofer, P., et al. The dose-response of caudal ropivacaine in children. *Anesthesiology* 90: 1339, 1999.
14. Armitage, E. N. Local anesthetic techniques for prevention of postoperative pain. *Br. J. Anesth.* 58: 790, 1986.
15. Brendel, J. K., Yemen, T. A., Berry, F. A. Intravenous injection of local anesthetic: Identification with isoproterenol and epinephrine in children during halothane anesthesia. *Reg. Anesth.* 18: 49, 1993.
16. Freid, E. B., Bailey, A. G., Valley, R. D. Electrocardiographic and hemodynamic changes associated with unintentional intravascular injection of bupivacaine with epinephrine in infants. *Anesthesiology* 79: 394, 1993.
17. Ahuja, A., Datta, A., Krishna, A., Bhattacharya, A. Infraorbital block for relief of postoperative pain following cleft lip surgery in infants. *Anaesthesia* 49: 441, 1993.
18. Giaufre, E., Dalens, B., Gombert, A. Epidemiology and morbidity of regional anesthesia in children: A one-year prospective study of the French-Language Society of Pediatric Anesthesiologists. *Anesthesiology* 83: 904, 1996.
19. Krane, E.J., Dalens, B.J., Murat, I., Murrell, D., et al. The safety of epidurals placed during general anesthesia. *Reg. Anesth.* 23: 433, 1998.

22 Obstetric Anesthesia

Several excellent textbooks of obstetric anesthesia detail the physiology and anesthetic management of the parturient (1–5). This chapter discusses briefly the required modifications in application of the previously described regional anesthesia techniques in the healthy pregnant patient. Specifically, the use of epidural, caudal, and spinal anesthesia for vaginal and cesarean delivery are reviewed.

Anatomy

The anatomic considerations for performing the blocks in the pregnant patient differ from those in the nonpregnant patient in some respects. Positioning is complicated by the presence of the distended uterus, which limits the mother's ability to flex the lumbar spine maximally. The bony landmarks can be obscured in patients whose weight gain has been generous or who have been at prolonged bed rest. Identification of the ligaments is further complicated by the hormonally induced softening of these tissues near term.

Increased abdominal pressure also influences the epidural and subdural mechanics. The epidural veins are now engorged and more frequently encountered. The epidural space itself is reduced and requires less anesthetic solution to produce satisfactory anesthetic levels during both epidural and caudal techniques. Spinal injections also produce higher than expected levels, and dosage is reduced for all of these techniques.

Circulatory changes also have an impact on anesthetic management. Cardiac output is increased, and intravascular injections rapidly produce toxicity. The weight of the gravid uterus in the supine position interferes with venous return from the lower extremities, and the uterus must be displaced off the pelvic vessels whenever a sympathetic block is produced or when resuscitation is performed, or whenever the patient is placed supine for cesarean delivery.

In general, these considerations indicate greater technical difficulty and greater risk in performing regional techniques in the parturient. Despite common practice in some institutions, the obstetric suite is not the ideal location for the novice to perform his or her first regional block. Familiarity with the techniques should be encouraged before attempting these blocks in "labor" situations, where the patient is frequently demanding speed and proficiency in attaining adequate pain relief.

Indications

The discomfort associated with delivery is manifest in one or more of three forms: (i) the pain of contractions in early labor, (ii) the stretching of the birth canal at delivery, (iii) or the surgical pain associated with cesarean delivery. The sensation of uterine contractions is mediated by nerve tracts that enter the spinal column at the 10th to 12th thoracic dermatome levels. Blockade of these pathways early in labor may transiently slow the progress of labor. Regional techniques are traditionally not applied until uterine contractions are well established and sustained, but there is no critical level of cervical dilation that dictates initiation of analgesia (6). The use of regional analgesia is not a significant factor in prolonging labor or increasing the need for instrumented or operative deliveries (7,8). As the fetal head descends the birth canal, vaginal distention is perceived by the sacral nerve roots innervating the perineum. Operative delivery involves the skin dermatomes of the lower abdomen, as well as visceral sensation, which require a dermatomal sensory blockade to the level of the second to fourth thoracic dermatomes. Each of these phases requires slightly different anesthetic management.

Lumbar epidural blockade is extremely useful in obstetrics, particularly for the uterine contractions of the first stage. Segmental analgesia can be produced for labor with minimal drug dosages, limited physiologic changes, and some retention of maternal mobility. Catheter techniques allow flexibility in duration and extent and density of blockade, so that the block can be extended for perineal anesthesia at the time of delivery or reinforced for cesarean delivery. The use of the epidural catheter increases the potential for intravascular or subarachnoid injection. Catheter insertion and injection also necessitate some time interval before analgesia is obtained. Nevertheless, on balance, epidural analgesia and anesthesia offer benefits for labor, delivery, and cesarean section that outweigh the risks (6).

Caudal (sacral epidural) blockade is also employed for obstetric analgesia and is particularly more effective for the delivery itself because of the superior anesthesia at the sacral roots. Caudal blockade requires a larger dose of drug to achieve analgesia than does lumbar epidural injection. The dense analgesia attained in the sacral area is not necessary for early labor. Caudal analgesia is also more likely to prolong the second stage by interfering with the "bearing down" or "pushing" reflex. This may be desirable when a slow, controlled delivery is sought, as in prematurity. Caudal anatomy is more variable than in the lumbar area, and thus this technique may be more difficult (see Chapter 8). For all of these reasons, caudal anesthesia is employed rarely.

Subarachnoid techniques have seen a resurgence of popularity because of the availability of the rounded-bevel needles, which significantly reduce the potential for postdural puncture headache in this susceptible population. Increased use of subarachnoid injection is also related to increasing familiarity with subarachnoid analgesia with narcotics for early labor (9,10). This technique relieves pain without motor or sympathetic blockade and can provide several hours of analgesia before epidural local anesthetics are employed. The simultaneous insertion of an epidural catheter (combined spinal–epidural [CSE] technique; see Combined Spinal–Epidural Technique, this chapter) allows later use of a more potent continuous infusion for the final stages of labor. Opioid analgesia can also allow greater mobility in early labor, and has contributed to the popular concept of a "walking epidural" during the early stages of labor. In later labor, subarachnoid injection of local anesthetic alone provides rapid onset of dense anesthesia, which is useful for vaginal delivery when rapidity of action and reliability are important, and thus is an appropriate alternative for rapidly progressing labor. This technique is limited to situations where delivery is imminent. Despite the potential for rapid onset of vasodilation and hypotension, saddle-block (low spinal) anesthesia remains the mainstay of obstetric anesthesia for vaginal delivery in many areas.

Cesarean delivery is the other common indication for anesthetic intervention. All of the techniques described so far can be employed, with the use of higher doses and concentrations of drug to provide the T2-4 level of sensory and motor anesthesia needed. An indwelling epidural catheter can be used to develop adequate anesthesia if time permits. Spinal blockade is frequently the technique of choice for cesarean delivery because of the rapid onset of dense anesthesia with this technique. The use of regional technique for operative delivery reduces the potential for inadequate airway maintenance associated with general anesthesia, and appears to provide a lower mortality in this situation in the United States (11).

Labor analgesia is also frequently requested for a patient who previously delivered abdominally. Vaginal birth after cesarean section (VBAC) represents an increased potential for risks, but is possible and safe if monitored appropriately to provide early detection of uterine disruption (12,13). This situation calls for the lowest possible density and height of epidural blockade, as well as intensified monitoring of mother and fetus while analgesia is present.

The use of regional techniques in other complicated obstetric situations is a complex decision. In the hypovolemic patient, regional anesthesia with its attendant sympathetic block may be contraindicated. In the hypertensive or preeclamptic parturient, early epidural analgesia may help reduce blood pressure elevations caused by pain perception, but it may be associated with more dramatic cardiovascular changes because these patients are frequently vasoconstricted and volume-depleted. In severe cases (diastolic pressure greater than 110 mm Hg), invasive hemodynamic monitoring may be necessary before instituting a sympathetic block. The use of regional techniques is not advised in the presence of coagulopathy. Breech presentation, multiple gestations, preeclampsia, or maternal cardiac disease all require more detailed modification of technique than is possible to discuss here.

One further presumed indication for regional anesthesia during pregnancy is for nonobstetrical operations. The choice of anesthetic must be dictated by the surgery and the patient's condition. Regional anesthetics are often favored because of the potential to provide the lowest exposure of the fetus to drugs, especially with a technique such as spinal blockade. Despite theoretical advantages, there is no clear evidence to support regional over general anesthesia. Whatever technique is chosen, there must be careful attention to maintenance of normal uterine perfusion and oxygenation. Intraoperative fetal monitoring is appropriate for surgery in later pregnancy.

Drugs

Although all of the local anesthetics are capable of providing anesthesia in the epidural space, there is concern about the effects of the drugs on the fetus and neonate if maternal blood levels and placental transfer are excessive. Mepivacaine particularly has been shown to attain high blood levels by accumulating in the maternal circulation. It is not well metabolized by the neonate, and prolonged epidural analgesia with this drug can produce measurable fetal blood levels and neurobehavioral changes. Etidocaine is not useful because of the long and profound motor blockade with this drug. Neurologic assessments have shown that chloroprocaine, lidocaine, and bupivacaine do not produce neurobehavioral changes in the newborn. In appropriate epidural doses, these drugs provide excellent analgesia with minimal motor blockade. In general, it seems wise to use the lowest practical dosage, both in concentration and total volume. Doses of 6 to 8 mL of 2% chloroprocaine or 1.5% lidocaine at the second lumbar level will give rapid onset of analgesia for labor. A similar dose of 0.25% bupivacaine is also appropriate, and is used more often when rapid onset is not needed. Successful analgesia has been achieved with 10 mL 0.125% bupivacaine with less motor blockade; this concentration is also effective as a continuous infusion. The success of this dosage supports speculation that pregnancy increases sensitivity to local anesthetics, and that lower doses are required. Levobupivacaine produces similar analgesia. Ropivacaine may be associated with less motor blockade at equal doses, but this may be related to a lower potency (14). The addition of narcotics (see below) provides significant potentiation of the lower doses of bupivacaine, particularly in continuous-infusion techniques (6).

The dose and concentration of drug must be increased for cesarean delivery. Generally, 15 to 20 mL 0.5% bupivacaine or 2% lidocaine will be required for epidural anesthesia for abdominal delivery. Although 0.75% bupivacaine or levobupivacaine or 1% ropivacaine will give excellent motor blockade, their use is not recommended for obstetric procedures. The primary concern is that systemic toxicity is more likely in the highly vascular epidural space, and cardiac toxicity has been seen with this higher mass of

Table 22.1   **Drug Dosage for Spinal Anesthesia for Delivery**

Drug	Saddle Block	Cesarean
Lidocaine 5%	25–40 mg	60–75 mg
Tetracaine 0.5%	3–6 mg	8–10 mg
Bupivacaine 7.5%	6–8 mg	10–12 mg

intravenous bupivacaine (see Chapter 3). Obviously, no drug is inherently safe, and very careful attention to test doses, incremental injection, and prevention of intravascular injection is critical when the lives of both mother and infant are involved.

For spinal anesthesia, the drug dosage also must be reduced when compared to that in the nonpregnant patient (Table 22.1). With the small doses used for subarachnoid blockade, neurobehavioral effects on the fetus are not a concern. All of the common spinal drugs are used, although lidocaine is less popular because of the concern regarding transient neurologic symptoms (TNS). The addition of opioids to bupivacaine may allow a further reduction of local anesthetic dose to as low as 5 mg, and decrease the frequency of hypotension (15).

Opioids alone have also been employed for analgesia for labor and delivery in both the epidural and intrathecal routes. Ideally, they can provide analgesia without motor or sympathetic blockade. Epidural doses have proved ineffective. Subarachnoid morphine offers prolonged analgesia, but it is not popular because of the long duration and significant incidence of pruritus (Table 22.2). Fentanyl and sufentanil have been shown to be effective as subarachnoid analgesics, especially for the early stages of labor. Doses of 25 µg of fentanyl or 10 µg of sufentanil will provide analgesia for 1 to 3 hours, allowing patients to ambulate comfortably until the denser analgesia of epidural local anesthetics is needed. If longer labor is anticipated, the addition of morphine (0.25 mg) can prolong the analgesia from fentanyl alone. It will prolong sufentanil analgesia less effectively, with a significant incidence of nausea and itching. Meperidine (15 to 20 mg) has also been used, and has the advantage of possessing local anesthetic properties of its own (16). This may produce some hypotension. The addition of 2.5 mg of bupivacaine

Table 22.2   **Spinal Narcotic Doses for Labor**

Drug	Dose	Duration	Comments
Morphine	0.25–0.4 mg	1–4 h	Side effects common: pruritus, nausea
Meperidine	10–20 mg	1–3 h	Local anesthetic effect: possible hypotension
Fentanyl	10–25 µg	1–2 h	
Sufentanil	10 µg	1–3 h	

to the opioid will also potentiate the analgesia and does not appear to produce motor or sympathetic blockade. With all of the intrathecal opioids, the previous use of intravenous agonist–antagonist opioids will reduce their efficacy.

Intrathecal opioids have not been as free of side effects as hoped. As noted, nausea and pruritus are common, and occur in as many as 50% of patients (17). Hypotension has also occurred in 7% to 20% of patients (9). Fetal bradycardia has also been described in 15% of patients, but did not result in significant problems with the fetus (16). The major difficulty is that subarachnoid narcotics alone do not always last long enough for regular labor and are often inadequate for analgesia in the second stage. Epidural infusions of local anesthetics are usually called for. Fortunately, the previous use of intrathecal narcotics appears to potentiate the efficacy of local anesthetics. Although the intrathecal route is not a panacea, it does appear to provide beneficial analgesia to a significant percentage of women in early labor, and may be worth the effort in selected patients, especially the patient experiencing severe discomfort with her first (presumably long) labor. In patients with severe cardiac diseases who will not tolerate sympathetic blockade (e.g., aortic stenosis, Eisenmenger syndrome) or those with local anesthetic allergy, a continuous infusion of subarachnoid narcotics represents significant advantages.

Opioids are more effective as adjuncts to epidural analgesia (6). The addition of 50 to 100 µg of the more lipid-soluble fentanyl to epidural 0.125% or 0.06% bupivacaine has been shown to improve the quality of analgesia and reduce the degree of motor blockade both in intermittent-injection and continuous-infusion techniques for labor. Neither maternal depression nor fetal neurobehavioral changes has been reported, although pruritus is present in 30% of patients. Sufentanil also has been used.

The use of spinal or epidural narcotics for postcesarean delivery pain appears to be more predictable and to possess a wider margin of safety. The addition of 0.1 to 0.25 mg of morphine to spinal anesthesia for cesarean delivery appears to provide safe and reliable postoperative analgesia. Usually, 3 to 5 mg epidural morphine will provide 12 to 18 hours of analgesia, which is frequently sufficient to allow conversion to oral analgesics. Epidural narcotics produce better analgesia than the use of patient-controlled analgesia (PCA) in the same situation. Unfortunately, the side effects of pruritus (80%), urinary retention (15% to 30%), and nausea are significant drawbacks to the epidural narcotics technique. Women usually prefer PCA to epidural analgesia because of these side effects and the greater ability to titrate their own level of analgesia with PCA. Nevertheless, spinal and epidural narcotic injections following cesarean delivery are highly effective.

The addition of epinephrine to epidural anesthetic solutions in laboring patients is controversial. As discussed in Chapter 7, there are several advantages, particularly in speeding the onset and increasing the efficacy of the analgesia, as well as the traditional role of prolonging blockade. The support of cardiac output and the use as a marker for intravenous injection also have been reviewed (18,19). Quantities absorbed systemically during epidural blockade may interfere with uterine contractions or blood flow. This does not appear to be a clinically significant problem in parturients having normal uterine perfusion with the doses of epinephrine contained in the usual 6 to 8 mL of a 1:200,000 solution. Transient fetal distress occurred in 2 of 10 patients in whom a standard 15-µg test dose was injected intravenously. A second issue is the reliability of the tachycardia response to the anesthetic test solution when trying to detect intravascular injection (18–20). Maternal heart rate varies considerably during labor, with as many as 50% of patients having cyclic elevations of heart rate of greater than 25 beats per minute. Changes due to epinephrine injection may not be detected in this setting. To circumvent this difficulty and to avoid the problems mentioned earlier, some obstetric anesthesiologists omit epinephrine entirely from their epidural solutions. In most cases, simple aspiration of a multiorifice epidural catheter is as reliable as the standard epinephrine injection (21). Also, dividing the usual epidural dose into two equal injections of 3 or 4 mL each will serve as an adequate technique to avoid systemic toxicity during epidural analgesia for labor. For elective cesarean delivery (without labor), the usual test-dose technique appears reliable. An alternative test dose of 1 mL of air (monitored with a precordial Doppler sensor or the usual fetal heart rate monitor) has been described. The appropriate tests for administering epidural doses to patients in labor about to undergo abdominal delivery remain controversial. Incremental injection, careful aspiration, and careful observation are clearly essential until a reliable alternative for epinephrine is found.

Epinephrine can also be added to subarachnoid injections. For cesarean delivery, it will potentiate the local anesthetic and prolong the duration of blockade. For labor analgesia, it will prolong the duration of opioids, but may increase the risk of motor block if local anesthetics are present (9). Clonidine in doses of 50 µg will also prolong analgesia, but with some sedation and hypotension, and thus neither of these additives has achieved popularity.

Techniques

There are essentially two clinical situations to which the obstetric anesthesiologist is asked to respond: vaginal delivery or cesarean birth. The anesthetic considerations merit separate discussions.

Vaginal Delivery

Intermittent Epidural Analgesia. For vaginal delivery, *intermittent-injection epidural analgesia* is a common approach and is performed as described in Chapter 7. There are several modifications •4• required in pregnancy.

1. The anatomic differences detailed earlier in this chapter increase the technical difficulty. The risks of aortocaval compression dictate that an intravenous route be established before an anesthetic is attempted and the mother is given an infusion of 500 to 1000 mL crystalloid solution.
2. For the patient in labor, local infiltration of the skin and deeper tissues can be performed between contractions or during a contraction.
3. The actual entry into the epidural space should occur between contractions, to avoid the risk of unintentional movement causing unwanted advancement of the needle. Ideally, the epidural space is entered, the catheter is threaded, and the needle is withdrawn between contractions so that the needle point is not in the narrower epidural space during a contraction.
4. The catheter is advanced only 3 to 5 cm into the space, and careful aspiration is performed. The drug dose is injected in 3- to 5-mL increments (depending on concentration) at 30-second intervals to reduce the chance of systemic toxicity from an intravascular injection. Standard heart rate monitoring is difficult but not impossible in the laboring patient. If epinephrine is used, injection of the test dose should immediately follow a contraction so as to avoid the misleading increase in heart rate usually produced by the onset of subsequent contractions. As discussed, some anesthesiologists will omit the epinephrine and rely on aspiration and incremental injection of two boluses to provide a margin of safety for labor epidural blockade.
5. If unilateral anesthesia is produced, the patient should be turned with the nonanesthetized side dependent for further injections. If more than 3 cm of catheter has been introduced, the catheter should be withdrawn in 1-cm increments until midline placement is attained, as indicated by analgesia on the opposite side.
6. Once epidural analgesia is established, the parturient is not allowed to lie supine, but must remain on her side to avoid aortocaval compression. Incremental injection is used with each reinjection of the catheter. The mother's blood pressure must be monitored at 5-minute intervals for at least 20 minutes following each injection. Hypotension should be treated with further fluid infusion and change of position. If severe, intravenous or intramuscular ephedrine is most effective in preserving uterine perfusion (22), although phenylephrine may have some use in normal pregnancies (20).

Constant-Infusion Epidural Analgesia. This technique avoids the periods of waning analgesia that often occur with the intermittent-injection technique and appears to provide better analgesia. After the initial dose injection of the epidural catheter, a syringe of local anesthetic mounted in a constant-infusion pump is attached to the catheter connector. Because of the resistance to flow in the catheter, a high-pressure volumetric pump with low-compliance tubing is required. The pump is then set to deliver 8 to 12 mL per hour of 0.125% bupivacaine or a mixture containing 0.06% to 0.1% bupivacaine and 1 to 2 μg per mL of fentanyl. If fentanyl is added to the infusion, 25 to 50 μg should also be added to the initial bolus injection of 0.25% bupivacaine. Ropivacaine 0.2% is also effective. Its interaction with opioids has not been well documented.

The analgesic level must be checked each hour to assess the correct infusion rate. If anesthesia becomes inadequate, a 3- to 5-mL bolus injection of 0.25% bupivacaine may be needed to restore the level while an increase in infusion rate is made.

This technique will avoid the risk of systemic toxicity, because the quantity of anesthetic injected at any time is insufficient to produce symptoms even if the catheter has penetrated a blood vessel. Complaints of diminishing anesthesia should be evaluated as possible indications of intravascular migration of the catheter. Likewise, the gradual development of denser anesthesia may indicate subarachnoid migration of the catheter.

Perineal anesthesia for delivery often will be inadequate with either the intermittent or continuous technique. A bolus injection of 4 to 6 mL 0.25% bupivacaine or 2% chloroprocaine with the patient in the semiupright position may be helpful.

Combined Spinal–Epidural Technique.   As described earlier in this chapter, this combination can be highly effective in providing analgesia with intrathecal narcotics alone without motor blockade in the early stages of labor, and providing denser analgesia with epidural local anesthetics for the second stage. Although this technique is not superior to standard epidural analgesia in most situations, it does provide a more rapid onset of relief (23) and a lower frequency of "break-through" pain later in labor (24). The technique is a simple combination of standard epidural and subarachnoid injection. It can be performed by separate injections at two levels or at a single level, but is most commonly performed by a "needle through needle" technique (10).

1. The patient is positioned and prepped as for a standard epidural injection, either in the sitting or lateral position, and the epidural needle is inserted into the epidural space in the standard manner.
2. A small-gauge rounded-bevel needle is inserted through the epidural needle to puncture the dura (Fig. 22.1). Several matching-pair sets are available commercially, with the spinal needle either extending beyond the tip of the epidural needle or through a special hole in the curvature of the bevel in line with the shaft of the needle, or even through a special side channel in the

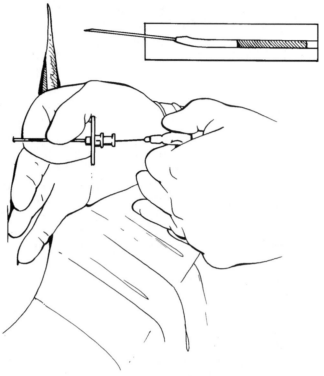

Figure 22.1   **Combined Spinal–Epidural Technique**
After identifying the epidural space in the standard manner, a small spinal
needle is passed through the epidural needle to perform a subarachnoid
injection before an epidural catheter is inserted.

   epidural needle shaft. The essential feature is that the spinal needle must be capable of extending 10 mm beyond the tip of the
epidural needle.

3. Once cerebrospinal fluid (CSF) is obtained, the dose of intrathecal opioid is injected and the spinal needle removed. The addition of 2.5 mg bupivacaine will prolong analgesia. If dural puncture is not easily obtained, the original needle may not be in the
epidural space, or may be angled tangentially to the dura. Repositioning of the epidural needle may be necessary.

4. An epidural catheter is inserted in the standard fashion and secured in place after the epidural needle is removed. When and if
the need arises, the catheter is tested for intravascular or subarachnoid placement in the standard fashion, and local anesthetic is injected. Injection of the epidural catheter will usually
produce higher levels of analgesia after a previous spinal injection, so lower doses may be prudent.

5. If the patient desires to ambulate after the initial subarachnoid
injection, they should first be monitored for 20 minutes to en-

sure the absence of hypotension or fetal bradycardia (9). Many units require some demonstration of adequate motor strength, such as ability to step up on a footstool, before allowing limited ambulation.

Caudal Anesthesia. This technique is performed as described in Chapter 8 and may be used in conjunction with lumbar epidural anesthesia to produce better perineal anesthesia for delivery. If used alone, analgesia for the first stage may be associated with more sacral anesthesia than the mother feels is desirable, but analgesia for delivery will be excellent. Because of the higher doses and denser anesthesia, this technique is used infrequently.

1. For the parturient, the knee–chest position of kneeling on the bed is often the easiest to assume. The lateral decubitus is another alternative.
2. The caudal catheter is advanced 8 to 12 cm into the canal, and incremental injection is used here also to avoid systemic toxicity. The usual dose is 16 to 18 mL of one of the standard local anesthetics for labor.
3. If the fetal head is well into the birth canal (just anterior to the sacrum), caudal blockade may be undesirable because of the risk of injection into the fetal scalp. If used, caution must be employed not to penetrate the sacrum during this block.

Spinal Anesthesia. This is also performed in a standard fashion, with the patient either in the sitting (to produce a classical saddle block) or the lateral position. A small-gauge (25 to 27) rounded-bevel needle is used to reduce the chance of headache, although this increases the technical difficulty and time required. Saddle-block anesthesia with local anesthetic is performed only after the cervical dilation is complete and delivery is imminent within 90 minutes; otherwise, a repeated block may be necessary.

Cesarean Delivery

In the event of a cesarean delivery, the choice of anesthetic is more complex. The degree of urgency must be clearly discussed with the obstetrician before choosing the appropriate technique. If the procedure is "urgent" but not emergent, a previously functioning *epidural blockade* can simply be augmented to produce the degree of anesthesia required or a new block can be instituted. If speed and reliability are desired, a *spinal anesthetic* is more appropriate, and with the current equipment and drugs, is a popular choice. If a true emergency exists, such as fetal distress or maternal hemorrhage, *general anesthesia* is required and should be instituted immediately in the manner described in standard obstetric anesthesia texts.

For each of the regional techniques, there are requirements beyond those for vaginal delivery alone. An upper level of anesthesia to the second to fourth thoracic dermatomes is usually required, as well as a denser motor blockade to provide adequate abdominal relaxation for the surgeon. Blood pressure changes will be more dramatic, and leftward uterine displacement is essential. The uterus must be displaced by a mechanical device or a pad under the right hip to ensure a 15-degree tilt until the fetus is delivered. The rapidity of blood pressure changes requires a previous intravenous infusion of 1000 to 1500 mL crystalloid solution immediately before the block. Ephedrine in doses of 10 mg intravenously or 25 mg intramuscularly may be needed. The fetal heart tones should be monitored up to the last possible moment before the incision. Supplemental oxygen to the mother is administered at least until the baby is delivered, with pulse oximeter monitoring. Blood loss is greater than with vaginal delivery (estimated at 1500 versus 500 mL), and careful intraoperative attention to the blood pressure is mandatory. Blood loss may aggravate hypotension and further increase the incidence of nausea. The potential for venous air embolism or amniotic fluid embolism is greater than with vaginal delivery. In addition to all of these factors, the probability of requiring resuscitation of the neonate is greater (because many cesarean deliveries are performed in the context of concern for fetal well-being). Ideally, a neonatologist or second anesthesiologist should be available for every cesarean delivery.

Complications

In general, the complications of these techniques are the same as in the nonpregnant patient and are handled in a similar fashion. Four complications deserve special mention.

Systemic Toxicity

Systemic toxicity is particularly devastating in the parturient. Intravascular injection occurs more readily with the venous engorgement of the epidural space, and the dynamic circulation produces rapid distribution to the brain with immediate signs of toxicity. Cardiovascular collapse appears to occur more frequently. This is usually related to aortocaval compression as the seizing patient is usually turned immediately to the supine position. Bupivacaine, a frequently used drug, is also associated with a narrower margin of safety with regard to depression of cardiac conduction. Cardiac resuscitation is more difficult because of the intruding mass of the uterus as well as the insufficient venous return resulting from aortocaval compression by the uterus. Urgent cesarean delivery may be needed to save the fetus if maternal cardiac decompensation occurs. Maternal acidosis will lead to fetal acidosis, which then increases the percentage of local anesthetic transferred across the placenta and "trapped" in the acidemic fetal blood.

Table 22.3   **Safety Measures during Obstetric Anesthetic Injections**

Procedure	Comment
Constant observation of mental status	
Gentle aspiration	May be unreliable in epidural space— better with multihole catheter
Epinephrine test dose	Unreliable in pregnancy
Local anesthetic test dose	Reliability not tested in pregnancy
Incremental injection	
Use of dilute solutions	
Replace catheter if block inadequate	Assume it is intravascular

Resuscitation is also more difficult in the family-centered labor room, where necessary equipment may not be available or may be stored in awkward drawers or cupboards in order to maintain the "homelike" environment. The full stomach increases the chance of vomiting and aspiration and necessitates immediate endotracheal intubation during resuscitation.

Prevention is a greater need than in the nonpregnant patient, and the use of test doses, incremental injection, and minimal effective concentrations, and constant careful attention to the patient's mental status and symptoms are essential (19) (Table 22.3). The use of these steps appears to have significantly reduced the frequency of this complication after 1983, and to have reduced the risk of mortality from regional anesthesia in obstetrics (11). The newer, less cardiotoxic amino-amides, ropivacaine and levobupivacaine, may be helpful in further reducing the risk of cardiac complications with cesarean delivery, although the quantities of anesthetic involved in analgesic infusions represent minimal risks.

Gastric Aspiration

Gastric aspiration during general anesthesia has been recognized as a major cause of maternal anesthetic mortality. All patients having regional analgesia must be considered potential candidates for general anesthesia and solids should be withheld during labor. If cesarean delivery is indicated, treatment with oral nonparticulate antacids and intravenous histamine (H_2) antagonists (and/or metoclopramide) is appropriate.

Postspinal Headache

Postspinal headache occurs more frequently than in the nonpregnant population. Although conservative management with fluids and bed rest following operative delivery may be effective, early aggressive treatment with epidural blood patch is indicated for the mother desiring to be discharged home to care for her new infant.

Instrumented Deliveries

One last "complication" to be mentioned is the issue of the increased incidence of instrumented deliveries when anesthesia is employed for labor. This is a frequent concern of mothers and a topic of conversation in many childbirth preparation classes. There is a higher incidence of the use of forceps after epidural anesthesia, but patients having analgesia are also those with prolonged (and perhaps less effective) labors (7,8). There is also not a clear connection with forceps and poor fetal outcome. There is no increased risk of cesarean delivery. The use of lower concentrations of local anesthetics (usually combined with low-dose fentanyl) may better preserve maternal expulsive forces, and reduce the incidence of instrumented deliveries. There are few studies that attempt to measure the benefits of stress reduction and pain relief and compare them to the risks of interfering with the progress of labor. This topic will remain controversial and, unfortunately, is colored by the emotional bias attendant on the current "natural childbirth" preference in the United States. Despite these emotional issues and the real challenges and increased risks outlined, appropriate anesthetic interventions can contribute to the successful conclusion of pregnancy with a healthy and happy mother and baby as long as the safety features outlined are followed.

References

1. Birnbach, D. J., Gatt, S. P., Datta, S. *Textbook of Obstetric Anesthesia.* St. Louis: WB Saunders, 2000.
2. Chestnut, D. H. *Obstetrical Anesthesia: Principles and Practice.* 2nd ed. St. Louis: Mosby, 1999.
3. Dewan, D. M. *Practical Obstetric Handbook.* St. Louis: WB Saunders, 2000.
4. Hughes, S. *Shnider and Levinson's Anesthesia for Obstetrics.* 4th ed. Philadelphia: Lippincott Williams & Wilkins, 2000.
5. Norris, M. C. *Obstetric Anesthesia.* 2nd ed. Philadelphia: Lippincott Williams & Wilkins, 1999.
6. Practice guidelines for obstetrical anesthesia: A report by the American Society of Anesthesiologists Task Force on Obstetrical Anesthesia. *Anesthesiology* 90: 600, 1999.
7. Chestnut, D. H. Does epidural analgesia during labor affect the incidence of cesarean delivery? *Reg. Anesth.* 22: 495, 1997.
8. Halpern, S. H., Leighton, B. L., Ohlsson, A., Barrett, J. F., Rice, A. Effect of epidural vs parenteral opioid analgesia on the progress of labor: A meta-analysis. *J.A.M.A.* 280: 2105, 1998.
9. Eisenach, J. C. Combined spinal-epidural analgesia in obstetrics. *Anesthesiology* 91: 299, 1999.
10. Rawal, N., Van Zundert, A., Holmstrom, B., Crowhurst, J. A. Combined spinal-epidural technique. *Reg. Anesth.* 22: 406, 1997.
11. Hawkins, J. L., Koonin, L. M., Palmer, S. K., Gibbs, C. P. Anesthesia-related deaths during obstetric delivery in the United States, 1979–1990. *Anesthesiology* 86: 277, 1997.

12. Flamm, B. L., Lim, O. W., Jones, C., Fallon, D., Newman, L. A., Mantis, J. K. Vaginal birth after cesarean section: Results of a multicenter study. *Am. J. Obstet. Gynecol.* 158: 1079, 1988.

13. Rageth, J. C., Juzi, C., Grossenbacher, H. Delivery after previous cesarean: A risk evaluation. Swiss Working Group of Obstetric and Gynecologic Institutions. *Obstet. Gynecol.* 93:332, 1999.

14. Polley, L. S., Columb, M. O. Comparison of epidural ropivacaine and bupivacaine in combination with sufentanil for labor. *Anesthesiology* 92: 280, 2000.

15. Ben-David, B., Miller, G., Gavriel, R., Gurevitch, A. Low-dose bupivacaine-fentanyl spinal anesthesia for cesarean delivery. *Reg. Anesth. Pain Med.* 25: 235, 2000.

16. Honet, J. E., Arkoosh, V. A., Norris, M. C., Huffnagle, H. J., Silverman, N. S., Leighton, B. L. Comparison among intrathecal fentanyl, meperidine, and sufentanil for labor analgesia. *Anesth. Analg.* 75: 734, 1992.

17. Grieco, W. M., Norris, M. C., Leighton, B. L., Arkoosh, V. A., Huffnagle, H. J., Honet, J. E., Costello, D. Intrathecal sufentanil labor analgesia: The effects of adding morphine or epinephrine. *Anesth. Analg.* 77: 1149, 1993.

18. Birnbach, D. J., Chestnut, D. H. The epidural test dose in obstetric patients: Has it outlived its usefulness? *Anesth. Analg.* 88: 971, 1999.

19. Mulroy, M. F., Norris, M. C., Liu, S. S. Safety steps for epidural injection of local anesthetics: Review of the literature and recommendations. *Anesth. Analg.* 85: 1346, 1997.

20. Santos, A. C., Pedersen, H. Current controversies in obstetric anesthesia. *Anesth. Analg.* 78: 753, 1994.

21. Norris, M. C., Ferrenbach, D., Dalman, H., Fogel, S. T., Borrenpohl, S., Hoppe, W., Riley, A. Does epinephrine improve the diagnostic accuracy of aspiration during labor epidural analgesia? *Anesth. Analg.* 88: 1073, 1999.

22. McGrath, J. M., Chestnut, D. H., Vincent, R. D., DeBruyn, C. S., Atkins, B. L., Poduska, D. J., Chatterjee, P. Ephedrine remains the vasopressor of choice for treatment of hypotension during ritodrine infusion and epidural anesthesia. *Anesthesiology* 80: 1073, 1994.

23. Hepner, D. L., Gaiser, R. R., Cheek, T. G., Gutsche, B. B. Comparison of combined spinal-epidural and low dose epidural for labour analgesia. *Can. J. Anaesth.* 47: 232, 2000.

24. Hess, P. E., Pratt, S. D., Lucas, T. P., Miller, C. G., Corbett, T., Oriol, N., Sarna, M. C. Predictors of breakthrough pain during labor epidural analgesia. *Anesth. Analg.* 93: 414, 2001.

23 Chronic Pain Management

James D. Helman

Anesthesiologists are frequently consulted in the management of pain problems. Their expertise in perioperative analgesia management makes this a natural role. Interventional procedures to alter or impede the transmission or perception of painful stimuli by patients are appealing. The application of diagnostic and, potentially, therapeutic neural blockade for the care of patients with chronic malignant or nonmalignant pain, when appropriately implemented, may reduce the patient's discomfort. However, numerous factors limit the successful application of interventional procedures. Pain is a subjective entity that poorly correlates with the severity of the patient's medical condition. The dynamic state of disease processes (e.g., growth or invasion of tumor) and anatomic variability may mitigate the technical success of interventional procedures. In addition, forces of psychological, sociologic, financial, and legal sources may confound the uncertain pathophysiology of pain mechanisms. Hence, Carron's astute observation, that "minimal pathology with maximum dysfunction remains the enigma of chronic pain," succinctly summarizes the predicament (1). However, information obtained from neural blockade may provide insight into the pathophysiology and location of nociception. The prior information is incorporated into a multidisciplinary approach to care of the patient with pain syndromes, which may include oral or parenteral medications, therapeutic blocks, or surgical procedures, complemented by psychological therapies (2).

Application and interpretation of diagnostic and therapeutic interventional neural blockade are difficult. Some of the techniques in this book can be applied successfully in chronic pain treatment. Regional anesthetic techniques, however, are not a panacea for all pain problems, particularly chronic nonmalignant pain syndromes. Limitations include the accurate selection of the diagnostic technique for the pain syndrome, the exact implementation of the technique, and the appropriate interpretation of the efficacy of the technique by both the patient and the practitioner (3). This chapter reviews some of the common applications of regional blockade to pain management, several of which are more traditional than effective (1).

Assessment

In an attempt to encourage standardization of methodology that can facilitate treatment outcome monitoring, it is imperative to perform a thorough evaluation of the patient who presents with a painful condition. Acquired information may be used for baseline assessment and subsequent interval responses to therapeutic interventions with waxing or waning of the pain disorder. The evaluation should include the acquisition of information through a medical pain history: (i) chief complaint and associated symptom characteristics of the pain condition (characteristics of pain; date of onset; conditions at onset; quality, severity, and persistence of the pain; associated symptoms; and provocative and mitigating factors); (ii) past medical history; (iii) medication history; (iv) systems review; (v) family history; and (vi) occupation and social history. The physical examination should include a thorough evaluation, and specifically, a focused evaluation of three particular areas: pain behavior during the examination, and neurologic and musculoskeletal structures. The inclusion of pertinent diagnostic modalities to include radiographic tests of structure, electrodiagnostic tests of somatic function, and tests of hematologic and metabolic status augment the formulation of a differential diagnosis.

The measurement of pain is a difficult task given its subjective variability among patients with similar disorders. Nonetheless, various tools and modalities are used in the assessment of pain and the subsequent impact of therapy. Single-descriptor pain measurement scales are simple to administer and include (i) numeric pain scales, (ii) visual analog scales, and (iii) facial drawings. These tools are easily understood by patients, easily used by pain clinic personnel, demonstrate reliability, and permit the assessment of analgesic efficacy. However, they are restricted by the limited response choices and occasionally by reduced comprehension by the elderly, mentally handicapped, and patients with poor communication skills. An additional complicating factor to the interpretation of interventional procedures includes a significant incidence of a placebo response. Patients obtain pain relief from placebo interventions in approximately one-third of acute pain conditions and in upward of two-thirds of chronic pain syndromes. Hence initial and subsequent pain assessment modalities are useful, but their interpretation must be cautiously individualized for each patient.

Adjuvant Agents and Modalities for Diagnostic or Therapeutic Intervention

Local Anesthetics

The structure and pharmacology of local anesthetics are reviewed in Chapter 1. The rationale for the use of local anesthetic nerve blocks in chronic pain patients is the consistency with which they interrupt nociceptive pathways. It is believed that neural blockade alters or interrupts nociceptive input, reflex mechanisms of the afferent limb, and the self-sustaining activity of the neuron pools and neuraxis. It is also believed that local anesthetics interrupt the pain–spasm cycle. Sensory nerve block thus obtained usually relieves pain and interrupts the afferent limbs of an abnormal reflex. With low concentrations of local anesthetic agents, one can block the A-delta, B, and unmyelinated C-delta fibers without clinically significant impairment of motor function. Notably, in early phases of chronic pain, local anesthetic nerve blocks can produce prolonged pain relief that outlasts the pharmacological action of the drug by days or weeks. The mechanism for this is not yet understood, but one can speculate that this may be due to a reversal of physiologic changes, which accompany chronic pain.

Intravenous (i.v.) administration of local anesthetics has been beneficial in managing such painful conditions as burns, postsurgical pain, central pain, deafferentation syndrome, Raynaud syndrome, phantom limb pain, causalgia, neuritis, and myofascial pain. Although the classic local anesthetic agent used has been procaine, the choice of drug has varied from chloroprocaine to tetracaine. When used for pain management, these local anesthetics have historically been administered in large, incremental dosages. However, techniques of administration have also used the flowmeter and the i.v. pump in an attempt to control the infusion rate of the local anesthetic agent. Examples of i.v. techniques include lidocaine (0.15%) administered at 4 mg per min using a pump for 1 hour, and chloroprocaine (1%) solution administered at a rate of 1.0 to 1.5 mg/kg/min until a total dose of 10 to 20 mg per kg is delivered. All infusions are conducted in a controlled environment where resuscitative equipment and drugs are immediately available.

Corticosteroids

Although corticosteroid injections are frequently utilized with the aim of reducing edema and inflammation around the nerve root, the efficacy and indication for this treatment continue to be debated. There is no consensus among the interventional pain management specialists with regard to type, dosage, frequency, total number of injections, or other interventions. Many studies have significant design flaws and systematic reviews have also presented varying conclusions. On the basis of the available literature and scientific application, the most commonly used formulations of long-acting steroids, which include methylprednisolone (DepoMedrol), triamcinolone diacetate (Aristocort), triamcinolone acetonide (Kenalog), and betamethasone acetate and phosphate mixture (Celestone Soluspan), appear to be safe and effective.

Side effects related to the administration of steroids are generally attributed either to the chemistry or to the pharmacology of the steroids. The major theoretical complications of corticosteroid administration include suppression of the pituitary–adrenal axis, hypercorticism, Cushing syndrome, osteoporosis, avascular necrosis of bone, steroid myopathy, epidural lipomatosis, weight gain, fluid retention, and hyperglycemia. However, Manchikanti et al., while evaluating the effect of neuraxial steroids on weight and bone mass density, showed no significant difference in patients undergoing various types of interventional techniques with or without steroids (4).

Frequency and total number of injections or interventions are a key issue, although controversial and rarely addressed. Some authors recommend one injection for diagnostic as well as therapeutic purposes; others advocate three injections in a series irrespective of the patient's progress or lack thereof; still others suggest three injections followed by a repeat course of three injections after 3-, 6-, or 12-month intervals; and, finally, there are some who propose an unlimited number of injections with no established goals or parameters. There are no quality studies available to reconcile this issue. On the basis of the present literature, it appears that if repeated within 2 weeks, betamethasone probably would be the best in avoiding side effects; whereas if treatment is carried out at 6-week intervals or longer, any one of the four formulations will be safe and effective (5).

Opioids

Opioids can provide analgesia either systemically or in neuraxial applications. The analgesic ladder method promotes prescribing oral nonopioid analgesics combined with adjuvant analgesics for mild to moderate pain, then adding oral opioids for moderate pain, and finally administering oral opioids (acute and sustained-release formulations) on a regular schedule for severe malignant and nonmalignant pain. Neuraxial opioids have been implemented in the treatment of malignant and nonmalignant chronic pain conditions for two decades. The effectiveness of spinal opioids is promising, but interpretation of different studies is difficult because of difference in inclusion criteria, outcome parameters, and duration of follow-up. Comparative data of epidural, subarachnoid, and intracerebroventricular opioids in patients with cancer pain suggest similar efficacy, with 60% to 75% of patients achieving excellent pain relief (6). In a retrospective survey of patients receiving intrathecal morphine for malignant and nonmalignant pain, the mean percent relief was 61% (7), whereas examination of patients with intrathecal opioids for failed back surgery syndrome or arachnoiditis reported limited efficacy (8). As with the use of oral opioids for chronic noncancer pain, the use of spinal opioids should be part of a multimodal and interdisciplinary pain management plan. The therapeutic objectives should include improvement in functional capabilities in addition to analgesic response. Combinations of opioids and nonopioid analgesics and occasionally local anesthetics may be more effective for the control of neuropathic or incident pain.

Tolerance refers to a phenomenon in which exposure to a drug results in the diminution of an effect or the need for a higher dose to maintain an effect. Tolerance to the analgesic effects of opioids after acute and chronic dosing has been clearly shown in man. Tolerance to the adverse effects of opioids also occurs and has positive benefit. There is a suggestion from animal research that ongoing nociception may modulate the development of tolerance to analgesic drugs. Many cancer patients with severe pain often have long periods of stable opioid dosage unless disease progression occurs. Clinical surveys of long-term opioid use in patients with noncancer pain, when an increasing nociceptive focus is unlikely, have not shown escalating drug dosage to be an inevitable clinical problem, although some dose increase is often observed over time.

Clinicians must evolve strategies for managing increasing analgesic dose and possible tolerance in the patient with chronic pain. Options for the management of tolerance include the following: (i) the "differential diagnosis" for declining analgesic effectiveness should be considered and treated, (ii) the dose of opioid can be increased, (iii) an alternative opioid can be substituted at a reduced dose, and (iv) alternative pain management strategies can be introduced with dose stabilization or reduction.

α_2-Adrenergic Receptor Agonists

α_2-Adrenergic receptor agonists, alone or in combination with other pharmacologic agents, are gaining increased utility in the management of perioperative and chronic pain. They affect neuronal excitability and transmitter release by the action of numerous G proteins at both pre- and postsynaptic neural membrane sites, both centrally and in neuraxial application. At neuroaxial locations (epidural or intrathecal techniques), the α_2-agonists inhibit A delta– and C nerve fiber-induced firing of wide dynamic range neurons in the spinal cord dorsal horn. The most favorable results for the use of α_2-agonists are in patients with deafferentation and sympathetically mediated pain in both malignant and nonmalignant states. Agents include clonidine, guanabenz, medetomidine, and dexmedetomidine. Monitoring for the principal side effects of hypotension, bradycardia, and sedation include assessment of mental status, heart rate, blood pressure, and pulse oximetry (if the dose exceeds 300 µg) (9). Chronic administration of α_2-agonists may result in the development of hypertension upon withdrawal of therapy. Gradual tapering of the α_2-agonists may mitigate this untoward development (10).

γ-Aminobutyric Acid Receptor Agonists

The amino acid γ-aminobutyric acid (GABA) is the dominant inhibitory transmitter of the spinal cord and brain. Three GABA receptor types exist and each has unique properties (GABA$_A$, -$_B$, and -$_C$). The receptor has discrete sites for binding numerous classes of sedative and hypnotic compounds to include GABA, picrotoxin, barbiturate, benzodiazepine, and neurosteroid sites (11). The greatest density of GABA$_B$ receptors is on monosynaptic Ia afferents and descending fibers. They mediate slow inhibition of polysynaptic potentials and act presynaptically to decrease the release of substance P and other primary sensory afferent transmitters. GABA receptors have minimal baseline activity until pathologic conditions arise (12). GABA agonists, such as baclofen, are effective analgesics in acute pain conditions but are inadequate for persistent pain syndromes. This inconsistency may be explained by the excess release and saturation of GABA, which are receptors in chronic pain syndromes. GABA agonists, such as baclofen, have been used for interventional pain procedures to suppress spasticity associated with spinal cord injury and multiple sclerosis (13,14). Baclofen inhibits excitatory amino acid release from spinal interneurons and primary afferents that result in muscle relaxation. It can be administered through an indwelling intrathecal catheter and implanted pump and reservoir. Adverse effects include weakness, nausea, emesis, drowsiness, dizziness, ataxia, and mental confusion. Abrupt withdrawal of baclofen may precipitate seizures. Monitoring during initial intrathecal baclofen trial includes serial neurologic evaluations of spasticity, and hemodynamic and respiratory function.

Techniques Available for Diagnostic or Therapeutic Intervention

Diagnostic Somatic Nerve Blockade

Peripheral nerve blockade is used as a diagnostic procedure to obtain a correct differential diagnosis by blocking a particular nerve or pathway (15). Therapeutic blocks with local anesthetics result in pain relief in accordance with the duration of the specific agents selected. Consequently, repetition of the procedure may be necessary. The beneficial effects of repeated infiltration of nerve may facilitate the implementation of physical therapy by relieving pain-induced immobilization.

Somatic nerve blocks are performed for diagnostic and therapeutic relief of chronic pain disorders. In addition, the procedure may determine the efficacy of neurolysis, cryoanalgesia, or surgical nerve division. Unfortunately, the nociceptive source of the pain may be proximal to the site of the diagnostic intervention and yield the incorrect diagnosis for the origin of the pain. In addition, neuroablative procedures demonstrate poor long-term relief despite resolution of pain with local anesthetic injection. Accurate needle placement may be confirmed by knowledge of the anatomy and adjacent structures, use of radiographic adjuncts, use of a nerve stimulator, or detection of paresthesias with needle placement.

The application of peripheral nerve blockade for either diagnosis or therapy must be interpreted cautiously because chronic pain may not be solely caused by a nociceptive mechanism (16). Chronic pain resulting from peripheral nerve damage may no longer be dependent on peripheral input. Spontaneous neural activity or altered spinal and supraspinal processing (central sensitization) of stimuli may produce the patient's pain syndrome. Subsequently, a partially successful diagnostic procedure may provide more uncertainty than information. In addition, peripheral nerve blockade has limited diagnostic utility to predict successful outcome for nerve transaction or neuroablative procedures. Therefore, diagnostic peripheral nerve blockade must be performed in the context of multidisciplinary assessment and management of chronic pain.

Sympathetic Plexus Blockade

Sympathetically maintained pain is pain that is maintained by sympathetic efferent innervation, or neurochemical or circulating catecholamine action (17). Pain relieved by a specific sympatholytic procedure (pharmacological or sympathetic nerve blockade) may be considered sympathetically maintained pain, although the duration of pain relief will only be temporary in some cases (18), and the degree of sympathetic dysfunction may not correlate with the degree of analgesia or response after sympathetic blockade. Because the sympathetic ganglia are separated from somatic nerves (except in the thoracic region), it is possible to achieve selective blockade of sympathetic fibers without effects on sensory and motor function. Sympathetic blockade has potential diagnostic and therapeutic effects in patients with chronic pain by the following:

1. Blockade of afferent visceral nociceptive fibers that may reduce or eliminate visceral pain;
2. Blockade of sympathetic efferent fibers that may interrupt the interaction between nociception and the sympathetic nervous system in sympathetically maintained pain states associated with complex regional pain syndromes (CRPS);
3. Producing vasodilatation that may provide relief of ischemic pain, and facilitate the healing of chronic ulceration in inoperable peripheral vascular disease.

Neurolysis

Neuroablative techniques have been utilized as an adjunct in the management of intractable pain secondary to malignancy and, infrequently, in nonmalignant pain syndromes. The application of lytic techniques should be restricted to pain that is discrete and expected to persist. Somatic and visceral origins of pain syndromes are more amenable to neurolysis than is neuropathic pain. The implementation of these techniques should be reserved for patients for whom trials of aggressive pharmacologic therapy and other conservative modalities have been unsuccessful. Neurolytic modalities include chemical, thermal, and surgical approaches. Surgical interventions are not discussed in this chapter.

Chemical Neurolysis. Neurolytic chemical agents used to treat pain syndromes include alcohol, phenol, and, infrequently, ammonium sulfate, chlorocresol, or glycerol. Absolute alcohol acts by extracting cholesterol, phospholipids, and cerebrosides from the nervous tissue and causes precipitation of lipoproteins and mucoproteins. Alcohol diffuses rapidly from the injection site after injection. The volume of the agent administered is usually small and hence the effects of ingested alcohol are not observed. However, complications, including local tissue injuries that range from irritation to cellulitis and necrosis, may occur. Alcohol neurolysis is occasionally associated with pain at the site of injection, neuralgia of variable duration (weeks to months), or hypesthesia in the distribution of the chemically lysed nerve(s). Appropriate patient counseling may mitigate the patient's distress if these conditions occur. Lumbar and sacral intrathecal alcohol administration may result in bowel and bladder incontinence. Appropriate patient positioning and the hypobaricity of alcohol may be considered to avoid this complication. Somatic neuralgia and paraplegia secondary to vascular spasm may occur during lumbar sympathetic neurolysis with alcohol. Preferential sites for administration of alcohol neurolysis include intrathecal, celiac plexus, lumbar sympathetic chain, cranial nerve, paravertebral, and epidural locations.

Phenol, or carbolic acid, is a monohydroxy benzene compound that is poorly soluble and diffuses slowly from tissues. Phenol acts by nonselective denaturing the proteins in axons and perineural blood vessels. Neural degeneration takes approximately 14 days and recovery occurs in 14 weeks. Phenol, in comparison with absolute alcohol, yields a less pronounced neurolytic block of reduced duration. Combined with glycerin or contrast solutions, phenol produces a hyperbaric mixture. Phenol acts as a local anesthetic at lower concentration and as a neurolytic agent at higher concentration. Hence it causes less pain with injection than does alcohol. Phenol's high affinity for vascular tissue must be considered when it is applied near major blood vessels (e.g., celiac plexus). The injury to blood vessels may be a factor in the pathogenesis of the neurotoxicity (i.e., paraplegia) inherent in the use of phenol. In addition, like alcohol, subcutaneous administration of phenol may cause ulcerations. Preferential sites for administration of phenol neurolysis include epidural, paravertebral, peripheral, intrathecal, and cranial nerves (19).

Monitoring during the administration of chemical neurolytic agents includes appropriate patient positioning with regard to agent baricity, precise attention to selection of injection site with serial aspiration through the needle to avoid intravascular or intrathecal injection (unless it is the proposed procedure), utilization of contrast agents and radiological modalities to verify needle position, and serial neurologic evaluations during and following the interventional procedure.

Cryolysis and Cryoanalgesia.   Neurolysis of variable duration can be achieved by hypothermia-induced nerve injury. The administration of cold results in the removal of pure water from solution. The subsequent formation of ice crystals causes changes in tissue osmolarity, cell wall permeability, and disruption of neural myelin (20). The axons are damaged at the site of injury with this process. However, the epineurium, perineurium, and endoneurium are preserved. The technique is quite safe, but unfortunately, the duration of analgesia may be variable.

Cryolysis can be applied to any nerve that can be precisely isolated. It can be utilized in the treatment of pain disorders involving peripheral nerves, pelvic pain, spinal facet pain, intercostal neuralgia, and facial pain. The nerves are initially blocked by the application of local anesthesia and then allowed to return to baseline function before lysis. This facilitates careful identification of sensory innervation in order to avoid motor nerve lysis. In addition, precise location of the distal tip of the cryoprobe may be facilitated by the use of fluoroscopy. Cryolysis equipment may leak along the shaft of the cryoprobe during the treatment and must be examined prior to use on the patient. Cryoprobe design includes insulation, but may be augmented by the placement of the probe through a large-gauge intravenous catheter. Finally, the application of cryolysis may be extremely painful during the initial freeze cycle. Patients must be appropriately counseled and, perhaps, may need analgesia and sedation. Hence monitoring for cryolysis includes careful isolation of the sensory nerve roots with nerve stimulation, fluoroscopy assistance to precisely position the cryoprobe, diagnostic application of local anesthetics, and utilization of appropriate hemodynamic and ventilatory monitoring if sedation is administered (21).

Radiofrequency Neurolysis.   Electrical current has been used to ablate neural structures and pain pathways. A radiofrequency-derived thermal injury occurs when the temperature of neural tissue exceeds 45°C. The increase in temperature is a product of frictional heat derived from molecular movement in a field of alternating current (AC). The current is derived from radio wave frequencies that form an electromagnetic field around an active electrode. The active probe is placed in the preferential location for neural lesioning, and a dispersive or indifferent electrode is placed to minimize current delivery across the heart. Heat is not generated by the active electrode itself, but from current movement through adjacent tissues. Gradually increasing the wattage results in the development of heat in the tissues and the thermocouple attached to the active electrode. The temperature is monitored and wattage adjusted to a desired temperature to produce the desired lesion size. The radiofrequency equipment specifications must include the ability to (i) measure impedance, amperage, and voltage; (ii) stimulate a wide range of frequencies; and (iii) accurately measure the duration of a specified probe tip temperature. Hence the needle–thermocouple apparatus used for radiofrequency ablation allows injecting, lesioning, and monitoring with one apparatus. Advantages include a low incidence of neuroma formation, a decreased incidence of adjacent tissue trauma due to temperature control of the lesion size and probe placement verification by prelesion electrical stimulation, the ability to perform the procedure under local or sedative anesthesia, and the ability to repeat the procedure if regeneration occurs (22–24).

Indications for radiofrequency ablation have included pain syndromes involving ganglia at all levels (stellate, sphenopalatine, trigeminal, cervical, thoracic, lumbar, and sacral) and facet joints from the cervical to sacral vertebral regions. Percutaneous cordotomy is a commonly used procedure for the treatment of cancer pain, especially for pain in the contralateral torso. Complications of radiofrequency lysis have included neuralgia, incomplete sympatholysis, pneumothorax, Horner syndrome, and motor paralysis. Monitoring to mitigate these complications (22–24) includes (i) inspection of equipment for potential fractures in the needle insulation that may cause tissue injury anywhere along the course of the needle, (ii) fluoroscopic or computed tomography (CT) guidance to facilitate placement of the needle, and (iii) stimulation with a wide range of frequencies to accurately position the tip of the probe and avoid motor nerve injury. Patients with sensing pacemakers represent a specific situation that warrants electrocardiogram monitoring. Patients with implanted stimulators may be at increased risk of injury with radiofrequency lesioning.

Neuromodulation of the Spinal Cord

Spinal cord stimulation was initially implemented for the treatment of chronic pain in 1967 (25). The original proposed mechanism of action was stimulation of large myelinated fibers (A beta) in the dorsal column of the spinal cord. Subsequently, additional proposed mechanisms have included activation of descending inhibitory systems, dorsal root modulation, antidromic stimulation, central inhibition of sympathetic efferent neurons, and activation of neurotransmitters (neuromodulators) (26). The success of this modality has improved with advances in the implantable electrodes (arrays of multiple electrodes), (27) computer-controlled pulse generators, and radiofrequency-coupled devices with appropriate patient selection (28). North et al. reviewed their clinical experience over two decades and noted that 52% of patients continued to report at least 50% pain relief with implanted spinal cord stimulators (7-year mean follow-up) (29). Patient factors that were associated with successful treatment outcomes in their review included (i) female sex, (ii) patients with deafferentation or neural injury (versus nociceptive pain), and (iii) those patients with fewer prior operations (29).

Other patient screening criteria prior to consideration of a percutaneous stimulation trial include objective pathologic findings, failure of all conservative therapies, and no evidence of major psychiatric illness or drug habituation. Presently, diagnostic indications for trial stimulation include (i) perineural fibrosis (postlaminectomy syndrome), (ii) sympathetically maintained pain, (iii) adhesive arachnoiditis, (iv) peripheral nerve injury (neuralgia), (v) peripheral vascular disease with ischemic pain, (vi) phantom limb pain, (vii) spinal cord lesions with defined segmental pain, and (viii) angina.

Patients who are considered candidates should have the area of pain clearly delineated, and a trial electrode passed into the epidural space (Fig. 23.1). The electrode is connected to a trial stimulator and the current adjusted to produce relief. If relief is satisfactory over a trial period, the lead can be tunneled under the skin and connected to a permanent stimulator unit implanted on the abdominal wall. These units can be programmed with an external device. Alterna-

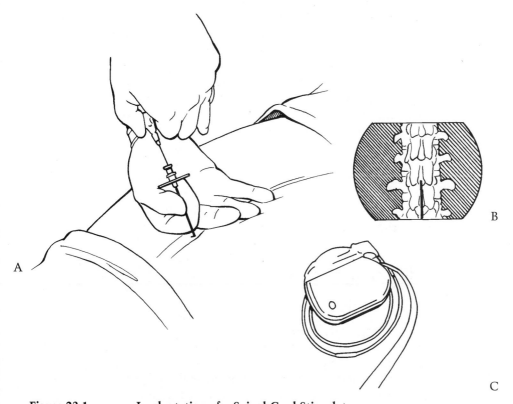

Figure 23.1   **Implantation of a Spinal Cord Stimulator**
A trial lead is inserted through an epidural catheter (**A**) and its location confirmed by fluoroscopy (**B**). If adequate pain relief is obtained, the lead can be tunneled subcutaneously and connected to an implantable programmable stimulator unit (**C**).

tively, if successful analgesia is obtained, larger, more durable leads can be implanted through a surgical incision and also tunneled to a stimulator unit.

The complications of spinal cord electrode and pulse generator or receiver implantation include wound infection, electromechanical failure (electrode, receiver, pulse generator), electrode migration, and, infrequently, catheter fibrosis (28). The neuromodulation modality may also fail if the patients are inappropriately screened during the percutaneous trial (adequate duration of trial to assess efficacy) or the patients have inappropriate expectations or comprehension with regard to the capabilities and effects of the technology (29).

Radiography

Fluoroscopy and, occasionally, CT are crucial adjuncts to the performance of interventional pain procedures in the cranial, cervical, thoracic, abdominal, and pelvic regions. Radiographic technology is most pertinent to the safe and successful completion of neuroablative procedures. In addition, the instillation of opaque contrast material augments the precision of needle (probe) placement provided by radiography. Contrast dyes used in radiography are either ionic or nonionic compounds formed from a triiodinated benzene ring. Nonionic formulations (iopamidol [Isovue], iohexol [Onmipaque]) have a lower risk of CNS toxicity when administered near the neuroaxis than ionic agents (diatrizoate meglumine [Renografin, Hypaque], iothalamate meglumine [Conray]). Ionic agents may be safely used when they are injected in regions other than the neuroaxis. However, contrast agents may cause local and systemic toxicity. Signs of toxicity may range from urticaria or skin ulceration (infrequent) to bronchospasm and possible anaphylaxis. Monitoring and treatments include therapies for hypoxemia, hypotension, and bronchospasm (30–32).

Approach to Specific Syndromes: Nonmalignant Pain Syndromes

Musculoskeletal Back Pain

Among the chronic pain problems, spinal pain, which includes pain emanating from cervical, thoracic, and lumbosacral regions, constitutes the majority of the problems. Spinal pain is inclusive of all painful conditions originating from spinal structures ranging from the vertebrae, intervertebral discs, spinal cord, nerve roots, facet joints, ligaments, to muscles. It is estimated that episodes of low back pain that are frequent or persistent have been reported in 15% of the U.S. population, with a lifetime prevalence of 65% to 80% (33). However, prevalence of neck pain, though not as common as low back pain, is estimated to be 35% to 40%, of which 30% will develop chronic symptoms (34). The duration of back pain has been a topic of controversy. It is believed that most of these episodes will be short-lived, with 80% to 90% of attacks resolving in about 6 weeks irrespective of the administration or type of treatment; and 5% to 10% of patients developing persistent back pain. However, this concept has been questioned, because the condition tends to relapse, so most patients will experience multiple episodes. Examination of other studies suggests a prevalence of low back pain ranging from 35% to 79% at 3 months and 35% to 75% at 12 months (35).

The history of the application of interventional techniques in back pain management dates back to 1901, when epidural injections for lumbar nerve root compression were reported. Since then, substantial advances have been made in the administration of epidural injections, and a multitude of other interventional techniques have been described. These interventional techniques include not only neural blockade, but also minimally invasive surgical procedures ranging from peripheral nerve blocks, trigger-point injections, epidural injections, facet joint injections, sympathetic blocks, neuroablation techniques, intradiscal thermal therapy, disc decompression, morphine pump implantation, and spinal cord stimulation (see Neuromodulation, this chapter).

The rationale for diagnostic and therapeutic neural blockade in the management of spinal pain stems from the fact that clinical features and imaging or neurophysiologic studies do not permit the accurate diagnosis of the causation of spinal pain in the majority of patients in the absence of disc herniation and neurological deficit. Further rationale is based on the recurring facts showing the overall rate of inaccurate or incomplete diagnosis in patients referred to pain treatment centers to range from 40% to 67%, and the presence of organic origin of the pain is mistakenly branded as psychosomatic in 98% of the cases (36). Finally, the most compelling reason is that chronic low back pain is a diagnostic dilemma in 85% of patients, even in experienced hands with all of the available technology. Thus, percutaneous injection techniques have been distinguished as the favored, and at times decisive, intervention in the diagnostic and therapeutic management of chronic painful conditions.

The general benefit of various types of injection technique includes pain relief exceeding the relatively short duration of pharmacologic action of the local anesthetics and other agents used. It is believed that neural blockade alters or interrupts nociceptive input, reflex mechanisms of the afferent limb, and the self-sustaining activity of the neuron pools and neuraxis. It is also believed that local anesthetics interrupt the pain–spasm cycle, whereas corticosteroids reduce inflammation either by inhibiting the synthesis or release of a number of proinflammatory substances. Various modes of action of corticosteroids include membrane stabilization; inhibition of neural peptide synthesis or action; blockade of phospholipase A_2 activity; prolonged suppression of ongoing neuronal discharge; suppression of sensitization of dorsal horn neurons; and reversible local anesthetic effect (5).

Although epidural corticosteroid injections are frequently utilized with the aim of reducing edema and inflammation around the nerve root, the efficacy and indication for this treatment continues to be debated. Many studies have significant design flaws and systematic reviews have also presented varying conclusions. If pain relief was achieved, it was only maintained in the short term, and there was no indication that epidural steroids were effective in the management of back pain without sciatica (37). A meta-analysis of 11 trials reviewed 907 patients with sciatica and clinical evidence of nerve root irritation or compression. Epidural injections varied in different studies with respect to the site of injection (lumbar or caudal), and also with respect to the steroid injected (methyl prednisolone, triamcinolone, or hydrocortisone) (38). Therefore, current data indicate short-term relief of leg pain, but minimal effects on back pain and function after epidural corticosteroid injection for herniated intervertebral discs (39).

Recently, Abram reviewed the use of epidural steroids for lumbosacral radiculopathy (40). There is extensive variation in belief and practice concerning the techniques of epidural steroid injection (e.g., caudal, lumbar, thoracic, cervical epidural, extraforaminal, transforaminal). Consensus suggests that pain associated with radiculopathy was the principal indication, particularly if there was an association with disk herniation, a dermatomal pattern of sensory loss, and positive sciatic stretch signs. Previous back surgery and long duration of symptoms seem to predict a lower success rate. Spinal stenosis also seems to be associated with a low, but not absent, success rate. He also opined that the needle must be placed at a level close to the affected nerve root. Those favoring transforaminal injection also cite this concept. However, in the presence of nerve root compression, this technique carries a risk of needle trauma to the nerve root and definitive data for risks/benefits are not available.

Finally, the chances of success with any therapy are much less if the pain is work related, is generating current disability compensation, or is related to a legal action (41). It must be emphasized that if epidural steroid injection is chosen, it is not definitive therapy. It can be employed to provide temporary relief of pain so that appropriate physical therapy can be instituted, and it should always be associated with an appropriate evaluation of the cause of the pain.

Myofascial Syndromes

Palpable, discrete muscle tenderness is characteristic of myofascial pain. The pain is associated with other painful disorders, which include radiculopathy and joint arthropathy. These painful disorders of muscle and fascia are examples of a "pain cycle" where initial muscle pain or strain elicits a spasm and possibly regional ischemia that then worsens the original pain and establishes a self-defeating and self-perpetuating cycle. The spasm can lead to abnormal posturing or gaits. In many instances, muscle or facial pain will lead to the development of one or more very localized trigger points, where pressure alone will precipitate an aggravation of the symptoms with reproducible "referral patterns." Ultimate therapy is vigorous physical rehabilitation and stretching of the muscle, which will restore function and reduce scarring and contractions. Restoration of normal function also will disrupt the pain cycle permanently in many patients.

The anesthesiologist can contribute to management of these patients by creating temporary relief of the cyclical pain and allowing physical therapy to begin. Relief can be attained by injection of the specific trigger points. Although relief from simple needle insertion into trigger points alone has been reported (42), it is more common to inject small quantities of long-acting local anesthetics at each trigger site. Careful examination is often needed to identify not only active sites but also latent trigger points. Some practitioners will include a depot corticosteroid preparation in the injections on the theory that chronic inflammation contributes to the activity of these points. The benefit of this therapy has not been demonstrated. Transcutaneous electrical nerve stimulation (TENS) therapy also may be useful.

Nerve-Entrapment Syndromes

A related form of chronic pain is a clearly delineated dysesthesia along the distribution of a single peripheral nerve. This frequently follows a surgical procedure where a nerve is unintentionally divided or sutured. The most common sites are hernia and thoracotomy incisions, where peripheral nerves lie close to the actual incisions. Pain is not usually acute but develops as the regenerating nerve forms a neuroma at the site of injury. Injection of local anesthetic along the nerve proximal to the site of pain will provide temporary relief and help confirm the diagnosis. Although some have claimed excellent relief of symptoms with injection of neurolytic agents, anesthesiologists probably have little to offer these patients beyond confirming the diagnosis, and surgical reexploration may be advisable (43).

Meralgia Paresthetica.   This is a specific entrapment syndrome of the lateral femoral cutaneous nerve below the inguinal ligament, as it emerges medial to the anterosuperior iliac spine. Patients complain of paresthesias and pain in the distribution of anterior or lateral thigh, usually aggravated by wearing a tight belt or other clothing or by prolonged standing. A diagnostic block of the nerve with local anesthetic will help confirm the diagnosis, but therapy is limited to recommendations for weight loss, clothing changes, and patience until the syndrome resolves.

Complex Regional Pain Syndrome

In the mid-1800s Claude Bernard and his neurological colleagues noted the association of pain with the sympathetic nervous system. Although the labels have changed over time (causalgia, reflex sympathetic dystrophy, CRPS), the challenge to practitioners has persisted. Although the original International Association for Study of Pain (IASP) criteria required only subjective and potentially only historical signs and symptoms, the suggestions for improving these criteria are that some objectification and observed evidence be included. It is recommended that the diagnostic criteria be modified to include at least one symptom in each of the four diagnostic categories derived by factor analysis: sensory (hyperesthesia), vasomotor (temperature and/or skin color asymmetry), sudomotor/edema (reports of asymmetrical edema in the affected limb and/or a sweating asymmetry), and a new symptom set which was identified by factor analysis: the motor/trophic set (reports of motor dysfunction or trophic objective sign changes) (44).

There is great heterogeneity of symptoms endorsed by patients with CRPS. It is essentially a disorder characterized by pain and dysfunction of the sympathetic nervous system. The symptoms most frequently mentioned by patients are spontaneous burning and stinging pain. The examining physician should seek evidence of altered central processing by looking for allodynia (innocuous stimulation that is now painful) or hyperpathia (slightly painful stimulation that is now significantly painful and/or painful for a prolonged period).

All treatments were focused primarily on functional restoration; the use of drugs, blocks, and psychotherapy was reserved for patients failing to progress in the functional algorithm. Interdisciplinary pain management techniques emphasizing functional restoration are thought to be the most effective therapy; they may work by resetting altered central processing and/or normalizing the distal environment.

Local anesthetic sympathetic blocks are commonly used in the management of CRPS (45). Early sympathetic blockade is advocated in the adult literature to reverse the autonomic changes (changes in blood flow, temperature, sweating, and edema) associated with CRPS and to provide analgesia, but controlled trials have not been conducted. A short trial of a limited number of nerve blocks with very clear goals and time limitations may be indicated ethically and may be cost effective if the patient fails to progress naturally in a functional restoration effort.

Intravenous regional anesthesia (IVRA) has been used for both diagnostic and therapeutic treatment of sympathetically mediated pain syndromes. Adjuncts utilized in IVRA include local anesthetics combined with guanethidine, bretylium, clonidine, or steroids. The purported mechanisms of action of local anesthetics via the IVRA technique are temporary and include (i) conduction impedance of small nerves and nerve endings, (ii) conduction impedance of nerve trunks at a proximal location, (iii) ischemia to neural structures, and (iv) direct compression of nerve fibers. IVRA application of guanethidine and bretylium demonstrates prolonged effects in patients with sympathetically mediated pain by inhibiting the release of norepinephrine from nerve terminals and by guanethidine's effect of depleting tissues of norepinephrine.

Herpes Zoster Infection (Postherpetic Neuralgia)

Painful infection with herpes zoster virus is occasionally referred to the anesthesiologist. This infection produces acute pain and vesiculation in the skin distribution of the involved cranial or peripheral nerve root. The acute infection is usually self-limited, but the pain can be incapacitating during the acute illness. More distressing, 30% to 50% of infected patients older than 50 years of age will develop a chronic pain perception in the involved dermatomal distribution. Anesthesiologists had been asked to perform sympathetic blocks in the past for pain relief or to reduce the potential for postherpetic neuralgia, but medical therapy appears to have eliminated this course. If neuralgia does occur, therapy with centrally acting drugs appears to be more effective. Neurolytic drugs have no role in this syndrome.

Phantom Limb Pain

Phantom limb pain is an example of neuropathic pain that develops in up to 60% to 80% of patients after amputation (46). The occurrence of phantom pain seems to be independent of age in adults, gender, or side of amputation, and the onset of pain may be early (greater than 75% of patients in the first few days after amputation). Many factors are likely to be involved in the transition from acute postoperative pain to long-term pain, but because a high proportion of patients have pain resulting from vascular insufficiency before surgery, this may contribute to a preoperative state of central sensitization and an increased risk of chronic pain. This hypothesis is supported by an early trial showing a reduction in the incidence of phantom limb pain after amputation by pretreatment with epidural local anesthetic and opioid (bupivacaine and morphine) for 72 hours before amputation (47). Since that time, a variety of regional analgesic techniques have been used to investigate the effect of perioperative analgesia on the incidence of phantom limb pain, with positive results for epidural techniques (48,49) and negative results for peripheral nerve sheath techniques (50).

There appears to be a series of mechanisms involved in generating phantom pains that include contributions from the periphery, spinal cord, and brain. The initial events occur in the periphery and continue with a series of events that recruit spinal and cortical pain processes. The presence of intense preamputation pain has been found to significantly increase the incidence of stump pain and phantom pain after 1 week and the incidence of phantom pain after 3 months (51). However, in a recent randomized trial, perioperative epidural blockade started a median of 18 hours before the amputation and continued into the postoperative period did not reduce the incidence of phantom or stump pain when compared with a control group receiving preoperative epidural saline and oral or intramuscular opioids (52). However, both groups received epidural bupivacaine and morphine in the postoperative period for a median duration of 166 hours. Currently available agents may not be sufficiently specific and potent (and blockade may have inadequate duration) to prevent development and persistence of central sensitization.

Approach to Specific Syndromes: Malignant Pain Syndromes

Pain of Malignancy

The management of acute pain syndromes is usually rewarding to the anesthesiologist, who is accustomed to rapid and clear results in daily practice. The management of chronic pain is often perceived as less rewarding. More time and effort are required to initiate therapy, and results are often delayed or dissatisfying. Cancer pain patients, however, are often grateful for whatever can be done. The use of epidural opioids and neurolytic blocks has been rewarding to patients and physicians willing to invest the extra time. Cancer pain arises from many sources (direct involvement, pressure, or even reactions to chemotherapy), and several therapeutic approaches may be useful.

Indwelling Catheters for Epidural or Spinal Opioids. Many patients with thoracic, abdominal, pelvic, or lower-extremity pain due to primary cancer or bony metastases reach a point where oral analgesics are no longer effective or produce unacceptable side effects, and can benefit from pain relief by epidural administration of opioids. The principles and mechanisms are the same as those discussed for acute postoperative pain, but the absence of mental obtundation is particularly rewarding in these patients. They also have a lower incidence of side effects (particularly respiratory depression) because they are usually already tolerant to the depressant effects of opioids. In fact, such patients are usually not referred for epidural therapy until large doses of oral or parenteral opioids no longer control their pain. Patients with direct spinal cord compression or neuropathic pain are poor candidates for opioid therapy (2), although infusions of local anesthetics can improve their pain. Coagulopathy or infections at the site are also contraindications.

A trial of epidural morphine can be conducted through a temporary catheter for 2 or 3 days. Ordinarily, the epidural dose is expected to be one-tenth of the current intravenous dose with morphine. However, calculation of the initial dose in these opioid-tolerant patients is difficult. Patient age, severity of pain, level of opioid use, and presence of neuropathic pain (resistant to opioids) are all factors (53). Obviously, adjustments must be made to the original dose. If pain relief is adequate, a permanent silicone catheter can be implanted surgically and connected to a second silicone catheter tunneled subcutaneously to the anterior abdominal wall (Fig. 23.2). Catheters can also be connected to a subcutaneous injection port for intermittent injections, which will reduce the problem of catheter infection and dislodgment. Percutaneous catheters can be connected to external continuous-infusion therapy, which can be adjusted more easily. Subcutaneous programmable

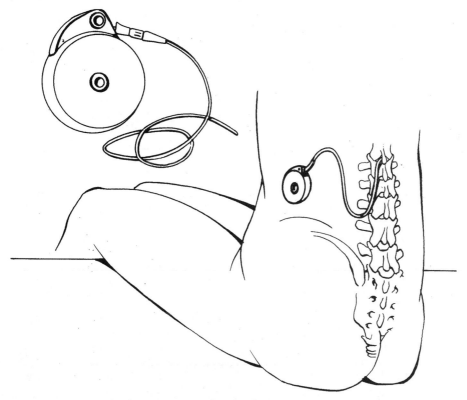

Figure 23.2   **Subcutaneous Epidural Infusion Pump**
A permanent silicone epidural catheter is inserted either percutaneously or through a surgical incision, and then tunneled laterally to be connected to a subcutaneously implanted pump. The pump has a central injection port for refilling the reservoir percutaneously.

continuous-infusion pumps are available, but their cost is quite prohibitive in these patients who are generally facing a limited life expectancy and frequently exhibit dramatic changes in analgesic requirements.

Patients can be discharged home to inject their own medication on the regimen established in the hospital, or they can be managed with a continuous infusion delivered from a portable infusion pump. Generally, local anesthetics are not added initially because of potential interference with ambulation, but their potentiating effect may be needed for patients with severe pain and high tolerance for opioids. Most recipients of this therapy have greatly reduced opioid requirements.

Side effects are minimal with opiate-tolerant patients. One major problem is the precipitation of opioid withdrawal symptoms when patients are shifted to the lower doses required for epidural administration. In the addicted patient, oral medication should be continued and tapered after the catheter is placed. Tolerance to epidural morphine will occur, and doses will gradually have to be increased or intervals between injections shortened. This is not a problem in the terminally ill. With severe intractable pain, hospital admission may be required to allow higher dosages of opioids or opioid and local anesthetic mixtures. The addition of 0.06% to 0.2% bupivacaine to a morphine infusion can enhance analgesia, but it may produce motor weakness and sympathetic blockade as the concentration is increased. Other adjuvants include clonidine, ketamine and, occasionally, steroids. Careful adjustment of dosage can maintain comfort for the terminally ill patient for a considerable time without mental obtundation. If the epidural route fails, there is also the alternative of intrathecal or intraventricular administration, with again a 10-fold reduction of dose requirements initially for patients taking high doses of epidural opioids. Local anesthetics can also be added to these infusions, but with greater risk of side effects (54).

Neurolytic Blocks

Malignant tumors can cause chronic pain by spreading to involve specific organs, peripheral nerves, bones, or the spinal cord itself. The dream of physicians for centuries has been the "silver bullet" that will selectively relieve such pain by destroying invasive growths or the involved nerves without affecting other tissues. Frequently, the anesthesiologist, with his or her focused needle points, is perceived in this role as able to inject a drug capable of abolishing localized painful sensation. Careful patient selection and informed consent are necessary. A trial injection with a local anesthetic is considered mandatory to document that neural blockade will relieve the symptoms and to acquaint the patient with the expected result. Confirmation of needle placement by paresthesia, local anesthetic injection, or radiologic localization is highly advisable before

Table 23.1   Neurolytic Agents

Agent	Concentrations Used	Clinical Uses	Comments
Alcohol	Absolute,[a] 95%,[a] 50%	Cranial nerve	Pain on injection
		Celiac plexus	Possible neuritis, motor block on peripheral nerves
		Subarachnoid	Longest, "best" block
			Best for nonsomatic nerves, terminally ill
Phenol	6%–8% in water	Peripheral nerves	Anesthesia on injection
	5%–10% in glycerine	Subarachnoid	Less profound, shorter than alcohol
	6%–12% in x-ray contrast (renograffin, metrizamide)	Epidural	Better for peripheral nerves
			More difficult to mix, handle

[a]Available commercially; all other solutions must be prepared by pharmacist.

injection of any neurolytic agent. Repeated injections may be needed, because the area of anesthesia tends to regress slightly during the first few days with most of these agents. The success rates are not impressive, ranging from 60% to 80% for most techniques. These blocks are not permanent, and they will wear off in weeks to months.

The agents commonly available in the United States for neurolytic block are alcohol and phenol (see Clinical Neurolysis, this chapter). Although frequently applied in cases of truly segmental pain, neurolytic agents available today are not without side effects and limitations. The side effects of motor dysfunction and other tissue damage are considerable. For each agent, there is a concentration-related potential for motor nerve damage (Table 23.1). A certain percentage of patients (ranging from 2% to 28% in published reports) may expect a painful neuritis or neuralgia in the treated segment. Neurolytic blocks are best reserved for patients with limited life expectancy and severe intractable pain who are clearly informed and willing to accept the risks of neuritis, bladder dysfunction, blindness, or paraplegia. There are many other medical and surgical alternatives that deserve careful consideration before neurolytic drugs are offered (55).

Celiac Plexus Block.   This is perhaps the most rewarding of the neurolytic blocks. It relieves the constant dull visceral pain in the middle or upper abdomen frequently associated with pancreatic cancer. Ninety percent of these patients will have excellent relief. Less satisfactory results are obtained with pain due to chronic pancreatitis (56,57). The block is performed in the manner described in Chapter 11. A diagnostic block with 50 mL 0.25% bupivacaine is usually performed first to confirm the effectiveness of the proposed therapy and give the patient a preview of possible side effects. Successful treatment will produce relief of pain and orthostatic hypotension lasting several hours.

The local anesthetic block can be performed using bony landmarks alone. Prior to actual alcohol injection, needle location at the anterior edge of the L-1 vertebral body should be confirmed. Fluoroscopy is the most effective method for monitoring and adjusting needle position. In difficult patients, a small amount of contrast media can be injected to confirm adequate positioning before injection of neurolytic drug. In any case, a permanent film documenting needle position should be obtained before final injection. In patients with severe anatomic deformity, CT may rarely be needed. A small volume of local anesthetic is injected first to reduce the discomfort. Then 25 mL of absolute alcohol is mixed with an equal volume of 0.5% bupivacaine, and 25 mL is injected through the needle on each side. The needle is cleared of solution before withdrawal by injection of 1 mL air.

Intravenous fluids should be administered to compensate for the expected orthostatic hypotension. The patient remains at rest for the first hour and then ambulates only with assistance during the next 24 hours. Oral ephedrine is sometimes useful in maintaining adequate blood pressure. Increased bowel activity and diarrhea may be expected. Occasional shoulder pain may be seen from diaphragmatic irritation from the alcohol. Pain relief may last from 4 weeks to 6 months.

Hypogastric Plexus Blockade. Patients with advanced pelvic tumors of gynecologic, colorectal, or genitourinary origin often have severe visceral pain perceived through the sympathetic afferent fibers from the hypogastric plexus. The hypogastric plexus can be blocked by a lumbar somatic block at the level of L5-S1 (58). The technique described in Chapter 11 is modified by insertion of the needles opposite the L4-5 interspace with a caudad direction. Location at the anterior border of the L5-S1 vertebral body is confirmed with fluoroscopy. As with celiac plexus block, a trial blockade with 0.25% bupivacaine is performed before injection of a neurolytic drug. Approximately two-thirds of patients treated with injection of 10% phenol will obtain excellent relief (59).

Other Locations for Sympathetic Blockade. Sympathetic blockade of other than the celiac plexus carries a higher risk of complications. Neurolytic stellate ganglion block is rarely indicated because of the potential undesirable spread of the neurolytic agent to several critical neighboring structures. Chemical neurolysis of the lumbar ganglia with 3 mL alcohol or phenol is more common, but it carries a risk of genitofemoral nerve neuritis or a 20% chance of a "sympathalgia" (sympathetic neuralgia) of the lower extremity.

Peripheral Neurolytic Nerve Blockade. Peripheral nerve blockade with neurolytic agents is generally limited to branches of the trigeminal nerve (see Chapter 18), where motor weakness is of minimal consequence. Radiofrequency ablation of the gasserian ganglion has largely replaced this type of injection (60). Blockade of the intercostal nerves (see Chapter 9) likewise involves minimal motor complications, but it carries the risk of neuritis. Transsacral nerve block of the S-2 or S-3 root has been used for painful spastic bladder problems. Block of the brachial or lumbosacral plexus roots is possible, but it is a rare patient who is willing to accept motor loss in an extremity in exchange for relief of pain. Phenol and alcohol give relief for 1 to 6 months.

Alcohol injections on peripheral nerves should be limited to 1 mL; and phenol should be limited to 0.5 mL. Larger quantities increase the risk of spread to other tissues, particularly in the head, where other cranial nerves (such as the optic nerve) are in close proximity. The final extent of analgesia is hard to appreciate immediately after injection. Twenty-four hours should be allowed before repeating an injection for an inadequate block.

Subarachnoid Neurolysis. Subarachnoid injections of 0.5 mL phenol or 0.7 to 1.0 mL alcohol are useful for blocks of selected roots from the cervical to the lumbar region (61). The patient must be positioned so that the injected solution will preferentially bathe the dorsal root fibers if sensory blockade is the goal. For (hypobaric) alcohol, the patient's spine is flexed laterally so that the affected dermatomal segment is uppermost, and the body is rotated 45 degrees forward from the lateral position (Fig. 23.3). For hyperbaric phenol, the affected root is placed lowermost and the body is rotated back so that the dorsal roots are lower than the ventral motor fibers (Fig. 23.4). Careful documentation of needle placement is performed, and a small quantity of local anesthetic may be injected to confirm appropriate location. This is important, because peripheral roots may enter the cord several segments above their foraminal exit from the spinal column. Exact localization of the segment producing the patient's complaints must be obtained before "permanent" blockade. The neurolytic agent is injected slowly in 0.1-mL increments, with the sensory loss evaluated every 10 minutes. After adequate relief or injection of the maximum volume, the patient remains in position for 30 to 45 minutes to avoid spread of the neurolytic agent. If multiple levels are to be blocked, each should be approached through a separate needle. No more than two levels should be blocked at any one time, and relief should be reassessed at 48 hours before further injections.

The area of immediate anesthesia will recede within the first 24 to 48 hours after injection, and many patients may recover some motor function in the affected segments over the next few weeks. Successful anesthesia can be expected in only 40% to 60% of patients. If pain recurs after 3 to 6 months, the block may be repeated, but success is less likely.

Bowel and bladder function frequently will be disrupted when a sacral subarachnoid block is performed. The close proximity of the

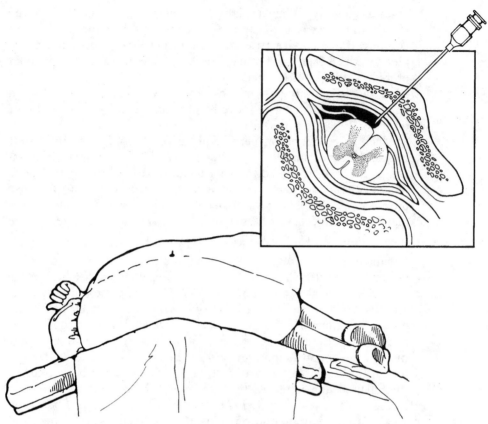

Figure 23.3   **Position for Spinal Alcohol Injection**
The patient is placed with the painful side up and rotated slightly anterior
so that the involved dorsal roots are uppermost and receive the bulk of
the hypobaric injection.

sacral and lumbar roots in the cauda equina makes selective blockade difficult in this region. Although injection of 1 to 5 mL alcohol
with the patient in the jackknife position can produce good sacral
anesthesia, this application should be avoided unless the patient already has diverting urologic and rectal surgical procedures or a permanent bladder catheter.

Epidural Neurolysis.   Epidural injections are less reliable than subarachnoid neurolysis. It is harder to localize the agent to a single
root, and it is difficult to gauge the extent of response at the time of
injection. Epidural neurolytic blocks are used in the management of
pain in the thoracic and cervical spine areas. Epidural alcohol is
more painful and may result in incomplete neurolysis and later neuralgia. Phenol may work better, but, in general, epidural injection is
less desirable than spinal or sympathetic block. If performed, the insertion of a catheter with multiple repeat injections may increase
the chance of success.

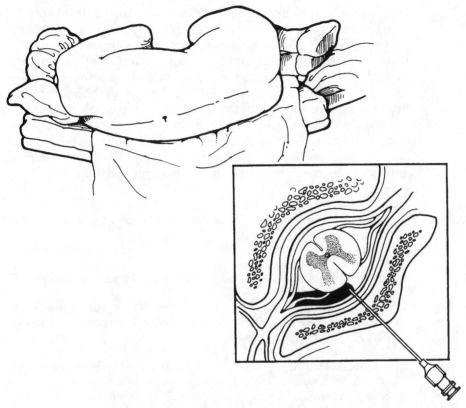

Figure 23.4   **Position for Spinal Phenol Injection**
Phenol is hyperbaric, so the patient is placed with the painful side down
and rotated posteriorly so that the injection will once again be
concentrated on the dorsal root nerve fibers.

Multidisciplinary Pain Clinics

The management of pain, whether acute or chronic, warrants careful technical implementation and cautious interpretation and application of interventional procedures. Pain, as defined by the IASP, is
"an unpleasant sensory and emotional experience associated with
actual or potential tissue damage or described in terms of such damage." In addition to pathophysiologic mechanisms for the generation of pain, subjective and affective processes modify perception of
pain. In dealing with these patients, the anesthesiologist acts as one
consultant in a multidisciplinary approach to management. Physical therapy, psychiatry, neurosurgery, and rehabilitation all may
play equal or more important roles. The anesthesiologist in independent practice who attempts to "solve" these patients' problems
with a regional technique alone is doing himself or herself and the
patient a disservice. Chronic pain of nonmalignant origin particularly may involve central mechanisms that elude treatment with

peripheral nerve blocks. In such situations, three points should be kept in mind. First, because such pain is multifaceted, a multidisciplinary approach is usually needed. Second, in any pain-control situation, a single physician must be clearly identified as the primary managing director of the group efforts. Third, in all pain work, there should be careful attention to avoid further harm to the patient. The interpretation of interventional procedures may be confounded by the improper use of pain measurement scales, placebo effects, incorrect clinician observations, and skewed patient expectations. Diagnostic or therapeutic regional block therapy can be considered only one adjunct in the treatment of many pain problems.

References

1. Carron, H. The changing role of the anesthesiologist in pain management. *Reg. Anesth.* 14: 4, 1989.
2. Rowlingson, J. C. Interventional cancer pain management. *Anesth. Analg.* 86: 106, 1998.
3. Hogan, Q. H., Abram, S. E. Neural blockade for diagnosis and prognosis. A review. *Anesthesiology* 86: 216, 1997.
4. Manchikanti, L., Pampati, V. S., Beyer, C. The effect of neuroaxial steroids on weight and bone mass density: A prospective evaluation. *Pain Physician* 3: 357, 2000.
5. Manchikanti, L., Singh, V., Kloth, D., Slipman, C. W., Jasper, J. F., Trescot, A. M. Interventional Techniques in the management of chronic pain (ASIPP Practice Guidelines). *Pain Physician* 4: 24, 2001.
6. Ballantyne, J. C., Carr, D. B., Berkey, C. S. Comparative efficacy of epidural, subarachnoid, and intracerebroventricular opioids in patients with pain due to cancer. *Reg. Anesth.* 21: 542, 1996.
7. Paice, J. A., Penn, R. D., Shott, S. Intraspinal morphine for chronic pain: A retrospective, multicenter study. *J. Pain Symptom Manage.* 11: 71, 1996.
8. Yoshida, G. M., Nelson, R. W., Capen, D.A., Nagelberg, S., Thomas, J.C., Rimoldi, R.L., Haye, W. Evaluation of continuous intraspinal narcotic analgesia for chronic pain from benign causes. *Am. J. Orthop.* 25: 693, 1996.
9. Kamibayashi, T., Harasawa, K., Maze, M. Alpha-2 adrenergic agonists. *Can. J. Anaesth.* 44: R13, 1997.
10. Eisenach, J. C., Kock, M. D., Klimscha, W. Alpha-2 adrenergic agonists for regional anesthesia: A clinical review of clonidine (1984–1995). *Anesthesiology* 85: 655, 1996.
11. Canavero, S., Bonicalzi, V. The neurochemistry of central pain: Evidence from clinical studies, hypothesis and therapeutic implications. *Pain* 74: 109, 1998.
12. Bowery, N. G. GABA-B receptor pharmacology. *Annu. Rev. Pharmacol. Toxicol.* 33: 109, 1993.
13. Kerr, D. I., Ong, J. GABA receptors. *Pharmacol. Ther.* 67:, 187 1995.
14. Penn, R. D., Savoy, S. M., Corcos, D. Intrathecal baclofen for severe spinal spasticity. *N. Engl. J. Med.* 320: 1517, 1989.
15. Arner S, Lindblom U, Meyerson BA, Molander C. Prolonged relief of neuralgia after regional anesthetic blocks: A call for further experimental and systematic clinical studies. *Pain* 43: 287, 1990.

16. Wall, P. D., Devor, M. Sensory afferent impulses originate from dorsal root ganglia as well as from the periphery in normal and nerve injured rats. *Pain* 17: 321, 1983.

17. Janig, W., Stanton-Hicks, M., *Reflex Sympathetic Dystrophy: A Reappraisal.* Seattle: IASP Press, 1996.

18. Stanton-Hicks, M., Janig, W., Hassenbusch, S., et al. Reflex sympathetic dystrophy: Changing concepts and taxonomy. *Pain* 63: 127, 1995.

19. Jain, S., Gupta, R., *Neurolytic Agents in Clinical Practice.* Philadelphia: WB Saunders, 1996.

20. Evans, P. J. D., Lloyd, J. W., Green, C. J. Cryoanalgesia: The response to alteration in freeze cycle and temperature. *Br. J. Anaesth.* 53: 1121, 1981.

21. Saberski, L. R., *Cryoneurolysis in Clinical Practice.* Philadelphia: WB Saunders, 1996.

22. Kline, M., *Stereotactic Radiofrequency Lesions as Part of the Management of Pain.* Orlando, FL: Paul M. Deutsch Press, 1992.

23. Lord, S. M., Barnsley, L., Wallis, B. J. Percutaneous radiofrequency neurotomy for chronic cervical zygapophyseal joint pain. *N. Engl. J. Med.* 335: 1721, 1996.

24. Taha, J. M., Tew, J. M. Treatment of trigeminal neuralgia by percutaneous radiofrequency rhizotomy. *Neurosurg. Clin. North Am.* 8: 31, 1997.

25. Shealy, C. N., Mortimer, J. T., Reswick, J. Electrical inhibition of pain by stimulation of the dorsal column: Preliminary clinical reports. *Anesth. Analg.* 46: 489, 1967.

26. Shetter, A. Spinal cord stimulation in the treatment of chronic pain. *Curr. Rev. Pain* 1: 213, 1997.

27. North, R. B., Ewend, M. G., Lawton, M. T. Spinal cord stimulation for chronic, intractable pain: Superiority of "multi-channel" devices. *Pain* 44: 119, 1991.

28. Holsheimer, J. Effectiveness of spinal cord stimulation in the management of chronic pain: Analysis of technical drawbacks and solutions. *Neurosurgery* 40: 990, 1997.

29. North, R. B., Kidd, D. H., Zahurak, M., et al. Spinal cord stimulation for chronic, intractable, pain: Experience over two decades. *Neurosurgery* 32: 384, 1993.

30. Cohan, R. H., Bullard, M. A., Ellis, J. H. Local reactions after injection of iodinated contrast material: Detection, management, and outcome. *Acad. Radiol.* 4: 711, 1997.

31. Gangi, A., Dietmann, J. L., Mortazavi, R. CT-guided interventional procedures for pain management in the lumbosacral spine. *Radiographics* 18: 621, 1998.

32. Thomsen, H. S., Bush, W. H. Jr. Adverse effects of contrast media: Incidence, prevention and management. *Drug. Saf.* 19: 313, 1998.

33. Manchikanti, L. Epidemiology of low back pain. *Pain Physician* 3: 167, 2000.

34. Bovim, G., Schrader, H., Sand, T. Neck pain in the general population. *Spine* 19: 1307, 1994.

35. Miedema, H. S., Chorus, A. M. J., Wevers, C. W. J. Chronicity of back problems during work life. 23: 2021, 1998.

36. Hendler, N. H., Bergson, C., Morrison, C. Overlooked physical diagnosis in chronic pain patients involved in litigation. *Psychosomatics* 37: 509, 1996.

37. Koes, B. W., Scholten, R. J. P. M., Mens, J. M. A., Bouter, L. M. Efficacy of epidural steroid injections for low back pain and sciatica: a systematic review of randomized clinical trials. *Pain* 63: 279, 1995.

38. Watts, R. W., Silagy, C.A. A meta-analysis on the efficacy of epidural corticosteroids in the treatment of sciatica. *Anaesth. Intensive Care* 23: 564, 1995.

39. McQuay, H., Moore, A., *An Evidence-Based Resource for Pain Relief.* Oxford: Oxford University Press, 1998.

40. Abram, S. E. Treatment of lumbosacral radiculopathy with epidural steroids. *Anesthesiology* 91: 1937, 1999.

41. Jamison, R. N., VadeBoncouer, T., Ferrante, F. M. Low back pain patients unresponsive to an epidural steroid injection: Identifying predictive factors. *Clin. J. Pain* 7: 121, 1993.

42. Cummings, T. M., White, A. R. Needling therapies in the management of myofascial trigger point pain: A systematic review. *Arch. Phys. Med. Rehabil.* 82: 986, 2001.

43. Massey, E. W. Sensory neuropathies. *Semin. Neurol.* 18: 177, 1998.

44. Bruehl, S., Harden, R. N., Galer, B. S. External validation of IASP diagnostic criteria for complex regional pain syndrome and proposed research diagnostic criteria. *Pain* 81: 147, 1999.

45. Breivik, H., Cousins, M. J., Lofstrom, B. J., *Sympathetic Neural Blockade of the Upper and Lower Extremity.* Philadelphia: Lippincott-Raven, 1998.

46. Katz, J. Phantom limb pain. *Lancet* 350: 1338, 1997.

47. Bach, S., Noreng, M. F., Tjellden, N. U. Phantom limb pain in amputees during the first 12 months following limb amputation, after preoperative lumbar epidural blockade. *Pain* 33: 297, 1988.

48. Jahangiri, M., Bradley, J. W. P., Jayatunga, A. P., Dark, C. H. Prevention of phantom limb pain after major lower limb amputation by epidural infusion of diamorphine, clonidine and bupivacaine. *Ann. R. Coll. Surg. Engl.* 76: 324, 1994.

49. Schug, S. A., Burrell, R., Payne, J., Tester, P. Pre-emptive epidural analgesia may prevent phantom limb pain. *Reg. Anesth.* 20: 256, 1995.

50. Elizaga, A. M., Smith, D. G., Sharar, S. R. Continuous regional analgesia by intraneural block: effect on postoperative opioid requirements and phantom limb pain following amputation. *J. Rehab. Res. Dev.* 31: 179, 1994.

51. Nikolajsen, L., Ilkjaer, S., Christensen, J. H. Randomised trial of epidural bupivacaine and morphine in prevention of stump and phantom pain in lower-limb amputation. *Lancet* 350: 1353, 1997.

52. Nikolajsen, L., Ilkjaer, S., Christensen, J. H. The influence of preamputation pain on postamputation stump and phantom pain. *Pain* 72: 393, 1997.

53. DuPen, S. L., Williams, A. R. The dilemma of conversion from systemic to epidural morphine: A proposed conversion tool for treatment of cancer pain. *Pain* 56: 113, 1994.

54. Deer, T., Winkelmuller W., Erdine, S., Bedder, M., Burchiel, K. Intrathecal therapy for cancer and nonmalignant pain: patient selection and patient management. *Neuromodulation* 2: 55, 1999.

55. Rowlingson, J. C. Management of malignant pain syndromes. *Anesth. Analg.* Review Course Lectures: 79, 1999.

56. Brown, D. L., Bulley, C. K., Quiel, E. L. Neurolytic celiac plexus block for pancreatic cancer pain. *Anesth. Analg.* 66: 869, 1987.

57. Thompson, G. E., Artin, R., Bridenbaugh, L. D., Moore, D. C. Abdominal pain and alcohol celiac plexus nerve block. *Anesth. Analg.* 56: 1, 1977.

58. Plancarte, R., Amescua, C., Patt, R. B., Aldrete, J. A. Superior hypogastric plexus block for pelvic cancer pain. *Anesthesiology* 73: 236, 1990.

59. DeLeon-Casasola, O. A., Kent, E., Lema, M. J. Neurolytic superior hypogastric plexus block for chronic pelvic pain associated with cancer. *Pain* 54: 145, 1993.

60. Loeser, J. D. What to do about tic douloureux. *J.A.M.A.* 239: 1153, 1978.

61. Hay, R. C. Subarachnoid alcohol block in the control of intractable pain: A report of results in 252 patients. *Anesth. Analg.* 41: 12, 1962.

24 Postoperative Pain Management

Traditional methods for the management of acute postoperative pain (intramuscular injections of opioids on a time- and dose-limited patient-request system) frequently result in long periods of inadequate pain relief. Fixed dosages ignore each patient's unique analgesic requirement and widely variable analgesic blood levels. It is not surprising that traditional intramuscular opioids have essentially been replaced with more effective modes that allow individual titration of medication, and, more recently, targeted delivery of analgesia to peripheral or neuraxial sites that avoids or reduces systemic side effects and complications. Anesthesia caregivers are most familiar with opioid effects, and are especially suited to employ this latter approach, with peripheral nerve and epidural catheters. It is natural that they have been involved in the development of the concepts of the "acute pain service" [1]. Several complete textbooks describe in extensive detail the application of these skills to postoperative analgesia [2–5]. This chapter will discuss the modalities included in a full range of postoperative pain therapy, starting with the development of patient-controlled analgesia (PCA).

Patient-Controlled Analgesia

A major improvement in postoperative analgesia was the development of a more appropriate delivery system, specifically, the use of PCA. This was first introduced with the intravenous route. It is superior to the traditional intramuscular route because effective blood levels are produced immediately with little overshoot. The on-demand patient control allows each patient to titrate the exact level that is needed for his or her analgesic requirement and to adjust that dosage to varying levels of activity. There are a multitude of pumps on the market that allow the patient to inject a small bolus of an intravenous opioid drug whenever he or she feels pain, and thus maintain the analgesic blood level in the range that is appropriate. Each of the machines has a "lockout" system, which provides an adequate delay time for the patient to achieve analgesia from each injected dose. Excessive dosing is avoided by the patient's own titration and, if inappropriate dosing occurs, the sedation that it produces during the lockout period usually prevents the patient from giving an overdose that would lead to respiratory depression. Because this delivery system only *maintains* a blood level, the initial production of adequate analgesia requires a bolus injection of an opioid, usually provided by a loading dose programmed for each patient.

One problem with this method is the need for constant reinjection to maintain adequate blood levels, most frequently resulting in interrupted sleep. Most machines will allow a continuous infusion mode that provides a constant background infusion of drug, which may alleviate this problem. The constant infusion mode does not reduce the total quantity delivered; it does increase the potential for respiratory depression by removing the patient control (6). Nevertheless, it may be useful for overnight setting, particularly on the first postoperative night. All standard PCA orders should include alternatives that allow the nursing staff to increase the incremental doses or decrease the lockout interval to meet the patient's needs. As with all opioid dosing schedules, age is a major consideration, and younger patients should be started at higher levels than the average.

Virtually all of the available opioids have been administered by this route (7) (Table 24.1). Morphine is the least expensive and often the drug of first choice. The development of side effects (pruritus, nausea, dysphoria) may require switching to an alternative. Meperidine is equally effective, but with a slightly shorter duration of action. Meperidine is less commonly used because of toxicity from its primary metabolite, normeperidine (7). Hydromorphone is an acceptable alternative in patients who experience intolerable side effects from other opioids. Fentanyl is more expensive, but it has also been used in patients with sensitivity to other opioids. The PCA delivery mode overcomes the usual disadvantage of the short duration of this drug, but the patient will need to inject more frequently.

As mentioned, the delivery systems appear to be safe. Mechanical problems are rare (7). Although central depression does occur (6), it is no more common than with any other delivery technique. The use of continuous infusions or the presence of advanced age increases the risk. The major problem with this modality has been when control of the device is shifted to a family member rather than the patient. Overall, this delivery system has been highly effective in providing appropriate analgesia for postoperative patients, usually with a lower total dose of opioid than was previously administered by the intramuscular route. It is very effective for peripheral and lower abdominal surgery, but neuraxial opioids appear superior

Table 24.1   Intravenous Patient-Controlled Administration: Drugs and Doses

Drug	Loading Dose (mg)	Increments
Morphine	5–20	0.5–2.5
Meperidine	50–250	10–25
Hydromorphone	1–2	0.05–0.25
Fentanyl	0.075–0.1	0.010–0.050

for upper abdominal and thoracic procedures (see Neuraxial Opioid Analgesia, this chapter). The PCA modality can be adapted to subcutaneous, perineural, and epidural catheters, and has been very effective with the targeted delivery systems discussed below.

Peripheral Nerve Analgesic Techniques

Several local and peripheral regional techniques are used to provide ongoing analgesia. The advantages of specifically targeting analgesia to one area include minimal limitations of mobility and reduction of systemic side effects such as sedation and nausea. Peripheral infusions usually employ low concentrations of local anesthetics, but opioids and alpha$_2$-agonists are also useful in some situations. The efficacy and popularity of continuous peripheral techniques have been enhanced by the introduction of new continuous catheter delivery systems and smaller portable pumps.

Surgical Wound Infiltration

Simple infiltration of the wound with dilute local anesthetic can provide 4 to 8 hours of analgesia, depending on the location. This technique is particularly useful in the pediatric patient, especially with the use of penile or groin blocks following urologic surgery (see Chapter 21). Local infiltration is also effective for adult outpatients (8), allowing them to be discharged without the side effects of systemic opioids. For inpatients, the analgesia in smaller wounds can be extended by the insertion of a multiorifice catheter and provision of a continuous infusion of solutions such as 0.1% bupivacaine or ropivacaine at 6 to 12 mL per hour (9). Orthopedic surgeons have used this technology with disposable pumps to provide 24 hours of analgesia after shoulder surgery for outpatients.

Another variation of this is injection of the knee joint following arthroscopic surgery. Bupivacaine will provide several hours of analgesia, and there is a suggestion that the addition of opioids such as morphine may prolong the analgesia considerably (10), although this remains controversial.

Peripheral Nerve Catheters

Peripheral nerve blocks provide excellent postoperative analgesia (11), which can be prolonged with continuous catheters. Femoral nerve catheters provide better pain relief after hip and knee procedures (12), and improve the recovery time and shorten the rehabilitation time following total knee replacement after inpatient surgery, compared to conventional opioids or epidural infusions (13,14). Some outpatient units have also employed continuous catheters for patients who remain in their overnight observation unit (15), demonstrating improved analgesia with interscalene catheters for shoulder surgery (16) and psoas compartment catheters for anterior cruciate ligament (ACL) repairs. The use of these catheters provides analgesia that is equivalent to that of epidural infusions, but peripheral nerve catheters have two advantages: they do not produce sympathetic blockade, and do not require the use of opioids to provide analgesia, as is commonly done with the epidural technique. Low-dose local anesthetic infusions are usually employed, although the addition of low-dose clonidine (17) and opioids appears to improve efficacy.

Intrapleural Catheters

Injection of local anesthetics through intrapleural catheters has been used to relieve postoperative pain. The technique is described in Chapter 10. For postoperative analgesia, 20 mL 0.5% bupivacaine can be injected every 6 to 12 hours, or a continuous infusion can be instituted. Satisfactory results have been reported in some patients with subcostal incisions for cholecystectomy as well as with thoracotomy patients. Other authors have found variable analgesia and a significant potential for systemic toxicity with the doses required. This technique is not as effective as epidural opiates for thoracotomy procedures (18).

Repeated Intercostal Blockade

Injection of the sixth to the eleventh intercostal nerves with 3 to 5 mL 0.25% bupivacaine with 1:200,000 epinephrine at 12-hour intervals will provide excellent continuous analgesia (18). It is utilized infrequently because of the personnel and time required to provide reinjections every 12 hours, compared to the ease and efficacy of epidural infusions. Insertion of a continuous catheter will reduce some of the technical and time problems. Its use is usually limited to the occasional frail patient requiring special attention, or the trauma patient suffering from multiple rib fractures in whom respiratory depression from systemic opioids is undesirable.

Cryoanalgesia

This approach to intercostal analgesia has been advocated for postthoracotomy pain, but, again, it is not as effective or popular as epidural opioids (18). Cryoanalgesia is accomplished intraoperatively by directly freezing the intercostal nerves with the tip of a commercial cryoprobe for up to 2 minutes. It may be associated with an uncomfortable dysesthesia in younger patients, who find the band of numbness unpleasant. (see Chapter 23)

Neuraxial Opioid Analgesia

The use of neuraxial administration of opioids has been the major advance in acute analgesic therapy (19,20). Opioids applied to the spinal cord are effective in blocking pain perception at the dorsal root entry zone in doses that are substantially smaller than those required to produce systemic analgesia. This effect is seen with both subarachnoid and epidural injection, although epidural application requires higher doses (by a factor of ten) to produce penetration of the membranes. The direct application of opioids to the specific receptor site reduces the systemic side effects of respiratory depression and sedation usually associated with intramuscular and intravenous injection. More importantly, this route has been demonstrated to produce superior analgesia compared to any other method for thoracotomy (18) and abdominal (21) procedures.

Choice of Opioids

Virtually all of the opioids have been employed in both the subarachnoid and epidural space. Initial clinical experience employed *morphine* in the epidural space. Because of its poor lipid solubility, morphine has a relatively slow penetration into the lipid layers of the spinal column (19) (Fig. 24.1). Although early investigators found they could overcome this by using higher doses, it was

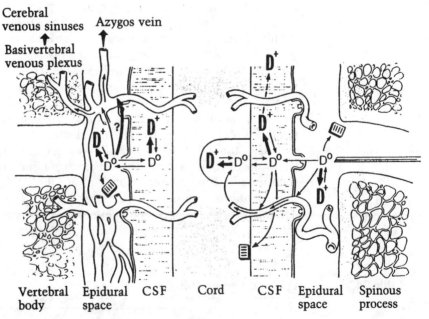

Figure 24.1   **Site of Action of Epidural Morphine**
A hydrophilic narcotic such as morphine is present primarily as the charged (D^+) form, and small amounts of the uncharged (D^0) form penetrate slowly to the sites of action in the cord. Much of the ionized form diffuses away from the site in the cerebrospinal fluid (CSF) or in the venous blood flow. (From Cousins, M. J., Mather, L. E. Intrathecal and epidural administration of opioids. *Anesthesiology* 61: 276, 1984, with permission.)

quickly discovered that these doses were also associated with a higher incidence of side effects, specifically the production of central sedation and respiratory depression as the water-soluble morphine diffused cephalad in the cerebrospinal fluid (CSF). Appropriate low doses [1 to 5 mg for most patients, based primarily on *patient age* (22)] will produce adequate pain relief with minimal side effects if a single dose is administered early enough to allow 60 minutes for the onset of action. Use of a continuous infusion of morphine avoids the peak and valley phenomenon of intermittent injections, and also appears to be associated with a lower incidence of side effects (Table 24.2).

Slow onset can be overcome by using direct subarachnoid injection of morphine, but the much narrower dose range may increase the risk of postoperative respiratory depression (Table 24.3). Subarachnoid injection remains an effective alternative (especially for patients receiving single-injection subarachnoid anesthesia and requiring only 24 hours of analgesia, such as cesarean delivery or hip surgery), but it needs to be used with caution.

The more lipid-soluble opioids diffuse less readily in the CSF. Historically, they were investigated in the hope that they would be less likely to move away from the site of injection and, therefore, produce a more localized segmental band of analgesia with less likelihood of centrally mediated respiratory depression and other side effects. *Fentanyl* is the prototype drug and has been shown to produce localized segmental anesthesia as required for postthoracotomy pain (18,20), with some suggestion of a lower side effect profile (23). There is significant uptake into the blood stream with the lipid-soluble drugs (24); however, and in several studies the blood levels attained with epidural infusion have equaled the blood levels with intravenous administration. Some have questioned whether there is really a direct spinal action at all, and whether these drugs have any use in neuraxial analgesia (25,26). Other data suggest that with small doses there is a local effect in the spinal cord, but only near the immediate area of injection. Despite the laboratory studies suggesting only systemic effects, there are two large clinical studies demonstrating a high degree of effectiveness with epidural fentanyl infusions (23,27). Both of these series demonstrate that the location

Table 24.2   **Epidural Opioid Infusions**

Drug	Loading Dose	Maintenance[a]
Morphine	1–3 mg	0.04 mg/mL, 4–8 mL/h
Meperidine	20–100 mg	1 mg/mL, 8–12 mL/h
Hydromorphone	1–2 mg	0.02 mg/mL, 4–10 mL/h
Fentanyl	75–100 µg	4 µg/mL, 8–16 mL/h
Sufentanil	50 µg	2 µg/mL, 8–12 mL/h

[a]Lower rates effective if local anesthetic added.

Table 24.3   **Spinal Opioid Doses for Postoperative Analgesia**

Drug	Dose	Duration
Morphine	0.1–0.3 mg	8–24 h
Meperidine	10–30 mg	10–24 h
Fentanyl	5–25 µg	2–6 h

of the catheter tip is critical; it must be located near the dermatomal source of pain. They also demonstrate that the combination with a local anesthetic is important for adequate analgesia with this opioid. If a large number of spinal segments are to be provided analgesia, higher doses (and systemic effects) may be required, and alternative opioids with a wider spread may be more desirable.

Even more highly lipid-soluble opioids such as *sufentanil* have been used in the epidural space. Because of its high lipid solubility, even higher doses are required. For effective analgesia, doses of sufentanil equivalent to the fentanyl dose are required. Although sufentanil may be an effective analgesic, there is nevertheless concern that its effects are also simply due to systemic blood levels. As with fentanyl, this has been confirmed when higher doses are used. The use of higher volumes of a more dilute solution for sufentanil infusions will improve its analgesic effects, but advantages of this drug over fentanyl are unclear.

The use of intermediate-solubility opioids such as *meperidine* or *hydromorphone* provides a spinal cord action with wider spread and duration than seen with fentanyl, and perhaps less frequent side effects (28–30). This class may represent an ideal balance of good spread with lower side effects, but as yet there are few large clinical series supporting their use.

Generally, there appears to be a relationship that suggests that drugs producing sufficient spread to provide excellent analgesia (morphine) do so at the price of side effects. The lower frequency of side effects of the lipid-soluble drugs is associated with lower efficacy, unless such high infusion rates are used that systemic levels are attained. This has led many to believe that the use of the lipid-soluble drugs should be limited to cases where the catheter is at or near the "epicenter" of a narrow band of painful dermatomes, such as thoracotomy incisions (and thus pain can be relieved with small doses). The more water-soluble opioids appear to be more appropriate for distant catheters (lumbar placement for thoracotomy pain) or wider incisions (abdominal cases) (Table 24.4). Unfortunately, there are very few comparative studies between the various opioids, and little clinical data to support the personal choice of drug.

All of the opioids have also been administered as subarachnoid injections. The doses required are significantly less than the epidural route, but the efficacy of this route is limited by the (usually) single

Table 24.4   **Postoperative Analgesic Regimens**

Surgical Procedure	Analgesic Regimen
Thoracic incision	Lumbar or thoracic morphine infusion or thoracic fentanyl infusion
Upper abdominal	Low thoracic or lumbar hydromorphone, morphine or fentanyl infusion
Lower abdominal	Lumbar hydromorphone, morphine or fentanyl infusion, or intravenous patient-controlled analgesia

injection. Morphine, with its long duration, is the logical choice of drug. Unfortunately, in these doses there is a narrow dose-response relationship, and a relatively high incidence of side effects. Although respiratory depression is the greatest concern, it is fortunately rare. More commonly, patients are disturbed by a high frequency of pruritus, ranging from 40% to 60% in reported series.

Addition of Local Anesthetics

The efficacy of epidural opioids is improved by the addition of a dilute concentration of local anesthetics, such as 0.05% bupivacaine. The addition of the local anesthetic provides a significant synergistic improvement in analgesia, especially with movement or coughing, which is particularly evident with the lipid-soluble opioids (20,31). Although higher concentrations of bupivacaine (0.1%) may occasionally be required, the maximum potentiation seems to occur in the 0.05% range. Higher concentrations may provide enhanced analgesia by providing some sensory analgesia, but the higher doses increase the potential for motor block and hypotension due to sympathetic blockade (23). Nevertheless, addition of local anesthetic appears to significantly increase the potency of epidural opioids and is a worthwhile adjunct therapy for both lipid-soluble and water-soluble (23,27,32) drugs, as long as appropriate monitoring is employed to prevent orthostatic hypotension or the development of pressure sores due to sensory anesthesia. In addition to potentiating the analgesia, the addition of local anesthetics is essential to speed the return of normal bowel function after abdominal surgery (33).

Other long-acting amino-amides are also effective, because all possess a good sensory–motor dissociation as well as the ability to potentiate the opioids. Levobupivacaine appears to act identically to the racemic mixture. Ropivacaine has been studied as a potential analgesic infusion without opioid. It produces less motor blockade than bupivacaine in the same concentrations, but still has a significant potential for motor blockade in the concentrations needed to produce analgesia without opioids. When combined with fentanyl in low concentrations, there does not appear to be a significant difference compared to equipotent mixtures with bupivacaine (20,34).

The alternative amino-amides have a lower potential for cardiac toxicity, but at the low concentrations and infusion rates used for postoperative analgesia, this advantage may not justify the additional cost.

Despite a plethora of published studies of almost every conceivable combination of opioid and local anesthetic for almost every type of surgery, there are no clear guidelines for the ideal proportion for combination therapy. Because of the synergism, any reduction in one component requires an increase of the other. Using a complex "direct search" method, Curatolo demonstrated this interdependence between bupivacaine, fentanyl, and clonidine dose (35). For practical purposes, it appears that the ranges of concentrations in Table 24.2 are useful, until further data are available to clarify this issue (20). A useful approach is to choose a "standard" opioid, and start with a combination with 0.05% bupivacaine. If analgesia is inadequate with patient-controlled epidural anesthesia (PCEA), the basal infusion rate can be increased a few times as a first step, and then concentration of bupivacaine increased to 0.1% as the next alternative. If a lipid-soluble opioid was the initial choice, conversion to a more water-soluble (wider spreading) drug is another alternative.

Other Adjuvants

Several other adjuvants show promise in potentiating epidural opioids or in having analgesic properties themselves, including alpha₂-agonists (clonidine, dexmetomidine), NMDA (N-methyl-D-aspartate) antagonists (ketamine), and other neurotransmitter modifiers. Ketamine has been shown to be effective, but its safety in the epidural space has not been confirmed. Clonidine appears to be the most effective, but at the price of a higher frequency of hypotension and sedation (20), which may limit the use of this drug to peripheral nerve infusions. Epinephrine has been shown to intensify analgesia with bupivacaine–fentanyl mixtures. At this time, most postoperative analgesia services appear to be interested in using the simplest combination of ingredients until there is more evidence of enhanced analgesia or reduced side effects with adjuvants.

Delivery System

As with the drug combinations, there are a number of reports, but a dearth of good comparisons. It does appear that the use of a thoracic epidural catheter for thoracic and upper abdominal procedures provides ideal analgesia with the lowest dose and lowest frequency of motor blockade (20,23), especially with the more lipid-soluble opioids. Although continuous infusions appear to have replaced bolus injection methods, the addition of a PCA component also improves analgesia and allows better titration to varying patient needs. PCEA does not appear to be effective without a background infusion, but that combination (as in Table 24.2) appears to provide the best analgesia with lowest side effect profile.

Multimodal Analgesia

Ideally, a single drug infusion would provide total analgesia without side effects or interference with ambulation or recovery of bowel function. This panacea does not exist. Two comments merit discussion. First, *combinations* of several modalities are more effective than a single-analgesic regimen (36,37). As just discussed, the synergism of local anesthetics plus opioids in the epidural space provides better analgesia than either alone and is also more effective in promoting return of normal bowel function than the use of opioids (either PCA or epidural) alone. In addition, the use of supplemental systemic analgesics that act by a separate mechanism provides additional synergism (38). Specifically, administration of nonsteroidal antiinflammatory drugs (NSAIDs) on a regular basis has been shown to improve analgesia while reducing opioid requirements in many procedures, and thus the potential for the side effects of respiratory depression or ileus is reduced. Most pain services now add NSAIDs to almost all regimens, and the introduction of the new cyclooxygenase-2 inhibitor (COX-2) class of drugs will widen the potential application. The use of acetaminophen on a regular basis has similar benefits, and is also included as a baseline in many pain services.

Second, there are other factors that determine final recovery in addition to adequate analgesia. The return of bowel function appears to be especially important, and accelerated recovery has been shown in patients who are treated with an analgesic regimen that reduces ileus combined with early feeding of low-fat diets. Nonpharmacologic treatment including early feeding and aggressive ambulation appears to be beneficial and is clearly an area for further study.

Preemptive Application

Animal data suggest that the *presurgical* application of neuraxial opioids will significantly blunt the phenomenon of spinal cord excitation usually associated with painful stimuli, and will reduce analgesic requirements for postinjury pain therapy (39). At this point, the human data are still unclear (40). Several reports suggest a reduction in postoperative analgesic requirements when epidural opioids are administered or local anesthetics are used for infiltration before skin incision. Others have not been able to confirm this, possibly because of the many factors that influence postoperative analgesic demands in human subjects. Although epidural opioids do not provide adequate analgesia for surgery itself, they may reduce anesthetic requirements by 30% to 40%.

A definite preemptive effect cannot be documented at this point. Nevertheless, it still appears to be worthwhile to consider initiating epidural analgesia early in the surgical course, perhaps by placing the epidural catheter before surgery and administering the anesthetic with a combined technique that includes local anesthetic and opioids for surgery. This allows a smooth transition to an epidural infusion for postoperative analgesia.

Treatment of Side Effects

Respiratory depression is the greatest concern. As mentioned, it is no greater risk than with intramuscular opioids or intravenous (i.v.) PCA if appropriate doses are employed (6,20) (Table 24.5). Nevertheless, all patients receiving neuraxial opioids should be monitored for signs of respiratory depression. Respiratory depression may occur 6 to 18 hours after initial injection or start of an infusion. Patients at greatest risk are the elderly, especially those who have received other systemic opioids or sedatives. Upper-abdominal and thoracic surgeries also increase risk. Patients receiving chronic opioid administration are more resistant. Mechanical monitoring devices have not proved useful (41). The development of increasing sedation coupled with a decreasing respiratory rate (less than 10 breaths per minute) is the best indication of impending respiratory failure and should be treated with an opioid antagonist. A single i.v. dose of naloxone is not adequate; depression will recur within 20 minutes as the naloxone effect dissipates. A continuous infusion of naloxone (5 μg/kg/hour) will reverse the respiratory depression without antagonizing the analgesia, and may even be an advisable prophylactic measure in high-risk patients. With appropriate education of nursing staff and patient monitoring, neuraxial opioids have been used successfully on patients in general hospital wards, and need not be limited to application in intensive care units (20,23,27,32,41).

Pruritus is the most common complaint with neuraxial opioids. It can be relieved with antihistamines, but histamine release is not

Table 24.5 **Risk Factors for Respiratory Depression**

Intravenous PCA	Epidural Opioids	Both
Continuous-infusion mode	Thoracic, abdominal incisions	Advanced age
Family interference	Dural puncture	Overdosage
Respiratory disease	Intrathecal vs. epidural	Other narcotics/sedatives
	Thoracic catheter	
	ASA status >3	
	Surgery >4 h	

PCA, patient-controlled administration; ASA, American Society of Anesthesiologists.

the mechanism of the symptom and more effective treatment is with an opioid antagonist. As with respiratory depression, a small dose of an antagonist will relieve the side effect without reversing the analgesia. This is true with pure antagonists, such as naloxone, or with agonist–antagonists, such as nalbuphine, which has been used in doses of 1 to 3 mg intravenously or 10 mg subcutaneously to relieve these symptoms (Table 24.6).

Nausea is less common, but also disturbing to the patient. Again, symptomatic treatment with any of the common antiemetic drugs is useful, or a low-dose antagonist or agonist–antagonist is appropriate. *Urinary retention* is the other troublesome side effect and, unfortunately, is not as readily reversed with antagonist therapy. Without good justification, many postsurgical patients treated with epidural opioids are simultaneously treated with an indwelling bladder catheter until the opioid infusion is halted.

Infection at the site of catheter placement is not a common problem. Epidural analgesia can be continued for several days or weeks, as long as the original dressing was placed in an aseptic manner.

Epidural hematoma is a rare but major complication. As discussed in Chapter 7, the performance of epidural injections (or removal of catheters) should be considered carefully in the presence of coagulation abnormalities. If there is any concern about the possibility of hematoma formation, it is best to remove any local anesthetic from the epidural infusion (to remove any ambiguity about motor weakness) and to institute evaluations of motor function every 2 hours.

Inadequate analgesia is an occasional problem, especially when low doses are chosen for the elderly or "standard" doses are used for young vigorous patients. A bolus injection of fentanyl (50 to 100 µg) or of the infusion solution itself will usually improve the analgesia for a few hours, but the basic infusion rate must be increased if a continued improvement in analgesia is desired. If repeated boluses and rate increases do not improve analgesia, the efficacy of the epidural catheter should be tested by injection of 5 to 10 mL 1.5% lidocaine or 2% chloroprocaine. This will usually produce analgesia

Table 24.6   Epidural Opioid Side Effects

Side Effects	Frequency	Treatment
Respiratory depression	Rare: <0.2%	Naloxone bolus followed by infusion
Pruritus	20%–60%	Mild: antihistamines Moderate: systemic nalbuphine, 1–3 mg Severe: naloxone infusion Reduced with infusions, lipid-soluble drugs
Nausea	6%–50%	Mild: antiemetics Moderate: opioid antagonist
Urinary retention	4%–40%	Indwelling catheter

for 2 hours and confirm that the catheter is in the appropriate location.

The most difficult patients to treat in this regard are those who have been habituated to opioid drugs preoperatively, and thus have a higher tolerance and perhaps even dependence. In this situation, use of a more potent opioid in the epidural space may be helpful (42). Another alternative is to use an epidural infusion of local anesthetic alone and provide the patient with an i.v. PCA of opioid to provide them with the "reassuring" signs of systemic effects, while allowing them to titrate to a level that meets their needs.

Outcome

All of the methods described, especially epidural opioid infusions, require some increased effort and imply some assumption of additional risks. It is important to place the use of regional techniques for postoperative analgesia in an appropriate risk–benefit perspective. Despite the risks of side effects and the effort involved, the use of epidural infusions of local anesthetics or opioids for postoperative analgesia has been shown to improve patient outcome in several significant areas (43). First, *pain relief* is superior, especially dynamic pain after thoracotomy (18) and upper abdominal (21) procedures. Postoperative *respiratory complications* are less frequent (44). Return of *bowel function* is more rapid (33). The usual hypercoaguable state of the perioperative period is reversed, leading to fewer complications with vascular grafts (45,46) and a reduction in *thromboembolic* complications (47). There is a trend toward reduction in the hormonal *stress response* to surgery (43), including a reduction in catecholamine release (48), which may be related to a trend to reduced *cardiac complications* (43). Data also confirms a reduction in cardiac morbidity, since optimal pain relief is obviously important in the high-risk group prone to ischemia (49). Finally, there is even an indication that use of optimal epidural analgesic regimens may reduce the potential for the development of *chronic postoperative pain* states (50). All of the above comments apply to epidural opioid–local anesthetic therapy: peripheral nerve blockade also confers advantages in pain relief and rehabilitation that were reviewed above (Peripheral Nerve Analgesia Techniques, this chapter) (13,14). With this growing body of data, it appears that the benefits of the analgesic regimens discussed here are significant, and merit use of these techniques.

Acute Pain Service

The use of these modalities is obviously complex and usually requires the creation of a dedicated anesthesia pain service (1,2). The major challenge of such a service is education of nursing personnel and surgeons about the limitations and complications of the therapies described. Expert coverage is also required to modify the dosages with these techniques and handle the unusual complications and, especially, the technical problems when epidural or peripheral nerve catheters appear to malfunction. These problems require that an experienced team of anesthesiologists be available on a 24-hour basis. Ideally, this team will round at least twice a day on the pain patients and be readily available for consultation. An essential component of the service is the development of standing orders that provide clear guidelines to ward staff about recognition and initial management of the complications and side effects discussed above.

The work of a pain service is greatly enhanced if a nurse specialist is included. This person is helpful in educating and supporting ward nurses, as well as in providing a more constant and consistent level of patient care. The use of standard protocols for administration of continuous analgesics is also helpful, as well as a set of standing orders for management of complications. The standing orders should specifically include the appropriate respiratory monitoring and the authorization for the nursing staff on the floor to initiate treatment (usually with naloxone) before the arrival of the pain team for evaluation.

This service requires the commitment by the anesthesia staff and, in larger hospitals, often requires a continuous in-house presence. It has been possible to provide coverage for pain services by at-home call in smaller community hospitals, but this requires intensive education of all the nursing staff and a thorough set of standing orders to cover eventualities. Overall, the institutions that have instituted the pain service have found that it offers significant advantages to the patients in their postoperative coverage.

References

1. Ready, L. B., Oden, R., Chadwick, H. S., Benedetti, C., Rooke, G. A., Caplan, R., Wild, L. M. Development of an anesthesiology-based postoperative pain management service. *Anesthesiology* 68: 100, 1988.
2. Ferrante, F. M., VadeBoncouer, T. R. *Postoperative Pain Management.* Philadelphia: WB Saunders, 1993.
3. Macintyre, P. E. *Acute Pain Management: A Practical Guide.* 2nd ed. Philadelphia: WB Saunders, 2001.
4. Rawal, N., Jones, R. M., Aitkenhead, A. R. *Management of Acute and Chronic Pain.* London: BMJ Publishing, 1998.
5. Sinatra, R. S., *Acute Pain: Mechanisms and Management.* St. Louis: Mosby-Year Book, 1992.
6. Etches, R. C. Respiratory depression associated with patient-controlled analgesia: A review of eight cases. *Can. J. Anaesth.* 41: 125, 1994.
7. Macintyre, P. E. Safety and efficacy of patient-controlled analgesia. *Br. J. Anaesth.* 87: 36, 2001.
8. Ryan, J. A., Jr., Adye, B. A., Jolly, P. C., Mulroy, M. F., II. Outpatient inguinal herniorrhaphy with both regional and local anesthesia. *Am. J. Surg.* 148: 313, 1984.

9. Rawal, N., Axelsson, K., Hylander, J., Allvin, R., Amilon, A., Lidegran, G., Hallen, J. Postoperative patient-controlled local anesthetic administration at home. *Anesth. Analg.* 86: 86, 1998.

10. Stein, C., Comisel, K., Haimerl, E., Yassouridis, A., Lehrberger, K., Herz, A., Peter, K. Analgesic effect of intraarticular morphine after arthroscopic knee surgery. *N. Engl. J. Med.* 325: 1123, 1991.

11. Allen, H. W., Liu, S. S., Ware, P. D., Nairn, C. S., Owens, B. D. Peripheral nerve blocks improve analgesia after total knee replacement surgery. *Anesth. Analg.* 87: 93, 1998.

12. Ganapathy, S., Wasserman, R. A., Watson, J. T., Bennett, J., Armstrong, K. P., Stockall, C. A., Chess, D. G., MacDonald, C. Modified continuous femoral three-in-one block for postoperative pain after total knee arthroplasty. *Anesth. Analg.* 89: 1197, 1999.

13. Capdevila, X., Barthelet, Y., Biboulet, P., Ryckwaert, Y., Rubenovitch, J., d'Athis, F. Effects of perioperative analgesic technique on the surgical outcome and duration of rehabilitation after major knee surgery. *Anesthesiology* 91: 8, 1999.

14. Singelyn, F. J., Gouverneur, J. M. Extended "three-in-one" block after total knee arthroplasty: Continuous versus patient-controlled techniques. *Anesth. Analg.* 91: 176, 2000.

15. Grant, S. A., Nielsen, K. C., Greengrass, R. A., Steele, S. M., Klein, S. M. Continuous peripheral nerve block for ambulatory surgery. *Reg. Anesth. Pain Med.* 26: 209, 2001.

16. Klein, S. M., Grant, S. A., Greengrass, R. A., Nielsen, K. C., Speer, K. P., White, W., Warner, D. S., Steele, S. M. Interscalene brachial plexus block with a continuous catheter insertion system and a disposable infusion pump. *Anesth. Analg.* 91: 1473, 2000.

17. Singelyn, F. J., Dangoisse, M., Bartholomee, S., Gouverneur, J. M. Adding clonidine to mepivacaine prolongs the duration of anesthesia and analgesia after axillary brachial plexus block. *Reg. Anesth.* 17: 148, 1992.

18. Kavanagh, B. P., Katz, J., Sandler, A. N. Pain control after thoracic surgery. A review of current techniques. *Anesthesiology* 81: 737, 1994.

19. Cousins, M. J., Mather, L. E. Intrathecal and epidural administration of opioids. *Anesthesiology* 61: 276, 1984.

20. Wheatley, R. G., Schug, S. A., Watson, D. Safety and efficacy of postoperative epidural analgesia. *Br. J. Anaesth.* 87: 47, 2001.

21. Liu, S., Carpenter, R. L., Neal, J. M. Epidural anesthesia and analgesia. Their role in postoperative outcome. *Anesthesiology* 82: 1474, 1995.

22. Ready, L. B., Chadwick, H. S., Ross, B. Age predicts effective epidural morphine dose after abdominal hysterectomy. *Anesth. Analg.* 66: 1215, 1987.

23. Liu, S. S., Allen, H. W., Olsson, G. L. Patient-controlled epidural analgesia with bupivacaine and fentanyl on hospital wards: Prospective experience with 1,030 surgical patients. *Anesthesiology* 88: 688, 1998.

24. Ummenhofer, W. C., Arends, R. H., Shen, D. D., Bernards, C. M. Comparative spinal distribution and clearance kinetics of intrathecally administered morphine, fentanyl, alfentanil, and sufentanil. *Anesthesiology* 92: 739, 2000.

25. de Leon-Casasola, O. A., Lema, M. J. Postoperative epidural opioid analgesia: What are the choices? *Anesth. Analg.* 83: 867, 1996.

26. Peng, P. W., Sandler, A. N. A review of the use of fentanyl analgesia in the management of acute pain in adults. *Anesthesiology* 90: 576, 1999.

27. Scott, D. A., Beilby, D. S., McClymont, C. Postoperative analgesia using epidural infusions of fentanyl with bupivacaine. A prospective analysis of 1,014 patients. *Anesthesiology* 83: 727, 1995.

28. Chaplan, S. R., Duncan, S. R., Brodsky, J. B., Brose, W. G. Morphine and hydromorphone epidural analgesia. A prospective, randomized comparison. *Anesthesiology* 77: 1090, 1992.

29. Liu, S., Carpenter, R. L., Mulroy, M. F., Weissman, R. M., McGill, T. J., Rupp, S. M., Allen, H. W. Intravenous versus epidural administration of hydromorphone. Effects on analgesia and recovery after radical retropubic prostatectomy. *Anesthesiology* 82: 682, 1995.

30. Paech, M. J., Moore, J. S., Evans, S. F. Meperidine for patient-controlled analgesia after cesarean section. Intravenous versus epidural administration. *Anesthesiology* 80: 1268, 1994.

31. Solomon, R. E., Gebhart, G. F. Synergistic antinociceptive interactions among drugs administered to the spinal cord. *Anesth. Analg.* 78: 1164, 1994.

32. de Leon-Casasola, O. A., Parker, B., Lema, M. J., Harrison, P., Massey, J. Postoperative epidural bupivacaine-morphine therapy. Experience with 4,227 surgical cancer patients. *Anesthesiology* 81: 368, 1994.

33. Steinbrook, R. A. Epidural anesthesia and gastrointestinal motility. *Anesth. Analg.* 86: 837, 1998.

34. Hodgson, P. S., Liu, S. S. A comparison of ropivacaine with fentanyl to bupivacaine with fentanyl for postoperative patient-controlled epidural analgesia. *Anesth. Analg.* 92: 1024, 2001.

35. Curatolo, M., Schnider, T. W., Petersen-Felix, S., Weiss, S., Signer, C., Scaramozzino, P., Zbinden, A. M. A direct search procedure to optimize combinations of epidural bupivacaine, fentanyl, and clonidine for postoperative analgesia. *Anesthesiology* 92: 325, 2000.

36. Brodner, G., Van Aken, H., Hertle, L., Fobker, M., Von Eckardstein, A., Goeters, C., Buerkle, H., Harks, A., Kehlet, H. Multimodal perioperative management—combining thoracic epidural analgesia, forced mobilization, and oral nutrition—reduces hormonal and metabolic stress and improves convalescence after major urologic surgery. *Anesth. Analg.* 92: 1594, 2001.

37. Kehlet, H., Dahl, J. B. The value of "multimodal" or "balanced analgesia" in postoperative pain treatment. *Anesth. Analg.* 77: 1048, 1993.

38. Dahl, V., Raeder, J. C. Non-opioid postoperative analgesia. *Acta Anaesthesiol. Scand.* 44: 1191, 2000.

39. Woolf, C. J., Chong, M. S. Preemptive analgesia—treating postoperative pain by preventing the establishment of central sensitization. *Anesth. Analg.* 77: 362, 1993.

40. Kissin, I. Preemptive analgesia. *Anesthesiology* 93: 1138, 2000.

41. Ready, L. B., Loper, K. A., Nessly, M., Wild, L. Postoperative epidural morphine is safe on surgical wards. *Anesthesiology* 75: 452, 1991.

42. de Leon-Casasola, O. A. Postoperative pain management in opioid-tolerant patients. *Reg. Anesth.* 21: 114, 1996.

43. Kehlet, H., Holte, K. Effect of postoperative analgesia on surgical outcome. *Br. J. Anaesth.* 87: 62, 2001.

44. Ballantyne, J. C., Carr, D. B., deFerranti, S., Suarez, T., Lau, J., Chalmers, T. C., Angelillo, I. F., Mosteller, F. The comparative effects of postoper-

ative analgesic therapies on pulmonary outcome: Cumulative meta-analyses of randomized, controlled trials. *Anesth. Analg.* 86: 598, 1998.

45. Christopherson, R., Beattie, C., Frank, S. M., Norris, E. J., Meinert, C. L., Gottlieb, S. O., Yates, H., Rock, P., Parker, S. D., Perler, B. A., et al. Perioperative morbidity in patients randomized to epidural or general anesthesia for lower extremity vascular surgery. Perioperative Ischemia Randomized Anesthesia Trial Study Group. *Anesthesiology* 79: 422, 1993.

46. Tuman, K. J., McCarthy, R. J., March, R. J., DeLaria, G. A., Patel, R. V., Ivankovich, A. D. Effects of epidural anesthesia and analgesia on coagulation and outcome after major vascular surgery. *Anesth. Analg.* 73: 696, 1991.

47. Rodgers, A., Walker, N., Schug, S., McKee, A., Kehlet, H., van Zundert, A., Sage, D., Futter, M., Saville, G., Clark, T., MacMahon, S. Reduction of postoperative mortality and morbidity with epidural or spinal anaesthesia: Results from overview of randomised trials. *Br. Med. J.* 321: 1493, 2000.

48. Breslow, M. J., Parker, S. D., Frank, S. M., Norris, E. J., Yates, H., Raff, H., Rock, P., Christopherson, R., Rosenfeld, B. A., Beattie, C. Determinants of catecholamine and cortisol responses to lower extremity revascularization. The PIRAT Study Group. *Anesthesiology* 79: 1202, 1993.

49. Beattie, W. S., Badner, N. H., Choi, P. Epidural analgesia reduces postoperative myocardial infarction: a meta-analysis. *Anesth. Analg.* 93: 853–858, 2001.

50. Perkins, F. M., Kehlet, H. Chronic pain as an outcome of surgery. A review of predictive factors. *Anesthesiology* 93: 1123, 2000.

Subject Index

Page numbers followed by f indicate figures; page numbers followed by t indicate tables.